# TEN YEARS YOUNGER

# TEN YEARS YOUNGER

## the amazing ten-week plan
### to look better, feel better, and turn back the clock

## STEVEN MASLEY, M.D.

BROADWAY BOOKS  New York

This book is not intended to take the place of medical advice from a trained medical professional. Readers are advised to consult a physician or other qualified health professional regarding treatment of their medical problems. Neither the publisher nor the author take any responsibility for any possible consequences from any treatment, action, or application of medicine, herb, or preparation to any person reading or following the information in this book.

PUBLISHED BY BROADWAY BOOKS

A hardcover edition of this book was originally published in 2005 by Broadway Books.

Published in the United States by Broadway Books, an imprint of The Doubleday Broadway Publishing Group, a division of Random House, Inc., New York.
www.broadwaybooks.com

Book design by Tina Henderson

Library of Congress Cataloging-in-Publication Data
Masley, Steven.
Ten years younger : the amazing ten-week plan to look better, feel better, and turn back the clock / Steven Masley.
p. cm.
Includes bibliographical references.
1. Rejuvenation. 2. Aging—Prevention. 3. Health. I. Title.
RA776.75.M366 2006
613—dc22
2005051331

ISBN: 978-0-7679-2171-8

PRINTED IN THE UNITED STATES OF AMERICA

5 7 9 10 8 6

First Paperback Edition

*To*
*my wife, Nicole,*
*and my boys, Lucas and Marcos,*
*for their love and support.*

# CONTENTS

# INTRODUCTION

What if I promised you that in only ten short weeks, you could give yourself a total body makeover, inside and out? What if you could get a fresh start without relying on plastic surgery, liposuction, fad diets, overpriced products, or weeks at an expensive spa?

What if I told you that typical aging is not inevitable and that I know the secret to looking and feeling healthier, sexier, and stronger than you have in a decade? That you can reclaim the energy you had ten years ago? That you can achieve younger bones and skin, a trimmer physique, a prettier figure, and an all-around fitter body? That you can restore sexual vitality and mental quickness? That you can not only lose pounds and inches and keep them off but also avoid the double bugaboos of aging—Type 2 (adult-onset) diabetes and heart disease?

What if I promised you that you could actually reverse the aging process and be *ten years younger* in just ten weeks' time?

Too good to be true?

Maybe. Until now.

You're about to discover my comprehensive, breakthrough, scientifically proven Ten Years Younger Program, which I've developed through decades of training, research, and clinical experience. I am a board-certified family physician, certified nutritionist, acupuncturist, health researcher, speaker, author, trained chef, and award-winning patient educator. I became active in longevity and cardiovascular disease research years ago as a clinical researcher for diabetic and cardiac rehabilitation. Since 1990, I've spoken before more than 600 groups of people young and old, including guests at the famed Canyon Ranch in Tucson, Arizona, about my anti-aging program, preventing heart disease and diabetes, promoting bone health, weight loss, supplements, and healthy cooking. I have helped thousands of patients in my clinical practice, as the medical director at the Pritikin Longevity Center® and in my current position as medical director for Carillon Executive Health in St. Petersburg, Florida, to slim down, get fit, and tap into unsuspected energy levels. In fact, my Executive Health Program there has been voted Best New Medical Idea for the 3-million-strong Tampa Bay metropolitan area in 2005. My work even made it to the television screen in 2003 in a multipart series for Discovery Channel called *Ten Years Younger.* I've also won acclaim for helping hundreds of patients reverse Type 2 diabetes and eliminate the symptoms of cardiovascular disease through lifestyle changes. If all of these people can be ten years younger, so can you!

It has given me joy to help so many people reclaim their lives with a program that has restored their physique, their health, and their zest for life. Although my life's work in anti-aging began with my desire to help my patients reverse the conditions that were holding them back, I quickly discovered that what works for cardiac and diabetes patients can also do wonders for healthy adults, young and old, who want even more out of life. Today I'm passionate about introducing everyone— including you—to the Ten Years Younger lifestyle. In my current research, I've taken great pleasure in watching the transformation of average, relatively healthy people from merely well to truly wonderful as they show off their new sexier shapes, their glowing faces, and their newly energetic presence.

Whether you're 30 or 70, whether you're healthy or not so healthy, the program in the pages that follow will help you turn back the clock so that you too can become more vibrant—younger, trimmer, and fitter—than you ever dreamed possible.

This is not a fantasy. Most of us believe that growing old is inevitable, that it's normal to lose function and good health as the years go by, that we're supposed to ache, get flabby, and gain weight. Even your doctor might comment, "What do you expect at your age?" But these are all myths. You don't have to succumb to love handles and wrinkles as the years go by. You can grow older and still feel terrific. Your choices today can make a big difference in how you live out your tomorrow. This book will show you how to make the right choices, and change the way you think about aging.

## The Accelerated Aging Syndrome

How can I make these promises? It's easy. Your body is capable of turning back the clock because these days, most of us are becoming old before nature intended us to. Americans on the whole are falling victim to what I call Accelerated Aging Syndrome—we're aging more rapidly than we're supposed to. In fact, our bodies from our skin to our bones are designed to last much longer than they generally do. Almost all of us, for a multitude of reasons, are victims of this Syndrome. Chances are you already know what it feels like:

- You follow the latest fad diet, but even though you might lose weight at first, the numbers on the scale are still creeping up over time.
- You find yourself dragging through your day. You just don't have the stamina you used to.
- Your cholesterol, blood pressure, weight, and/or blood sugar levels are on the rise. Your doctor warns you that you're "pre-diabetic," but you're not sure what that means.
- Your thighs have become flabby, your belly paunchy, and your muscles saggy.
- Your skin looks dry, rough, and blotchy.
- You don't enjoy sex the way you once did.
- You frequently need to retrace your steps because you can't remember why you walked into a room.
- You *feel* as if you're getting old, even if you're only in your 30s!

Maybe you've even thrown up your hands in frustration and said, "What can I do about it? My mother had high cholesterol; my father had diabetes. It's in my genes!" But that's not necessarily true. In this book, I'll present you with other options. You can eat fast food three meals a day, lie on the couch watching TV, gain 50 or even 100 pounds over five to ten years, acquire diabetes and heart disease, and become disabled with arthritis. This is one expression of your genetic potential. Another possibility? You exercise or play sports for an hour daily; you eat healthy seafood, veggies, fruits, and whole grains; you form intimate relationships in your personal and professional life. You feel fabulous, full of vitality, and mentally sharp. You're sexy, trim, and fit to boot! A bonus, of course, is that you're unlikely to have many medical problems. This, too, is your genetic potential.

I've treated patients who are in their early 40s but act and feel more like 60. Their joints ache, their blood pressure is elevated, and they don't have the stamina to keep up with their kids. But I've also treated hundreds of others in their 60s who act and feel years younger than their peers. Age is not just chronological. It's also a matter of lifestyle, health, activity, energy, weight, and the steps we take to further our own mental well-being.

We'll discuss the phenomenon of accelerated aging much more in Chapter 1. But for now, let's just establish that it's another way of saying we're all growing old before our time. The effects of accelerated aging are readily apparent every single day. We are a nation that's growing soft, smooth, and round. Go anywhere in America—grocery stores, airports, malls, amusement parks—and you'll see people with ballooning waistlines and shrinking muscles instead of the shapely and muscular bodies they could have. And that's just on the outside. While you can't observe it, these same people may not think as sharply as they used to. Chronic low-grade inflammation may be setting them up for clogged arteries and perpetual weight gain. Toxins and a poor diet may be working to cause premature wrinkling and the deterioration of brain cells.

Even our children are now falling victim to accelerated aging; they're being diagnosed with diabetes, obesity, and high blood pressure in frightening numbers. In fact, according to an alarming 2005 article in the *New England Journal of Medicine*, for the first time in history our children may have shorter life spans than we, their parents, do.

The Ten Years Younger Program is specifically designed to combat accelerated aging. And since accelerated aging affects us all from the moment we're born, the program can work for you, no matter what your age. If you're in your 30s, it will put the spring back in your step, renew your mental clarity and focus, discourage fine lines and wrinkles from forming, and revive those sexy curves that are starting to turn into pockets of fat around your waist. If you're in your 50s, the Ten Years Younger Program can help you stave off age-related diseases like Type 2 diabetes and heart disease, as well as shed those extra pounds that you've been struggling with, and it can dramatically tone, strengthen, and sculpt your muscles, making you ten years fitter. If you're in your 70s, the program will reverse that climb in your blood pressure and cholesterol, add sharpness to your wit and shapeliness to your limbs, and put some zip back into your romantic life.

An 80-year-old can't go back to being 20—that would be physiologically impossible—but he or she can be the equivalent of a 70-year-old who is mentally sharp, energetic, and fit. And a 50-year-old can have the strength, energy, and appearance of an athletic 40-year-old. Unless you are one of the rare few who have followed an excellent diet, exercise, and stress management program for years, a reversal of ten years is achievable for everyone. No matter what your starting point, you will get the Ten Years Younger result.

Starting today, right now, you will be improving your age and your life. It won't always be easy—some of it is hard work! But the results you'll get after only a few short weeks will keep you motivated. In fact, you'll feel so good that you'll never want to give up the program! Not only will you be turning the tables on Accelerated Aging Syndrome, you'll also be saying yes to a lifestyle that will add years to your life—and life to your years!

## The Ten Years Younger Program

The Ten Years Younger Program is an integrated, comprehensive, scientifically proven method to help you reverse accelerated aging. My approach doesn't just focus on your wrinkles or your fat—it involves your *whole body*. Built around three pillars—the Ten Years Younger Diet, Age-Busting Fitness, and the Relaxation Routine—the program teaches you how to gently phase in lifestyle changes that will rapidly start to turn back the clock. I've tested the specific combination of diet, fitness, and relaxation recommended here in multiple clinical trials and research studies to confirm that what I advocate really works. And I've used this program with thousands of patients successfully over the past fifteen years in my medical practice.

My customized nutritional supplement and skin care plans will also help you meet your unique needs. Although I recommend that everyone take a multivitamin, I'll be recommending additional supplements for particular conditions. I'll also help you choose skin products that actually work—and they may not be the ones sold at glitzy department store counters in fancy tubes. The products and foods I recommend will not only improve your skin's outward appearance but make your skin structurally younger, too, from the inside out.

So, how do you get started? First, you'll do the self-tests in Chapter 3 to assess your fitness level, strength, body shape, cholesterol, and mental performance. These simple tests look at biological markers that predict aging, and they'll tell you how old you *really* are, no matter what your birth certificate says. Then you'll be able to compare your results to those of average people your age to see where you rank. This will help you determine if you're suffering from Accelerated Aging Syndrome and provide the baseline for your lifestyle changes.

I'll then outline the steps you need to take to start turning back the clock. The first two phases of the Ten Years Younger Program, which focus on learning to incorporate anti-aging foods and building your fitness capacity, span two weeks each; they prepare you for Phase Three, the full-blown anti-aging regimen of diet, exercise, and relaxation. And by following the three phases for ten weeks, the average person will be ten years younger.

And here's an unexpected bonus: Unlike so many other lifestyle and diet programs that are based on cutting out entire food groups—most fruits and vegetables, beans, and whole grains—especially during that difficult first phase, the Ten Years Younger plan does something much more appealing. Rather than denying yourself the certain foods your body needs, you'll be gradually *adding* foods and activities that have proven anti-aging benefits. You won't go hungry on the diet; in fact, I've even built in what I call Rescue Snacks for times when you just have to have something to eat.

However, the program may also require your limiting or avoiding choices that are clearly *harmful*, especially some bad fats that have been touted in popular low-carb/high-saturated-fat diets. Certain kinds of fats and carbs will age you, and clearly those have to go. You'll hardly miss them, though, because you'll be feeling so good.

While I worked as a physician with Group Health Cooperative in Olympia, Washington, I met one of my breakthrough longevity patients. When we became acquainted, Jack was a 57-year-old engineer who lived alone. His wife had passed away ten years earlier, but with children and grandchildren living in the area, he didn't lack companionship. Jack had a great sense of humor and always had a joke to share when he came for office visits. Unfortunately, as time went on he began to develop elevated cholesterol and blood pressure, and his list of medications slowly grew. His energy was dropping from visit to visit, and one day he failed to bring a joke. I took this as an ominous sign. Now, at the young age of 60, Jack was rapidly getting old.

Together, we looked back over Jack's medical history during the three years since we'd first met. He had gained 25 pounds, mostly around his waist, and whereas he used to walk every day on his lunch break, he now hadn't taken a walk in six months. Living alone, he was eating mostly fast or prepackaged foods. And despite adding two blood pressure medications, his blood pressure had risen 10 points in three years, and his cholesterol level had jumped alarmingly, from 220 to 280. His medications made him feel tired, and he had lost his libido as well as his drive to exercise. Two flights of stairs left him gasping for breath. He also seemed to be visiting with friends and family less frequently.

It was clear to me that Jack had a choice: He could continue on this path and face more serious problems, or he could try to undo the damage before it was too late.

I had been conducting research at our medical center with groups of patients who suffered from diabetes and cardiovascular disease. In each of my studies, the people assigned to my group-visit programs had implemented a series of dietary and lifestyle changes, and met monthly for educational and discussion sessions. Their cholesterol and blood sugar levels had plummeted on the program, and their energy and quality of life had improved as well. Every study I conducted saved our clinic money, because even though there were costs for the extra educational visits, the patients weren't as ill and consequently used fewer health care resources. I had developed twenty-eight days' worth of recipes with shopping lists and cooking plans, exercise regimens, and supplement recommendations. And I suspected that the program could help Jack if he was up to the challenge.

But Jack was hesitant—it sounded like a lot of work. So I asked him a few questions about his grandson's soccer team, since he'd loved bragging about how well the boy did in his position as goalie. He frowned and shrugged as if to indicate he hadn't been to a match in a while. We sat in silence. Finally, Jack said, "Okay, Dr. Masley, I'm interested. But what do I have to do?"

I gave Jack a month's worth of shopping lists and recipes. "Clean out your cupboards and drop off everything not on this shopping list at the local food bank," I advised. I also started him on an exercise regimen that got him active for sixty minutes each day. I asked him to plan a minimum of two social events each week: He could cook dinner for friends, go to a movie or a game—anything that was fun and healthy. I also told him that I wanted him to visit with his family at least once a week.

One month later, Jack showed up in my office for his regular visit with a joke and a smile. He had lost 10 pounds and his muscle tone was much improved. He was cooking dinner every night after work, his blood pressure had fallen by 12 points, and his cholesterol had dropped back to 220 from a high of 280. Best of all, he was feeling more positive about himself and had begun enjoying life again.

Six months later, Jack came to his appointment holding hands with a female companion. He looked great—at least ten years younger. He had lost another 25 pounds, his cholesterol was at 170, and his blood pressure now stood at 120/70. We were able to discontinue all of his medications except for a daily baby aspirin and some supplements. And he was back to attending all of his grandson's soccer matches.

Two years later he was married—happier, healthier, and feeling years younger than his age.

Over the years, I have worked with thousands of individuals just like Jack. Young or old, they've bounced back from the effects of accelerated aging, and you can too!

## The Three Pillars

Let's take a closer look at the different components of the Ten Years Younger Program so you'll understand what's in store in the pages ahead.

### The Ten Years Younger Diet

The essential secret behind the Ten Years Younger Diet is that what we eat dramatically impacts the way we age—and it's not just about unwanted pounds. The wrong foods will age you prematurely, but the right foods work to rejuvenate your heart, mind, skin, and bones. They detoxify your body. They help you lose weight and keep it off. They ward off diabetes and lower your risk of heart disease and cancer. They build muscle and give you energy. When you combine the right foods in the right quantities, they can actually help you get younger and younger.

What are the "right foods"? They are those that are rich in anti-aging compounds (they act as powerful antioxidants, a term I'll explain and expand upon in Chapters 1, 4, and 5). I call these Vitality Foods, and they include brightly colored fruits and vegetables, fresh seafood, beans, soy, whole grains, nuts, flaxseed, spices and herbs, red wine, and even chocolate. Red wine in moderation protects your blood vessels, improves blood pressure, decreases your risk of Alzheimer's, and helps control blood sugar. And dark chocolate is packed with anti-aging, heart-healthy, stress-relieving compounds. So chocolate lovers, rejoice! Certain Vitality Foods like green tea and tomato paste are even great for rejuvenating your skin. (No, you don't smear them on your face. You eat them!)

In each phase of the program, you'll find myriad delicious recipes to help you integrate these diet recommendations into your daily life. Relying on my background as a trained chef and world traveler, I've developed a varied menu for you, including American, French, Chinese, Japanese, Spanish, Mexican, Thai, Italian, Indian, and Middle Eastern cuisines. You'll never be bored! And some of the desserts, like Chocolate Mousse with Grand Marnier, are simply outstanding.

## Age-Busting Fitness

We all know that exercise is a must for weight control and that it helps every part of you, from your skin to your abs, look toned and fit. But did you know that your muscles also provide an enormous reserve of protein for tissue repair and to fight infections? These proteins also serve as building blocks for the hormones that regulate many aspects of your biochemistry. That's why muscle mass is the best predictor of your ability to live free of disability as you age.

Most of us are aware that of all the therapies available for preventing and treating cardiovascular disease, the single most effective one is exercise. People who work out regularly have 40 percent fewer heart attacks and strokes. It's also the first line of defense against diabetes— walking has been cited as the best therapy and prevention for this ever more prevalent disease. Research has also shown that maintaining adequate muscle mass can lower the risk of hip fracture. It also improves your ability to survive pneumonia, major surgery, and cancer.

The section on Age-Busting Fitness will guide you in determining which activities in particular will help you lose weight most efficiently. I'll teach you to find your optimal heart rate during your workouts so you maximize the return on your exercise-time investment. I'll also share the twelve best muscle-building, age-defying activities that you can do at home or at the gym. These will supercharge your metabolism and wake up your muscles so that you burn more calories even while you're resting. I'll show you how to customize the program to match your level of fitness in order to get fast results, no matter what level you begin at. And as these activities get ramped up over the three phases of the program, you'll feel so good that they'll become a welcome habit, not an obligation!

## The Relaxation Routine

By now, we all know that too much stress is bad for our health. But it's actually an enormous factor in how we age. Excess stress hormones (like adrenaline and cortisol) circulating in your body boost your blood sugar levels and raise your blood pressure. They also increase the fat on your belly, which is a sign that you're also collecting fat around your liver and heart—a dangerous development. As I'll explain in Chapter 7, high cortisol levels also injure your hippocampus, the part of your brain associated with memory, thereby increasing your risk of Alzheimer's disease. Moreover, too much of these hormones will cause the breakdown of muscle and bone tissue.

To make matters worse, when you're under stress, you may turn to food for comfort. And comfort food usually doesn't take the form of fruits and vegetables! Fries, chips, ice cream, pizza, doughnuts, cookies, and other junk foods are usually on the menu when we're feeling stressed. Unfortunately, this kind of eating feeds your sense of guilt as well as your gut, and you're likely to be even more stressed out when you discover that you've put on a couple of extra pounds.

On the other hand, managing your stress will lower your levels of stress-related hormones, thus slowing the aging process. Naturally, it would be impossible to completely remove stress from your life, but adding simple stress management activities daily will soothe your soul and promote a general sense of well-being. You'll also find that you think more clearly, have more energy, and sleep better. Deep breathing, meditation, various forms of massage, and listening to relaxation tapes can all be very helpful, as can simple activities such as lighting candles, soaking in a hot bath, playing gentle music, or watching a sunset. Your goal? Find time for ten to thirty minutes of inner peace and quiet every day. The Ten Years Younger Program will help you do just that.

## Building on the Three Pillars: Supplements and Skin Care

Despite what some health books would have you believe, supplements can't make up for a risky lifestyle. They won't compensate for gorging on junk food, smoking, drinking to excess, burning the candle at both ends, or your after-work job as a couch potato. But if you eat well, exercise regularly, manage your stress, and control the toxins in your environment, they can help you reach your goal of being ten years younger.

Eighty percent of Americans are nutrient deficient. Yes, we get plenty of calories (far too many, some would say), but we don't get enough nutrients. The most common vitamin deficiencies are in folic acid, $B_6$, $B_{12}$, C, D, and E. Frequent mineral deficiencies include zinc, calcium, magnesium, and iron. Furthermore, most Americans don't eat enough fiber or omega-3 fats—all excellent Vitality Foods. So a major part of your Ten Years Younger goal is to add these nutrients back into your diet.

Everyone should start by taking a one-a-day multivitamin, but even these can't meet your needs perfectly. So how do you know which supplements to take from the hundreds that are out there? The best plan is to create a personalized program that accounts for your health history and current lifestyle. Medications, diet and activity level, and health conditions all determine which supplements will best slow the aging process. In Chapter 10, I'll help you choose the supplements that are right for you. We'll also discuss your skin and the products you can buy that can help revitalize and rejuvenate your appearance. The anti-aging foods in the Ten Years Younger Diet will also help renew it from within.

## How Do We Know the Program Works?

Others who have written bestselling lifestyle books make exciting claims about weight loss or other benefits but may not have had any hard scientific data backing their programs when they wrote their books. I do!

As a medical student, I was keenly aware that more than half of my hospitalized patients were dying of acute cardiovascular disease—strokes and heart attacks. When I looked outside the hospital, I could also see that 40 percent of Americans were victims of this disease. And even if they didn't die, they suffered long-term disability: impaired speech, thought, or movement; limb amputations; disabling chest pain; wounds that wouldn't heal; permanent loss in erectile function for men.

My initial desire was to become a specialist in international medicine, so I was fortunate enough to work in a number of foreign countries during my early medical career, including Jamaica, Guatemala, Kenya, China, India, and Pakistan. Although we often think of these countries as poverty-stricken, developing nations, I was astonished to see that undernourished people who were active were often healthier than the average, affluent Americans whom I'd treated during medical school.

Even more surprising was my discovery that unless a resident of a third-world country had adopted a Western lifestyle, that person did not develop Type 2 diabetes or heart disease. Later, while working in hospitals in Switzerland and Australia, I noted that the same diseases we struggle with in the United States were emerging there.

The bottom line from my overseas experiences? I theorized that if you could avoid foods that were high in bad animal fat or were highly refined and processed, and if you stayed physically active, you could avoid Accelerated Aging Syndrome. But I needed to prove this theory scientifically, and that's exactly what I set out to do.

In the 1990s, as a physician and lifestyle researcher with Group Health Cooperative, a multispecialty clinic in Olympia, Washington, I worked with groups of people with coronary disease and Type 2 diabetes. There, I developed a lifestyle program—the one that eventually evolved into the Ten Years Younger Program—that reversed the disease process for many. For instance, in my studies with diabetics, I had great results with high cholesterol levels. My subjects had a whopping 29.5 percent drop in their ratio of total cholesterol to healthy cholesterol (HDL) levels, from 6.1 to 4.3. (I'll discuss the importance of this ratio in Chapter 2.) It wasn't a quick fix; my subjects were able to sustain the change even after two years. My patients' blood sugar levels also dropped from terrible to very good control, and this 25.3 percent plunge in average blood sugar level was sustained over two years. In fact, the subjects in this study who followed my program closely went from having a poorly controlled disease with medications to having normal blood sugar levels without medication. In essence, even one to two years later, they no longer had diabetes. Much to everyone's delight, I soon realized that while this program had restored my patients' health, it also gave them slimmer, shapelier figures and increased their zest for life.

More research brought me to Clearwater, Florida. As a clinical researcher for diabetic and cardiac rehabilitation, I was appointed principal investigator for studies sponsored by the American Heart Association at Morton Plant Hospital with the Florida Geriatric Research Program, one of the nation's largest long-term studies on geriatric groups. I studied how and why older people develop heart attacks and strokes that could lead to death.

In addition, my position as the medical director of the Pritikin Longevity Center in Miami gave me the opportunity to help thousands of cardiac and diabetes patients reclaim their lives with a program that gave them back their health. It was there that I also discovered that lifestyle changes for adolescents could work wonders in reshaping young people's lives, too.

In fact, at Pritikin, we performed an intervention with nineteen teenagers who stayed at the center for two weeks. I believed the children wouldn't tolerate the ultra-low-fat, low-salt Pritikin regimen, so we adjusted the usually austere Pritikin Eating Plan to something much more akin to my Ten Years Younger Diet. I increased the fat and salt to a range that lies within my Ten Years Younger recommendations: 20 to 30 percent of calories from fat and less than 2,400 mg of sodium daily. I figured this would make meals tastier and more appealing. The participating adolescents experienced statistically significant changes that were later presented at the 2003 American Heart Association's Epidemiology meeting: a 30 percent drop in total cholesterol, a 25 percent drop in their ratio of total cholesterol to healthy cholesterol, a 33 percent drop in bad cholesterol (LDL), and a 48 percent drop in triglycerides (these are tiny beads of fat that are part of the total cholesterol in the bloodstream). These kids averaged 6.6 pounds of weight loss during the two weeks. And at a six-month follow up, they had continued to get trimmer and fitter.

But I was puzzled. Back in 1991, the Pritikin Center had published studies showing that its ultra-low-fat diet plan produced an 11 percent decrease in the ratio of total cholesterol to HDL. Not bad. But why were my results with these teenagers so much better?

I didn't get the opportunity to research the answer, but I did ask Dr. Antonia Demas (Pritikin's nutrition consultant hired for the adolescent study, who had developed several of the recipes for the children) why she thought the kids had done so well. She suggested that the healthy fats added to the teenagers' diets (in the form of nuts and healthy oils) may have improved upon the Pritikin protocol.

Add the results from all these studies together and you can see how I've discovered that what works for patients with diabetes, heart disease, and obesity can also do wonders for healthy adults, young and old, who want even more out of life. My ten years working in a primary care, family medicine clinic in Olympia, Washington, my years as the medical director of the Pritikin Longevity Center, and my current position as medical director at Carillon Executive Health in St. Petersburg, Florida, further cemented my faith in the Ten Years Younger Program. *It works for everyone who is willing to commit to it.*

During the spring of 2003, I had the pleasure of bringing my breakthrough work to millions of people with the help of a wonderful television director, James Bates, and a terrific producer, Paula Goodburn. They were filming a five-part series entitled *Ten Years Younger* with a British film company that was broadcast on Discovery Channel in 2003. For the show, they selected five adults (three women and two men) from the Miami area, ages 35 to 52. James and Paula recruited me as one of their key longevity doctors. They had been drawn to me on account of my experience in prevention, nutrition, cooking, medical research, and writing. They showed me the candidates' pictures, briefly described them, and then asked, "Can we make these five people younger in just ten weeks?" They also asked me to create medical tests we could use to show progress over a ten-week period.

Initially, I spent an hour with each of the five adults in a detailed interview and intake exam. For this group, we chose several age markers that I have used in my clinical practice for many years, including endurance and fitness level tests while running on a treadmill, maximal heart rate achieved with exercise, cholesterol levels, pulmonary function tests, body composition, and strength and flexibility markers established by the American College of Sports Medicine. (You'll be working with many of these in Chapter 3.) We met the following week to review results and developed a ten-week customized plan for each of the participants. Each received a diet, exercise, and stress management plan drawn from the same anti-aging program I'd been succeeding with for many years. I conducted several additional follow-up visits over the ten-week course and a detailed final evaluation at the end.

Over the ten weeks, we threw out the junk food in the participants' kitchens and sent them to fitness trainers for endurance and strength training. They were massaged, stretched, and tested. They were also fortunate to have counseling with a terrific local physician and psychiatrist, Andrew Levinson, M.D. His goal was to deal with their stressors and to aid in their detoxification. To enhance their skin appearance, they worked with Leslie Bauman, M.D., a cutting edge board-certified cosmetic dermatologist at the University of Miami. The film crew spent days creating a long list of challenges that the age-busters endured while the crew captured their disappointments and triumphs on film.

After ten weeks, we retested the participants, and I compared their progress on the objective markers for aging with their initial numbers. The results were phenomenal! It showed the group as a whole to be 10.5 years younger. Not only were they physiologically younger, but they looked and felt noticeably better, too. Four of the five had needed to lose weight, and lose weight they did—their average loss was 10 pounds each, and the most motivated and compliant person in the group dropped 30 pounds! In particular, this group slimmed down at their waistlines—on average over 4 inches in just ten weeks. (I'll explain in Chapters 1 and 2 why this is so important—and it's not just an issue of vanity or fitting into your favorite pair of jeans.) Lastly, they didn't just lose fat; most of them gained muscle mass during the ten weeks, too. The one woman who was underweight added 8 pounds of lean muscle mass over the ten-week period.

Prior to accepting this challenge, one of the age-busters had been on track to hurt both his health and his active career as a fireman. Despite participating in a regular exercise program in the past, Abel's terrible diet had yielded a marked weight gain, and he was obese based on body mass index measures. His cholesterol profile was poor, and sadly, at the young age of 40, he was already clogging his arteries. The initial medical evaluation I performed became a startling wake-up call for him. Adhering to nearly all of my recommendations, he became our star age-buster. Thanks also in part to counseling with Dr. Levinson, his mental outlook improved immensely. At the end of 10 weeks, his fitness level was that of a 20-year-old, he'd lost 30 pounds, he'd dropped 7 inches from his waistline, he was stronger, and his cholesterol level had fallen 40 points.

This age-busting experiment as well as my work with Jack and hundreds of other patients like him clearly shows that if you are motivated to make the effort, you can become physiologically 10 years younger—and armed with the program in this book, you're on your way.

## The Ten Years Younger Study

Following my work on the Discovery Channel program, I decided to see if I could replicate these remarkable results in a controlled study, and that's when Younger, Trimmer, Fitter—The Ten Years Younger Study was born. My aim was to enroll healthy men and women ranging in age from mid-20s to mid-60s and to follow them over ten weeks as they engaged in the Ten Years Younger Diet, Age-Busting Fitness, and the Relaxation Routine. Funded by St. Anthony's Health Care, we conducted our research at the state-of-the-art Carillon Outpatient Center, where I work. (It was voted Best New Gym by *Tampa Bay Magazine* in 2004.)

Fifty-eight adults joined my study at the outset. Like the participants in the television show, all were assessed for their aerobic endurance, muscle strength, cholesterol, body composition, and brainpower (I'll explain these measures more fully in Chapter 3). Half were randomly assigned to a control group; they simply continued on with their current lifestyle. The other half spent ten weeks following the Ten Years Younger Program.

The subjects who followed my recommendations for ten short weeks were able to:

- *Increase their aerobic fitness level by 29.2 percent.*
- *Increase their strength.* Abdominal strength nearly doubled, rising 91 percent; push-up strength shot up by 79 percent; flexibility increased by 30 percent.
- *Decrease their fat mass by 12.8 percent.* Those who were overweight on average lost 10.6 pounds of weight, of which 10 pounds consisted of pure fat (that's about 2.5 footballs of fat volume), without losing lean muscle mass. That means the average person who needs to lose weight will drop an orange-sized pound of fat every week on this program.
- *Lower their cholesterol ratio (total cholesterol to HDL) by a solid 12.7 percent.* In contrast to my earlier studies with diabetics, most subjects in the Ten Years Younger Study had normal and sometimes very good cholesterol levels to start with. But based upon my many years of experience with this program, if you have an elevated cholesterol level, you can expect to see a 10 to 25 percent drop in your cholesterol profile by following the Ten Years Younger Program.
- *Improve their executive thinking function by 24.6 percent and increase their span of attention by 44.3 percent.*

But the numbers don't tell the whole story. As Doris, a busy radiation therapy specialist and mother of two active teenage boys, told me with lots of enthusiasm after the ten weeks were over, "I feel like I have a lot more energy. Definitely my muscle tone is a lot better—the arms and legs. Those are the two biggest things that changed physically. And my husband dropped a ton of weight. He *feels* a lot better. He had some pretty terrific results!" And 53-year-old Jill told me, "In the very beginning, I thought, 'Okay, what am I going to get out of this? Maybe I'll lose a few pounds.' Well, I started sleeping better. There was an overall better general feeling. After going through the whole program, I had more energy, I was mentally better at my job. I even look better. I put on a pair of jeans that were a size 6 that I haven't been able to wear for three years."

What could be better than that?

# Ten Weeks Is a Long Time.
## What If I Can't Stay on the Plan?

Yes, ten weeks is a long time. And yes, there are a lot of different pieces to the program. But don't worry—you don't have to do everything 100 percent perfectly all the time for the plan to work. If you slip a little on the diet, if you miss a day of exercise, it's not the end of the world. The path toward the new you is a continuum; this isn't an all-or-nothing proposition. If you adhere to the plan 90 percent of the time, you will still be making progress. In fact, once you reach the maintenance stage, if you manage to stay on the program for twenty-five days a month, that's usually good enough. This way, you can enjoy holidays, birthdays, and other special occasions without feeling guilty. Besides, unlike other diet plans, there's no punishing first phase to slog through again. With Ten Years Younger, you just hop right back on the wagon wherever you fell off.

So turn the page and let's get started!

# PART I

# OLD BEFORE YOUR TIME?

# CHAPTER 1

# The Accelerated Aging Epidemic

Today, nearly half of all Americans are getting old before their time, suffering all kinds of age-related symptoms at alarmingly younger ages. I call this Accelerated Aging Syndrome, and it is fast becoming an epidemic in this country. Quite simply, accelerated aging is a faster-than-normal deterioration in the functioning of your body and mind. In my practice, I've seen it begin with a subtle shift in body shape—an expanding waistline or shrinking muscles—caused by indulgent eating, lack of exercise, and yo-yo dieting. Your energy decreases while your cholesterol, blood sugar, and blood pressure levels climb. You're tired and achy all the time. Your libido dwindles, your muscles sag, and your skin looks dull. You just don't feel like you can keep up with your job, your kids, and your routine the way you used to. Perhaps most upsetting are symptoms of memory loss, which only add to your level of discouragement and distress. You realize that you *feel* old—even if you're not!

So why is this happening to so many of us these days? Unfortunately, changes in the American diet and lifestyle have conspired to make us age more rapidly. Before we can begin the process of becoming ten years younger, we need to understand these aging enemies—what I call aging accelerators—and how they impact our daily lives.

## Aging Accelerator #1: Oxidative Stress

Catherine, a 36-year-old woman living in Olympia, Washington, seemed to be sick all the time. If she wasn't fighting upper respiratory infections, she was in my office complaining of sinus headaches or intestinal cramping. She couldn't think clearly; she seemed depressed; she ached all over. I saw her once every three weeks for a whole year for one issue or another.

"It's because of that darned office building," she told me. "It's one of those sick buildings—you know, the kind that has no windows. We're all breathing the same air all the time. We're constantly passing colds on to each other." It never occurred to Catherine that the fact that she never exercised and ate poorly could be the source of her illnesses. She was always looking for a quick fix for her problems, requesting prescriptions for antibiotics and anti-inflammatory medications.

Although I could appreciate her frustration, I believed Catherine's workplace had nothing to do with her situation. She was suffering from a disorder that often lies hidden and goes undiagnosed—a condition called oxidative stress. At first she resisted my suggestions that a healthier lifestyle might be her ticket to a better life. But after a frustrating year of illness, Catherine finally agreed to try the Ten Years Younger Diet for a month and to work out at the local gym at least four days a week.

A month went by, and to my surprise, Catherine hadn't called once. After about two months of silence, I became concerned. I called her, to be sure nothing terrible had happened.

"How have you been?" I asked Catherine. "I haven't seen you for a while, and I was worried."

Fortunately, my fears proved unfounded. "Oh, Dr. Masley, I feel wonderful," Catherine responded. "I haven't felt this well in ten years!"

What is oxidative stress—the mysterious ailment that laid Catherine so low for so long? It's a natural process in our bodies that underlies much of what ages us. In fact, many of the suggestions I've included in the Ten Years Younger Program are meant to fight this thief that robs you of your energy, good health, and longevity.

Oxidative stress is the result of your body's inability to process free radicals, which are a by-product of your body's natural energy production. Every process that creates energy also makes waste products. Take your car, for example. It burns gas and oxygen to make energy, and exhaust is created as a by-product. These pollutants must be removed from the engine so that it can run well; that's what the tailpipe is for. The exhaust that comes out of the tailpipe is packed with pollutants—you certainly wouldn't want to breathe it in.

Your body is no different, only in this case free radicals are the chemical exhaust. These biochemical compounds damage your living cells. But in addition to the free radicals you produce naturally, you also encounter others from outside sources: pesticides, drugs, pollutants, cigarettes, fumes, smog, tobacco smoke, lead, mercury, and cadmium. Every cell in your body takes between 10,000 and 100,000 aging hits from free radicals every day, and these micro-attacks injure your cells.

If your lifestyle doesn't protect you against the onslaught of free radicals—oxidative stress—you'll almost certainly suffer premature aging. Oxidative stress is the result of an imbalance: You generate or encounter too many free radicals without taking in enough antioxidants, anti-aging biochemical compounds that are found in foods. They turn off free radicals the way a fire extinguisher puts out little fires, thus slowing aging and enhancing your health. These essential nutrients counteract the harmful free radicals your body encounters, and play a critical role in promoting a long and healthy life.

So how do free radicals make you age? They attack not only your cell membranes—the outer walls of each cell in your body—but also your DNA, causing mutations that impact the function of your cells. This assault may even transform a normal cell into one that is cancerous. In fact, most cancers develop from normal cells whose DNA has been damaged by free radicals and oxidative stress. Free radicals will also age your skin by destroying its structure and speeding the creation of wrinkles. In fact, many of the aging scenarios I'll cover in Chapter 2 are due directly to the effects of oxidative stress. If you're healthy, however, you will have enough antioxidants to extinguish free radicals, and the limited DNA damage that does occur can be easily repaired.

The Ten Years Younger Program will help you change and/or reverse the damage caused by oxidative stress and will continue to protect you in the future so that you remain healthy as the years go by. In Chapter 4, I provide a list of Vitality Foods with high antioxidant activity, and The Ten Years Younger Diet and recipes in Part III are rich in antioxidants as well. The Age-Busting Fitness regimen and the Relaxation Routine will also decrease your level of chronic oxidative stress. It is possible to overcome it, and I'll show you how.

## Aging Accelerator #2:
## Low-Carb, High-Protein, High-Fat Diets

Sharon had been on a popular low-carb diet for three months. The first month, she was delighted to find that, after giving up her cookies, coffee cake, and other high-carb treats, she had lost about 6 pounds. "Only 24 pounds to go," she told herself, happily pulling on a size 12 dress for the first time in a year.

Her delight turned to disappointment two months later when she'd lost only another 7 pounds. "You're on a plateau," a fellow dieter reassured her, but try as she might, she couldn't shed another pound. What she did notice, though, was that her energy was flagging and she wasn't thinking as clearly as she used to. Then, to add insult to injury, her boyfriend, Teddy, complained that she had terrible breath. Even worse, once Teddy started his own low-carb diet program, he lost all interest in sex. Sharon didn't know why. Was it because she was tired all the time? Was it the bad breath? Maybe he didn't find her attractive anymore. Or was it him? Had the low-carb diet diminished his libido?

Soon, given all the unpleasant changes in her life, Sharon's favorite doughnuts were calling her name. And one day, discouraged, she answered. From that moment on, her low-carb diet was history. Sharon went on to regain all the weight she'd lost, plus an extra 5 pounds.

For the past few years, we've been living in the "Age of Atkins," and low-carb consciousness has become a way of life for dieters and non-dieters alike. Many of you will be aware of two studies conducted by Frederick Samaha, M.D., and Gary Foster, Ph.D., that were published in the *New England Journal of Medicine* in 2003 and showed that an Atkins-like diet did in fact yield short-term modest weight loss in obese patients, but only when compared against an average American diet that was rich in refined sugar, low in fiber, and lacking in healthy fats. And within the year the results of the conventional diet and the Atkins diet were about the same. Furthermore, the fact that the Atkins diet did not succeed in achieving even a 10 percent weight loss in obese patients in either study suggests that this type of dietary intervention is a failure. To top it all off, the dropout rate in the studies was extremely high, as most people find it next to impossible to sustain this type of eating over the long haul.

But the effects of the low-carb diet are even more serious than most people realize, because it's not just pounds we're talking about. The truth is that yo-yo dieting (on one day, off the next) strongly contributes to accelerated aging. Not only are these diets difficult to tolerate, but they are actually dangerous and will make you old before your time. *Rather than melting away the pounds, these regimens are melting the years from your life!* Here's why:

- *Low-carb diets lack the fiber necessary to lower cholesterol and blood sugar.* Low-carb diets are notorious for pushing high-fat meats and cheeses, which have no fiber at all! Every day your body needs at least 30 grams of fiber (found in fruits, whole grains, vegetables, beans, and nuts). Fiber lowers your cholesterol by binding to it in your gut and preventing it from being absorbed into your bloodstream. It also slows the absorption of sugar from your intestines. This prevents insulin surges after meals and protects you from developing diabetes. Fiber also helps to remove toxins from your digestive tract that can cause low-grade inflammation throughout your body—another major age accelerator (see below).
- *Low-carb diets lack antioxidants.* As I explained before, antioxidants are health-promoting biochemicals found in edible plants that actually slow the aging process in your cells. For instance, fibrous Vitality Foods such as apples, grapefruit, broccoli, and cauliflower prevent damage to your cells that can lead to cancer.

These antioxidant-rich foods extinguish free radicals before they do damage to your body. But low-carb diets shun these nutrient-rich foods, for reasons that defy true scientific thinking. Diets low in antioxidants also allow cholesterol to be quickly converted into artery-clogging plaque (I'll explain how in Chapter 2), and actually promote the death of brain cells. The 1 to 2 cups of salad allowed on low-carb diets just doesn't cut it—and vitamins marketed to low-carb dieters supply only a tiny fraction of the vast array of nutrients found in high-fiber foods.

- *Low-carb diets are often loaded with saturated fats.* Some low-carb, high-protein diets encourage you to eat lots of red meat, bacon, and high-fat dairy products such as whipped cream, cheeses, and butter. These all contain high levels of saturated fats that clog your arteries. Clogged arteries are associated with an increased risk of heart attack, stroke, amputation, and loss in brain function—and you don't have to be over 50 to experience these very negative side effects. Furthermore, foods that are loaded with saturated fats are also often high in additives and pesticides that elevate your cancer risk.

- *Low-carb diets shrink your muscles and weaken exercise performance.* If you shed more than 2 to 3 pounds a week, you can be sure that you're losing more muscle than fat. Why? Because to burn fat, you need an enzyme called lipase, which only allows you to burn at most 2 to 3 pounds of fat a week. If you lose any more than that, you're clearly losing lean muscle mass instead. But when you yo-yo, as Sharon did, and go off the diet, you'll most likely gain back only the fat, not the muscle! A cycle of rapid weight loss (losing more muscle than fat) followed by weight regain (gaining more fat than muscle) leaves you with a higher percentage of body fat and a lower percentage of muscle mass. If you cycle on and off these diets several times, you may get flabbier, fatter, and weaker over time—definitely *not* the desired result!

- *Low-carb diets can cause ketosis.* Very-low-carb diets can induce ketosis, a dangerous physical state that occurs with prolonged fasting and the eating of a diet restricted to high-fat, low-carb foods. When you're in a state of ketosis, you're essentially pouring battery-acid-like compounds into your bloodstream. Not surprisingly, this makes you feel ill, and it also suppresses your appetite—part of the gimmick behind the Atkins weight-loss claims. Unfortunately, ketosis is quite dangerous. It can destroy your brain cells as well as your kidneys (see below). And since ketosis increases acid production, it changes the pH level or acidity of your blood, which can further dull your brain function.

- *Low-carb diets can cause kidney failure.* Animal protein in moderation won't hurt your kidneys, but the sheer volume of animal protein in some low-carb diets can put significant stress on them. Excess protein is difficult to process, and while most kidneys can manage the added work, some can't. In particular, if you have diabetes or signs of metabolic syndrome (see Aging Accelerator #3, on page 12), your kidneys are more likely to be injured by excess protein. And ketosis appears to worsen this problem considerably. I've seen patients who've pushed themselves into ketosis over and over again in their attempts to lose weight and were later diagnosed with kidney failure. Although these patients did eventually drop the low-carb, high-protein, high-fat diet, their kidney function never recovered. Now they're facing kidney transplants.

- *Low-carb diets speed bone loss (osteoporosis).* Low-carb diets are usually deficient in calcium and magnesium, two minerals critical for the health of your bones. But that's not the whole story. Excess animal protein (more than 6 to 8 ounces of meat, poultry, or fish daily) can also deplete calcium from your bones. Here's how: Animal protein is acidic, and the extra acid you take in from a diet high in animal protein can make your blood acidic too. Your body has a wonderful built-in mechanism to prevent this from happening: It sucks calcium from your bones to neutralize any changes in your blood's acidity. Unfortunately, the calcium that's now in your blood is passed out of your body in the urine, ultimately weakening your bones. Considering that average Americans don't come close to consuming enough calcium, people with a lifetime history of excessive animal protein intake risk spending their final years disabled in nursing homes with hip or spinal fractures.

- *Low-carb diets expose your body to deadly toxins.* Fully 80 percent of the pesticides in the American diet come from meat, poultry, and dairy. These toxins stress your body and can create or intensify illness when your body is weakened. They can also contribute to chronic low-grade inflammation and further speed aging.
- *Low-carb diets can cause severe digestive problems.* As we've shown, low-carb diets fail to provide enough fiber, which deprives you of important antioxidants. But fiber is also essential for proper digestion. A lack of it leads to a breakdown in the motility within your intestines. And that, in turn, gives rise to and can aggravate a combination of constipation, irregularity, loose stools, and abdominal pain and cramps—a condition called irritable bowel syndrome. Worse, starving your intestinal tract of fiber produces an environment in which healthy bacteria, which rely on fiber as a food source, can't thrive. When healthy bacteria dwindle, bad bacteria associated with increased inflammation flourish, and the potential for bodywide autoimmune flare-ups, such as inflammatory bowel disease (Crohn's disease and ulcerative colitis), increases. Perhaps most frightening, over the long haul diets that are low in fiber and high in animal protein heighten your risk for colon cancer.
- *Low-carb diets can prematurely age your skin.* Low-carb diets that drastically restrict fruits and vegetables and are therefore low in antioxidants likely speed skin damage from the inside. They also limit your intake of nutrients that normally slow skin aging—such as lycopene, found in tomatoes, red peppers, and other red and yellow vegetables.
- *Low-carb diets decrease sexual performance.* Many scientific studies confirm that low-carb, high-saturated-fat diets are associated with spasms in your blood vessels that result in decreased blood flow. When this happens, you reduce the amount of blood flowing not just to your heart—which is bad enough—but also to your genitals. The flow of blood to your sex organs is what makes them sing! Though Sharon was taking it personally, the truth about Teddy's loss of interest in sex may be as simple as this: No blood

flow, no turn-on. And to compound the problem, these diets can give you appallingly bad breath—something akin to rotting meat!

## Why Atkins-Type Diets Deceive Us—At First

Yes, high-fat, low-carb diets are effective for short-term, rapid weight loss. They may even lower your cholesterol levels at first. But the initial gains may not last. Dr. Richard Fleming, whose research appeared in the *Journal of Preventive Cardiology*, was the first to publish cholesterol and weight loss results after one year on each of three diets: a high-fat, high-protein, low-carb diet; a moderate-fat, moderate-fiber diet; and a very-low-fat, high-fiber diet. Early in the study, the high-fat, high-protein dieters lost significant weight and their cholesterol levels improved. But after the weight-loss honeymoon was over, these same subjects regained the weight and their cholesterol worsened. The moderate-fat, moderate-fiber dieters only had modest improvements. The very-low-fat, high-fiber dieters had the greatest weight loss and best cholesterol improvements at the end of the one-year study.

Long-term weight loss—taking it off and keeping it off—should be your Ten Years Younger goal. And as you can tell, your long-term health will *not* benefit from following an Atkins-like diet in the long run. In fact, this type of plan may worsen the plaque in your arteries, even at a young age, despite an initial decrease in cholesterol. To understand why, let's take a closer look at how these diets actually work.

Your muscles store excess energy from carbohydrates in the form of glycogen chains. These chains form in your muscles when energy resources are abundant and are then used when energy is required. If you need energy quickly, your glycogen stores are ready to provide your body with the fuel it needs.

But glycogen chains also bind to water. A 154-pound person has about 5 to 7 pounds of water attached to the glycogen in his or her muscles. Therefore, if you avoid eating carbohydrates for four to five days, you will deplete all of your glycogen stores, and you will also lose 5 to 7 pounds of *water*. If you're an average person wanting quick weight loss, you will likely find this big drop on the scale exhilarating. You assume you're losing fat. But the truth is, over the first week you're mostly losing water!

Buoyed by the first blush of success, you may want to continue on this diet. So what happens if you stick with it for another month or two? After the water loss, you may continue to lose weight quickly. That's what has made these diets so wildly popular. But if you can lose only 2 to 3 pounds of fat a week and you've already depleted the water in your cells, where is the weight loss really coming from? The alarming answer is your muscle mass. And that, as I've already explained, can have dire consequences for your overall long-term health.

As you can see, the very regimen that you've been using to try to take off those extra pounds may be sabotaging your health in more ways than one. So if there's one thing you'll learn in *Ten Years Younger*, it's this: Carbs are not the enemy! Rather, just as there are good fats and bad fats, there are good carbs and bad carbs. The trick is to choose the right ones. The more fiber and antioxidants you eat, the better and younger you'll feel—and the more weight you'll ultimately lose. The Ten Years Younger Diet, described in Chapters 4 and 5, will help you choose these life-enhancing foods and design an eating plan that will keep you slim—but not at the expense of getting old before your time.

## Aging Accelerator #3: The Metabolic Syndrome

The only exercise Phil got each day was the short walk from the parking lot to his office. An engaging 39-year-old African American, he was too busy with his accounting practice to work out, despite his girlfriend's encouragement. Phil freely indulged his passion for hamburgers and fries, Cocoa Puffs, pizza, and onion rings. Fruits and veggies were rarely part of his meals, and he preferred Diet Coke to bottled water.

But when a life insurance company asked him to take a physical, Phil was in for a rude awakening. He'd hit a lifetime high of 181 pounds—dangerous for a man who stood only 5 feet 7 inches. His blood pressure was way up, and his waist measured an alarming 42 inches.

Further tests revealed normal blood sugar and triglycerides but low HDL (healthy) cholesterol.

Phil learned that because of his high blood pressure, growing waistline, and low HDL, he had a precursor to diabetes called metabolic syndrome. He desperately needed to change his lifestyle or face not only the onset of full-blown Type 2 diabetes but the other ravages of rapid aging as well.

Unfortunately, Phil isn't alone. A shocking 47 million Americans have developed metabolic syndrome—the result of an imbalance between how many calories we consume and how many we actually burn through daily activities. The first sign of metabolic syndrome is weight gain, and in particular an expanding waistline.

Unlike diabetes, if you have metabolic syndrome, your blood tests may show normal blood sugar levels. However, your body is working so hard to keep these levels normal that the syndrome is causing you harm in other ways.

Gerald Reaven at Stanford University was the first scientist to identify, categorize, and make public the signs and potential damage of this condition. He called it Syndrome X and characterized its signs as mildly elevated blood sugar, high triglycerides, elevated blood pressure, an increased waistline, and low HDL (good cholesterol) levels. People with this syndrome also tend to have an "apple" body shape (with excess weight around the belly, as opposed to a "pear shape," with weight around the hips and thighs) and to have lost muscle as they gained weight. With time, we've discovered that people with metabolic syndrome also have increased inflammation, higher insulin levels, and abnormal hormonal metabolism.

Metabolic syndrome is actually a problem of blood sugar regulation. When you eat a meal, your body converts the food into its nutrient components: fats, proteins, and carbs. The carbs (sugars) then enter the bloodstream to be used as energy. However, when you eat more calories—and thus take in more sugars than you are able to burn—the hormone insulin sends a message to your cells to store energy for future use. If your blood sugar levels are constantly elevated from fatty, high-calorie foods, your insulin levels will be constantly elevated as well, and eventually your cells become resistant to the hormone. Indeed, insulin resistance is the first step in developing metabolic syndrome. As insulin rises to abnormal levels trying to compensate for the cells' lack of response, so do other hormones—in particular the stress hormones cortisol and adrenaline, which try to counterbalance insulin's effects.

These additional hormones can have negative side effects as well if they are constantly present in your bloodstream. Too much cortisol burns muscle and bone mass and is harmful to your brain cells. Adrenaline increases your heart rate and blood pressure and impairs blood vessel function. These high hormone levels also build belly and organ fat. The combined effects speed aging and lead to the multiple problems associated with this syndrome.

Technically, you have metabolic syndrome if you develop any three of the following five criteria:

- Your fasting blood sugar level (your blood sugar first thing in the morning, before breakfast) is more than 100 mg/dl.
- Your blood pressure is higher than 130/85.
- Your triglyceride levels are greater than 150 mg/dl.
- Your waist is larger than 35 inches for women and 40 inches for men. (Don't be fooled. Men's pant sizes in the United States are usually 3 inches less than the actual waist measurement. So a 40-inch waist actually correlates to a size 37 pants.)
- Your good cholesterol or HDL levels are less than 40 mg/dl for men or 50 mg/dl for women.

If even one of these five criteria applies to you, I suggest you see a doctor. If you have two of these, it is likely you are already experiencing accelerated aging. Once you have three of the five signs, you clearly fit the profile for accelerated aging and metabolic syndrome. While the metabolic syndrome can develop into Type 2 diabetes, what is most worrisome about this common condition is that it can kill its victims from heart attacks or strokes even before they reach the diagnosis of diabetes.

The good news is, you can prevent and even reverse both metabolic syndrome and Type 2 diabetes by following my Ten Years Younger Diet and other aspects of the Ten Years Younger Program.

# Aging Accelerator #4: Physical Inactivity

At the age of 40, Dave had been promoted to a great new position as VP of marketing at the Fortune 1000 company where he worked. Though he'd never been athletic, he had been active, walking his dog, riding his bike, and playing racquetball with some college buddies from time to time. But with his new responsibilities, he began working sixty hours a week, and all of these other activities fell away. He was chained to his desk, and not surprisingly, his weight started ballooning, his belly began expanding, and his mental acuity plummeted.

Dave was so wrapped up in his job that he hardly noticed these changes. But one day his boss looked at him and said, "Dave, what happened to you? You look like hell!"

Despite the fact that Dave's cholesterol was soaring, he didn't see the connection between his increased job responsibilities and his new health problems. Even though he was now only 42, he just thought it was all part of "getting old." Still, within two years, he'd become a medical train wreck.

When I consulted with Dave in my office at Carillon Executive Health, I showed him his test results: high cholesterol and body fat, soaring blood sugar, low fitness scores, and diminishing cognitive performance. That really grabbed his attention. He made a commitment to follow the Ten Years Younger Program. Within ten weeks he'd lost 20 pounds and corrected his cholesterol, blood sugar, and mental function.

Like Dave, you can get old by just sitting still! With our affluent American lifestyle and all of our labor-saving devices—cars, elevators, drive-through windows—as well as video games and other passive entertainments, our activity levels have plummeted. You hear it talked about all the time: Far too many of us are becoming couch potatoes—or, as in Dave's case, desk potatoes. And this lack of activity is making us old before our time. Not only do we lose muscle mass and pack on the pounds when we don't exercise, but we increase our risk for cancer, heart attacks, joint pain, blood clots, broken bones, metabolic syndrome, and diabetes.

Our bodies have got to move to stay young, and any diet or lifestyle book that ignores this important part of your life does you a great disservice. You might lose weight in the short term without exercise, but almost no diet will work in the long term if it doesn't include activity. The good news? Consistent exercise, even if it's only three or four days a week, increases certain enzymes that boost your ability to recharge the antioxidants that already exist in your body so they can remove more free radicals. And that enhances your ability to control oxidative stress. By exercising every day, you produce more efficient antioxidants that continue to protect you even while you're resting. And if you exercise moderately six days a week, your resistance to illness will be even higher.

According to the Harvard Study of Adult Development, regular exercise is one of the top six factors that predict healthy aging. With regular exercise, you will:

- Lower inflammation levels and reduce joint pain (see Aging Accelerator #7)
- Enhance the function of your blood vessels and circulation
- Lower your risk of blood clotting, thereby decreasing your risk of heart attack and stroke
- Improve your thinking power
- Enjoy better weight control and physical fitness
- Lower your free radical levels
- Increase your muscle mass
- Reduce your chances of developing metabolic syndrome

If you are inactive, you are likely missing out on all of these benefits, and accelerated aging is probably already taking place. In fact, the loss of muscle mass is one of the most critical aging problems. Although we often assume that muscle mass depletion is part of the normal aging process, the truth is that you can reverse it at any age. You can maintain and even gain muscle if you're 30, 50, or even 70 years of age.

Muscle protein is enormously important because it is constantly being broken down into amino acids for the body to use for tissue repair, immune activity, and many other everyday functions. Your muscle mass drops about 1 to 2 percent a year after age 50, and if you don't exercise to build new muscle, this important protein reserve becomes depleted. Not only will you be physically weakened, but your body will also lack the resources to carry out the tasks described above. At the same time, unfortunately, between the ages of 30 and 60, your fat mass naturally increases 2 to 4 percent a year.

Because idleness can speed aging, the Age-Busting Fitness component of my program includes activities to help you raise your heart rate for 30 to 60 minutes daily with brisk walking, jogging, or some other form of aerobic activity. Even 30 minutes a day will benefit you substantially. But not everyone can start even at this level; you may need to begin with ten to twenty minutes of moderate walking. To build muscle mass, my Age-Busting Fitness regimen also advocates strength training two or three times a week for 20 to 30 minutes. Stretching daily for as little as 5 minutes a day is also a great way to prevent injuries and enhance your performance. Besides, there's nothing like a toned, muscular body to help you feel ten years younger!

## Aging Accelerator #5: Chronic Stress

Jenny's life was filled with stress. A 35-year-old reporter with a major newspaper, she'd been attracted to the high-energy environment when she took the job right out of college. But as the years passed, her satisfaction began to ebb as she struggled to make increasingly tighter deadlines and keep up with the demands of her tough-as-nails editor while juggling her new role as mom.

When she began to suffer recurrent headaches and stomach pains, I suggested that she might need a better approach to manage her stress. Her quick-grab lunches of cookies and two cups of coffee were creating an acidic environment in her body, and she had begun popping Gas-X capsules several times a day. Soon after experiencing a panic attack at her desk, she quit her job and became a freelance writer.

While leaving the security of a known job for the risk of a new one was certainly challenging, Jenny's choice was a wise one. As her stress level decreased, her body began to heal. Her symptoms have never returned, and she looks forward to each new assignment. She began an exercise program, and today her friends tell her that she looks better than she has in years. She's much more vibrant and can devote that energy to her growing family and her new career.

There's no doubt about it—we live in a difficult world. The constant background noise of terrorism, political strife, continuing economic insecurity, and the local issues and problems that unfold on our nightly news all gnaw at our well-being and conspire to keep us on edge. That, coupled with normal, everyday life—a fight with your boss or spouse, nonstop demands at work, coping with teenage kids or elderly parents, a computer breakdown or car accident, that jangling cell phone, even the effects of bad weather—can push you to the limit and test your resiliency.

But as most of us know, too much stress can play a major role in how we age. When you're upset, the stress hormones adrenaline and cortisol travel all over your body, causing your heart to beat faster, your blood pressure to rise, your muscle cells to break down to release amino acids for fuel, and your fat and liver cells to release fat and sugar for quick energy—all great if you face a life-threatening situation. Adrenaline and cortisol even encourage blood clotting, a neat evolutionary trick designed to help us cope with wounds and injuries, the kinds of stress our ancestors worried about.

But what if these fight-or-flight reactions are a constant part of your everyday life? Your pulse and blood pressure stay high. You run a higher risk of stroke or heart attack. Bone and muscles erode. High levels of stress hormones also injure brain cells, especially in your memory center. They cause insulin resistance, emotional fatigue, depression, weight gain (especially around your waist) with its associated health problems, an elevated risk for Alzheimer's, metabolic syndrome, and Type 2 diabetes.

Stress also depletes your immune system, which can lead to many illnesses, including cancer. Too much long-term stress decreases the function of your white blood cells, limiting your ability to fight intruding microbes and emerging cancer cells. We now know that trouble in your immune system can also hurt your heart and blood vessels through increased inflammation that irritates your arteries and leads to more plaque formation. Yes, it's true—unmanaged chronic stress can and does age you prematurely and may even shorten your life.

An important part of the Ten Years Younger Program is getting your cortisol and adrenaline levels down by adopting a proactive approach to relaxation. I realize that that may sound counterintuitive—after all, is it really relaxation if you have to schedule a time to do it? But in my plan, you're aiming for any activity that brings peace and pleasure—whether it's listening to a symphony on tape, gazing at a sunset, working in the garden, cuddling with a loved one, attending a prayer group, reading a bedtime story to your child, or taking the dog for a walk in the park. For some, the solution may be a practice such as yoga or meditation, which have proven calming, balancing effects. As an important stress management tool, I also recommend that you enjoy a massage two to four times per month while you work hard at turning back the clock—you'll see it suggested in my Ten Years Younger Program. What's important is that any activity you choose makes you feel relaxed and refreshed. If you choose a hot bath by candlelight, that could be wonderful, but if you spend your bath time yelling at the children who are trying to bang down the door, that doesn't count as peace and calm!

The Relaxation Routine in Chapter 7 will help you carve out ten to thirty minutes daily to enjoy the special beauty of each day. Creating this kind of simple healing can do wonders for your anti-aging efforts.

## Aging Accelerator #6: Toxins

Scott had just popped the question, and he found himself in my office after his fiancée insisted that he have a complete physical before announcing their engagement. Becky was worried about Scott's health. A 30-year-old landscaper, Scott looked fit, but he seemed sluggish. He complained of recurrent headaches and stomachaches. On top of that, he was drinking more alcohol than he used to—at least three or four beers every day.

After speaking with Scott, it became clear to me that he had an alarming exposure to pesticides at work. In fact, he seemed quite casual about how he handled them, refusing to wear a mask for protection. I concluded that the accumulation of chemicals he used daily, aggravated by his drinking, explained his many symptoms. Beyond the headaches and stomachaches, I feared Scott was putting himself on the road to brain injury or cancer. Pesticide exposure has a strong relationship to Parkinson's disease and many other neurological disorders, as these poisons have the potential to accumulate and damage fatty nerve tissue in the brain over time. And, of course, many of them are carcinogenic.

I set to work, trying to help Scott overcome his health problems. First, I stressed to him the importance of his using all the safety equipment available to him to minimize his exposure. Then I put him on the Ten Years Younger Program. Within two months of following my recommendations, which included adding Vitality Foods to his diet, taking antioxidant supplements (turmeric in pill form and a cruciferous vegetable extract), and limiting his alcohol consumption to one to two servings daily, Scott's headaches and abdominal pains subsided. His energy level has never been better. And Becky is thrilled with their new romantic life.

Toxins of any kind can speed the aging process. Smoking, drinking too much alcohol, eating barbecued meats (which are packed with heterocyclic amines, chemicals that cause colon cancer), and exposure to pesticides and other industrial agents like dry cleaning fluid—all common toxins in our environment—contribute to Accelerated Aging Syndrome. They age your skin, damage your liver, harm your brain, and cause inflammation, allergies, asthma, and even cancer.

You don't have to be exposed to chemicals on a daily basis like Scott to suffer the age-accelerating effects of toxins. If you imbibe more than two servings of alcohol daily (two 12-ounce beers, two 5-ounce glasses of wine, or two 1½-ounce shots of hard liquor), you increase your cancer risk substantially. Not only does alcohol block your liver's ability to remove carcinogens from your system, but it also decreases folic acid levels, which is strongly associated with an increased cancer risk. In the Ten Years Younger Program, I recommend that you take the following steps to minimize the aging effects brought on by toxins:

- *Avoid all exposure to tobacco.* Even breathing in secondhand smoke for thirty minutes a week is harmful to your health.
- *Limit alcohol to no more than one to two servings daily.* One or none is best!
- *Enjoy at least one cup of cruciferous vegetables—broccoli, kale, cauliflower, cabbage, bok choy, or Brussels sprouts—a day.* As I explained above, these will enhance your liver's ability to remove toxins from your body. (You'll find more information on this process in Chapter 8.) If you cannot partake of these vegetables for whatever reason, consider taking some of the supplements I discuss on my Web site, www.tenyearsyounger.net.
- *Minimize your exposure to pesticides and industrial chemicals.* Decreasing the amount of meat, poultry, and dairy you eat is the most important step you can take. Since the 1980s, we've known that meat and poultry contain 40 percent of all the pesticides in the American diet, and dairy accounts for another 40 percent. If you eat these foods often, make sure you buy organic products. Rinsing all fruits and vegetables and choosing organic produce whenever possible will also help.
- *Limit mercury in your diet.* This means choosing seafood carefully. A rule of thumb is that the bigger the mouth of a fish, the higher its mercury contamination. Avoid bluefin tuna, swordfish, king mackerel, and shark. Instead, enjoy wild salmon, trout, sardines, sole, cod, oysters, mussels, and other shellfish that are low in mercury. (More specific advice on these choices follows in Chapter 4.)
- *Eliminate trans fats (hydrogenated fats) from your diet.* The food industry created this type of industrial fat (found in solid shortening, margarine, and many processed foods, including packaged chips, cookies, and crackers as well most fried offerings in fast-food restaurants, such as french fries, chicken, and fish fillets) to increase the shelf life of its products. Sure, they retard spoilage, but trans fats may also actually extend the time it takes a cadaver to decompose, increasing our shelf life at the morgue! Unfortunately, they also shorten your life—increasing your risk of heart attacks,

strokes, and cancer. Read food labels to ensure that you aren't eating partially hydrogenated fats.

- *Minimize how much refined carbohydrates (table sugar, white flour, and corn syrup) you eat.* These "bad carbs" are toxic to you. When you eat them, you get a sugar surge in your bloodstream. The excess sugar actually sticks to your proteins, including your red blood cells. I like to say that it sugarcoats the protein in your body, metaphorically speaking. When you sugarcoat your proteins, they burn up more quickly, and you age faster; it is the equivalent of pouring gas on a log before you set it on fire. High-fructose corn syrup, an ingredient in thousands of processed food products and most sugary soft drinks, is one of the most common age-accelerating toxins in the American diet today.

## Aging Accelerator #7: Inflammation

Joe, a 50-year-old accountant, came to see me regarding pain in his right foot. His ankle and big toe had been mildly swollen and tender for weeks. But I soon discovered that this was just the tip of the iceberg. Joe complained of feeling achy and tired all the time, and in recent years he'd gained nearly 40 pounds, making him clearly overweight. He admitted that he no longer exercised due to his general state of exhaustion and soreness, and his diet was just plain terrible—chock full of refined carbs and unhealthy fats. His idea of a great meal was a Big Mac and fries washed down with a milk shake. He was shackled to his desk all week and then, despite his wife's pestering, he lounged on the couch all weekend watching sporting events, without ever setting foot in the state-of-the-art gym to which he continued to pay dues each month.

After taking a careful history and conducting a few blood tests, it became clear to me that Joe and I needed to address several problems at once. His cholesterol profile suggested he had metabolic syndrome. Moreover, he was also insulin resistant, which can cause inflammation throughout the body and lead to aches, swelling, and fatigue. I followed up with a C-reactive protein (CRP) test (a measure of overall body inflammation) and found that Joe's blood level for this protein was in fact quite high. It seemed that metabolic syndrome and chronic inflammation were at the root of his problems.

The Ten Years Younger Program contains specific Vitality Foods, fitness activities, and supplements that lower inflammation, so I put Joe on my Ten Years Younger Diet and suggested that he start to exercise to bring his insulin resistance under control. I also added a fish oil supplement—a potent anti-inflammatory—to decrease the level of inflammation in his body.

Joe was quite surprised when his toe and ankle pain disappeared in less than two weeks. But even better, as he continued on the program he felt less tired and achy. And as his overall condition improved, he became more energetic and began visiting his gym on the weekends and after work a couple of nights a week—creating a positive, healing cycle that began taking off the pounds as well as the years.

Inflammation is a protective reaction to an irritant or invading host. For instance, when your body encounters harmful bacteria, your blood vessels dilate, and white blood cells (also called immune cells) rush to the site like a SWAT team flying to the scene of a crime. These white blood cells produce powerful chemical compounds (cytokines and free radicals) that are designed to kill invaders. Cytokines, while useful in fighting an infection, also trigger inflammation, which manifests in the swelling, redness, or pain that accompanies an injury or illness.

Immune cells are constantly traveling through our respiratory and intestinal tracts and a nearly infinite corridor of blood vessels, searching for a diverse range of enemies. Microbes enter our bodies and penetrate our outer defenses by the thousands with every breath and bite we take. Cancer cells also develop from within our own living tissues. The responsibilities of the immune system are enormous.

Still, the power of immune cells must exist within a delicate balance. If we don't have enough immune cells to fight off invaders, we die of infection or cancer. But when we have too many, or when our immune system is constantly being stimulated by factors other than actual disease—poor dietary habits, environmental toxins, and even excess weight—we're setting ourselves up for chronic low-grade inflammation at the cellular level.

Inflammation can occur in the cells lining our arteries (contributing to cardiovascular disease), brain (contributing to Alzheimer's), lungs (contributing to asthma and bronchitis), intestines (contributing to inflammatory bowel disease, including Crohn's disease and ulcerative colitis), joints (manifesting in osteoarthritis as well as rheumatoid arthritis), and skin (causing dermatitis). Indeed, many diseases are associated with inflammation. Chronic, excessive inflammation accelerates aging because it, like oxidative stress, can increase the breakdown of tissue in organs throughout your body.

Many internal and external factors can increase inflammation. Internal causes often relate to your lifestyle, including excessive oxidative stress, insulin resistance, and obesity. Surprisingly, fat cells can pump cytokines into your system, which will cause inflammation and make you tired and achy, further limiting your activity and discouraging you from exercising, which will lead to the growth of more fat cells. Thus remaining active and controlling your body fat are vitally important to controlling inflammation and stopping this downward spiral.

External triggers can also increase inflammation. The typical American diet is low in omega-3 fats (found in seafood, flaxseed, soy products, nuts, and canola oil) and high in omega-6 fats (found in corn and other grain oils and in land animal protein sources such as meat and poultry). Omega-6 fats increase inflammation at the same time that omega-3 fats reduce it. The imbalance in the average American diet—with nearly a 20:1 ratio of omega-6 fats to omega-3 fats—appears to increase inflammation substantially.

Many elements of the Ten Years Younger Program—weight loss, reversing insulin resistance, modifying your food choices, and adding specific dietary supplements—will help you decrease inflammation and thus slow tissue injury and aging. You'll increase your intake of anti-inflammatory Vitality Foods and omega-3 fats while decreasing omega-6 fats. You'll eat less land animal protein and more seafood. You'll choose olive or canola oil over corn or other oils. Like Joe, you may benefit from supplements that have anti-inflammatory activity, such as fish oil, turmeric, ginger, and/or rosemary. In fact, adding 2 to 4 grams of fish oil daily can have a dramatic impact on autoimmune diseases such as rheumatoid arthritis and inflammatory bowel disease. I'll expand on this in Chapter 10.

Ginger also has significant anti-inflammatory activity. It can relieve joint pain and arthritis symptoms if used regularly over several weeks. And, in contrast to anti-inflammatory medications, it does not increase the risk of stomach or intestinal ulcers. This wonderful spice has been a great boon for people who have arthritis and gastrointestinal complaints. You'll find many delicious recipes containing ginger in Part III of this book.

Now that you know what your aging enemies are, you'll be able to avoid them using the Ten Years Younger Program. The good news is that my program will help you not only avoid these harmful aging accelerators but reverse much of the damage they've already done. Now let's take a closer look at how your body ages.

CHAPTER 2

# How the Body Ages

Everything ages—that's just a part of life. But aging can be accelerated or slowed down, if you know how.

Before you begin your anti-aging regimen, it's important to
understand how different parts of our body are influenced by the aging
accelerators we examined in Chapter 1 and look at how they can all
work together to keep you young. Although you might like to think
of your body's many different systems as independent, in truth they are
all linked to one another and integrated in amazing ways. And because
they are so interconnected, if you neglect one system, you're likely hurt-
ing others as well. The Ten Years Younger Program yields a total body
transformation and is designed to rejuvenate all your systems, top to
bottom.

Some of you may be eager to go ahead and get started on the diet,
and if so, feel free to skip ahead to Chapters 4 and 5. It's not necessary
to understand all the ins and outs of aging for the program to work. But
I do believe that the more clearly you grasp how all the choices you make
on a daily basis impact your own aging process, the more likely you'll be
to stick with the program. So if you'd like to know more about how and
why we age, and how my program can help, read on.

# Your Heart and Blood Vessels

As I explained in the Introduction, my experience working in third-world countries taught me that cardiovascular disease is not a given as we get older. You absolutely can prevent and even reverse it by changing your lifestyle. Food in particular plays an incredible role in the health of your heart and blood vessels. One kind of meal can deliver anti-aging nutrients to your cells that will clean your arteries and promote circulation and energy; another meal, one low in nutrients and packed with nasty fats and refined carbs, will form plaque in your blood vessels and constrict your circulation. Let's take a closer look at how this works.

## The Cholesterol Factor

Your arteries, the blood vessels that carry oxygen-rich blood from your lungs and heart to all of your cells, should be as wide open as an eight-lane freeway at two A.M. When your arteries are healthy, blood cells, nutrients, and cholesterol bubbles (composed of proteins and fats) should float easily downstream. And when you exercise, these arteries naturally dilate to increase the flow of blood to your lungs and muscles. But if you have cardiovascular disease, your arteries will look as if they're suffering from rush-hour traffic—obstruction and congestion. When you exercise, these clogged arteries don't open—they spasm, putting you at risk.

Although many of us have grown used to viewing cholesterol as a dangerous thing, it's important to understand that we all need *some* cholesterol in our bodies. Cholesterol is a fatty substance that helps cell walls remain flexible, is used as a raw material to make hormones and vitamin D, and sheaths nerves (like the plastic covering on wires that prevents short circuits). Cholesterol is also converted into bile acids (secreted by your gallbladder to digest fat) and thus plays an important role in digestion. Because our blood is mostly water, fatty nutrients (like vitamin E) don't dissolve in it. Like oil and water, they don't mix. They need to be carried some other way. Bubbles of cholesterol convey these fat-soluble nutrients from your intestines to the rest of your body.

Even with all the good it does, cholesterol has become everyone's favorite aging bugaboo. This is because not all cholesterol is created equal. There are three main kinds, and they affect your body in different ways:

- LDL (low-density lipoproteins)—or, as I like to think of it, lousy cholesterol—is the largest cholesterol component and is essentially a bubble full of fat and protein. LDL can clog your arteries the way that piles of garbage would disrupt traffic on a narrow city street. This is the kind of cholesterol that we need to worry about.
- Triglycerides are small beads of fat that fill the inside of LDL cholesterol bubbles and your fat cells and travel through your bloodstream. In excess, they cause problems. The higher your triglycerides, the higher the risk of clogging your arteries.
- HDL (high-density lipoproteins)—or healthy cholesterol—is like the garbage truck of the bloodstream. It travels around cleaning up loose garbage—namely, cholesterol and triglycerides—in your bloodstream, keeping your arteries clean. Clearly, you want more of that.

When you go for a physical, your doctor will give you a number that indicates your cholesterol level—for example, 186 or 225 or 300 mg/dl. That's your total cholesterol. But that single number doesn't tell the whole story. You need to know your specific HDL, LDL, and triglyceride levels. And what's even more important than the individual numbers themselves is the ratio of total cholesterol to your healthy, HDL cholesterol. That usually appears as the abbreviation TC/HDL.

To understand this TC/HDL ratio, think again of a large city with narrow streets. Your HDL acts like a garbage truck, hauling away excess bad cholesterol to your liver. If more garbage is produced than the garbage trucks can clean up, traffic is blocked. Your ratio reflects the proportion of total garbage to garbage trucks. When you lower your LDL and raise your HDL, your ratio improves, and your body—particularly your heart and blood vessels—is healthier.

But let's focus a bit more on the LDL cholesterol. The problem is

| TEN YEARS YOUNGER TARGETS | AVERAGE | YOUR MINIMAL GOAL | TEN YEARS YOUNGER GOAL |
| --- | --- | --- | --- |
| Total cholesterol | 200 | Less than 180 | Less than 160 |
| LDL | 130–160 | Less than 130 | Less than 90 |
| HDL (men) | 45 | More than 40 | More than 55 |
| (women) | 55 | More than 50 | More than 65 |
| Triglycerides (TG) | 100–150 | Less than 150 | Less than 90 |
| Total cholesterol/HDL ratio | 4.8 | Less than 4.0 | Less than 3.0 |
| Triglyceride/HDL ratio | 4.0 | Less than 3.0 | Less than 2.0 |
| Homocysteine | 10–11.4 | Less than 10 | Less than 9 |
| Blood pressure | 130/80 | 120/80 | 110/70 |
| hs-C-reactive protein | 1–1.5 | Less than 1.0 | Less than 0.5 |

not so much in the LDL itself but the way that it contributes to the creation of plaque or blockages in your arteries. The formation of hard plaques or lesions on the walls of your arteries is strongly related to inflammation (see Chapter 1). How does this happen? Free radicals, those exhaust products from energy production, attack LDL floating in your bloodstream. They oxidize the LDL, making them irritating to your cells and causing inflammation. Your white blood cells—the soldiers of the immune system—sense this abnormal LDL and come to your defense to remove the irritant, essentially swallowing the oxidized cholesterol.

You'd think that would be the end of the problem, but in this case, your white blood cells compound the situation. Poisoned by the oxidized cholesterol, the white blood cells die and slip into the lining of your arteries, where they accumulate, creating more inflammation and pus within the lining of your artery—essentially a pimple. A fibrous material forms around the dead cells and then hardens, turning into plaque within the lining of your artery. This arterial plaque builds up over time and blocks the flow of blood within the arteries. Continued inflammation can make this plaque pop like a pus-filled pimple—and that can lead to heart attack or stroke, especially since inflammation also increases the stickiness of your blood, making it clot more easily. When triglycerides are high in your blood, they increase plaque formation as well.

Lower levels of arterial plaque can have dangerous consequences, too. A 30 to 50 percent plaque obstruction doesn't sound like much. In fact, it doesn't block enough of the normal blood flow to cause symptoms like chest pains (angina) or give you an abnormal stress test. You may be totally unaware that it even exists. But if this relatively small obstruction ruptures, it can release inflammatory chemicals into the artery that could cause a large blood clot, blocking an entire artery and leading to a stroke or heart attack, or sudden death from an irregular heart rhythm. In fact, research has shown that 80 percent of heart attacks occur when little plaques (blocking less than 40 percent of the opening) have popped. This is why you'll occasionally hear stories of relatively young individuals in their forties who suddenly drop dead of a heart attack without any previous "history" of heart disease.

## CRP and Homocysteine

Several other factors may tell you about the state of your heart and arteries. For instance, C-reactive protein (CRP), recently in the news, can also predict your risk for cardiovascular disease. In fact, in some women it may be more accurate than cholesterol levels in determining the risk of a future cardiovascular event.

What is CRP? It is a protein produced by the liver in response to the amount of inflammatory compounds your body makes. Just as your home thermostat measures temperature, CRP is a measure of your body-wide inflammation. The more inflamed you are, the higher your CRP level and, as I just explained, the higher your risk for a cardiac event.

Homocysteine is an amino acid (protein building block) that is formed while the body is converting other amino acids into anti-aging proteins. It is another important marker for cardiovascular disease, and it appears to be toxic to brain cells as well as the cells that line your arteries. It also increases oxidation of LDL into plaque, and high homocysteine levels make your blood sticky, increasing your risk of a stroke or heart attack. People with high homocysteine levels develop more cardiovascular disease, suffer from greater memory loss, and have higher rates of Alzheimer's disease as well as blood clots in their limbs.

Your body is designed to use a mixture of B vitamins and enzymes to keep your homocysteine levels low, but people who either lack these enzymes or are deficient in B vitamins may have higher homocysteine levels and may be setting themselves up for dire results. The Ten Years Younger Diet combined with my supplement recommendations will help lower your homocysteine to a safe level.

## How Food Fits In

Poor eating habits, including low-carb, high-saturated-fat diets, can encourage plaque to form over time. But, shockingly, even a *single* low-carb, low-nutrient, high-saturated-fat meal can increase your immediate risk of a heart attack and/or stroke.

Here's how: If you eat whole-wheat pasta for lunch with a delicious sauce of vine-ripened tomatoes, garlic, and basil and a green leafy salad on the side with vinaigrette, your intestinal tract absorbs the nutrients from the food and delivers them to your blood. As I explained above, the fatty nutrients need to be carried to your cells by LDL cholesterol.

But here's where it gets interesting. Those same fat-soluble vitamins and nutrients that came from the healthy lunch I just described actually shield your LDL cholesterol from free radical damage, and thus from ultimately being converted into plaque. Every time you eat a healthy meal, you ensure that your LDL is "protected," so to speak—it will not become oxidized, irritate your arteries, or do you harm by fostering the creation of arterial plaque.

So what happens when you eat unhealthy foods that have no fat-soluble nutrients? To begin with, foods packed with refined carbs (white bread or pasta, sugary sweets) cause your HDL levels to drop and your triglyceride levels to leap. But more important, without nutrients to protect it, the LDL becomes oxidized. Not only will it begin forming plaque in your arteries, but the oxidized cholesterol will almost immediately begin to irritate your blood vessels, making them constrict. Studies have actually shown a 20 percent decrease in the diameter of arteries after an unhealthy breakfast (say, a stack of white-flour pancakes slathered in butter and syrup with pork sausage on the side) as compared to a healthy one (a bowl of oatmeal with blueberries and nonfat milk). I guess that's what they mean by the expression "a heart attack on a plate"!

This spasm occurs within twenty minutes of your meal and lasts for six to eight hours. The reduced circulation partially explains the stuck-in-your-chair feeling that's common after an unhealthy meal. If you block blood flow to the heart in a person who already has substantial artery plaque, that's the recipe for a heart attack, stroke, or sudden death.

Your Ten Years Younger goal is to stop making plaque and to dissolve some of the plaque you might have formed. The Ten Years Younger Diet as well as other aspects of the Ten Years Younger Program will normalize your cholesterol, triglyceride, CRP, and homocysteine levels. The program will help you revitalize your circulation so that you feel more energetic and full of life. In fact, the lifestyle changes I propose appear to be much more effective in preventing heart attacks, strokes, and death than medications, supplements, and cardiac procedures.

The best news is that when you decrease the oxidation of your LDL, you also extend your healthy life span, since, as we saw earlier, oxidation itself is an aging process.

## Your Metabolism

Diabetes is an age accelerator that can rob you of energy, health, and peace of mind. Most people think of it as a disease of high blood sugar, but it's really a problem of blood sugar regulation or metabolism. Over time, these problems destroy the function of your organs and clog your arteries. During its end stages, diabetes can even be a cause of death.

Yet diabetes is only the tip of the iceberg. As we saw in Chapter 1, beneath the surface lies a much bigger issue, metabolic syndrome—the early phase of diabetes, which causes weight gain and rapid aging despite normal blood sugar levels. It is nearly as devastating and much more common. Forty percent of us are afflicted with it by the time we reach 65. The Centers for Disease Control have estimated that 47 million Americans already have metabolic syndrome. One-third of Americans born in 2000 will develop it *and* Type 2 diabetes within their lifetime. Unless we do something right now, by the year 2050, the rate of this rapid-aging syndrome will have tripled.

It's entirely possible that you may have early symptoms of metabolic syndrome and not know it. If so, you are already aging rapidly, just like a diabetic, and it's only a matter of time before your body lets you know.

## How We Develop Metabolic Syndrome and Diabetes

When you're healthy, you have normal blood sugar, insulin, cholesterol, and hormone levels. Your weight is stable. Your blood sugar and fats do increase some after meals—this is normal—but all the calories you've eaten are burned. However, when you eat more calories than you use, you can begin that long downward spiral toward metabolic syndrome and Type 2 diabetes. Here's how the condition progresses.

*Stage I.* Your muscle cells are designed to store sugar (or energy) as glycogen. A beautiful rhythm exists between activity and eating—energy is packed away in your muscles following a meal and then burned away with activity. Insulin is the hormonal messenger that prompts your muscle tissue to store energy, and it is produced by the pancreas in response to eating. But if more calories are coming in than your muscles can burn, your tissues stop listening to insulin as a messenger. The extra energy is stored not in your muscles but now in fat cells, and you gain weight.

At first, your insulin and blood sugar levels remain normal. But over time, your muscle cells become more and more resistant to insulin's message to store that extra sugar. Insulin levels rise, causing fat to build around your heart, liver, and kidneys and at your waistline. In fact, an expanding waist is a strong indicator of insulin resistance. It's one of the first signs that you're developing metabolic syndrome and suffering from accelerated aging.

*Stage II.* Insulin levels continue to rise, still managing to keep blood sugar levels normal, but your muscle and fat cells become increasingly resistant to their message. Now your liver is forced to convert the extra sugar floating in your blood into fat in the form of triglycerides, so your triglyceride levels increase. At the same time, your poor overworked liver is less able to handle the responsibility of producing healthy HDL cholesterol, so your HDL levels drop. High insulin levels are harmful, especially because they trigger the increase of other hormones (cortisol, adrenaline, and glucagon) that normally counterbalance their effects.

These hormones boost your heart rate and blood pressure and cause abnormal blood vessel function. They also build belly and organ fat. This stage reflects rapid aging, often years before a diagnosis of Type 2 diabetes is confirmed. In fact, here's where the diabetes–heart disease connection comes in.

*Stage III.* Not only do your muscle and fat cells remain resistant to insulin, but now your liver balks. When it fails to convert all the extra energy into triglycerides, your blood sugar levels begin to rise, resulting in an increase in fatty acids in your blood. These acids are toxic to beta cells, the cells in your pancreas that produce insulin. As your beta cells start to die, insulin production drops, causing a quick spike in blood sugar.

*Type 2 diabetes.* As insulin levels drop, blood sugar levels now rise. Diabetes is the end result. Although it seems to come on suddenly, this process has usually been going on for at least ten years before the diagnosis is made.

Now here's the good news. You can prevent and even reverse the various stages of metabolic syndrome and Type 2 diabetes by following the Ten Years Younger Program—a lifestyle tailored for your genes. Your food and activity choices will help you. The Vitality Foods in the Ten Years Younger Diet, such as leafy greens, rye and barley, nuts and other high-fiber foods, and seafood high in healthy omega-3 fats, will help to naturally regulate blood sugar levels and unhealthy fats. And the exercises and muscle-building activities I emphasize in Age-Busting Fitness will get to the root of the problem—the imbalance between how many calories you eat versus how many you burn. Supplements can help in this regard as well.

While I do prescribe medications for my patients to treat full-blown Type 2 diabetes when necessary, I encourage (and they prefer) a Ten Years Younger lifestyle that reverses the process completely!

## Your Muscles

You know that you need muscles to plant flowers, pick up your baby, chew your dinner, and dance the night away. You need them to drive a car and even turn the pages of this book. But did you know that your muscles are essential for life?

Muscle protein is dynamic. It's constantly being broken down and converted into amino acids, the building blocks that your body uses for a variety of functions. Amino acids are used to repair tissue and build immunoglobulins that fight infections. They provide the primary fuel for cells that line the small intestine and regulate most of your nutrition. They carry oxygen to your cells in the form of hemoglobin, transport calcium and iron in the blood, and perform countless other functions essential to life. Muscle mass also provides a reserve of protein during times of stress. If you think about your muscle mass as an organ that builds and maintains a protein reserve, it becomes the largest organ in your body. Nearly 8 to 12 percent of your muscle tissue is turned over every day. Of your total need for protein, about 75 percent comes from this kind of internal recycling and only 25 percent comes from your diet.

However, as time goes on, more muscle protein is withdrawn from your protein bank than is deposited back into your muscle account. This means that you gradually but consistently lose muscle tissue. All things remaining equal, you can expect to gain at least a pound of fat and lose half a pound of muscle a year. That's a 15-pound drop in muscle mass and a 30-pound gain in fat between the ages of 30 and 60!

The beef industry would describe this transformation as a change from free-range to prime beef—from lean and tough to highly marbled. While some might think this makes for tasty eating, what this change really means is that your body tissue is now packed with fat!

Although this process is normal to some degree, it's also a major factor in accelerated aging. Less muscle and more fat at any age means more inflammation (because excess fat produces excessive amounts of cytokines) and thus more joint pain, more plaque in your arteries, weaker muscles and bones (with a greater risk of disabling fractures), and less strength and stamina. Plus the added cytokines and loss in blood sugar regulation further increase inflammation, thus elevating your risk of clotting (upping the danger of heart attack and stroke), and raise your risk of memory loss. The drop in muscle mass (and the normal supply of amino acids used to build immune-fighting compounds) also results in a greater risk of cancer.

Sadly, the shift toward more fat and less muscle turns into a nasty downward spiral, with more weight gain and a greater chance of developing metabolic syndrome and diabetes. The long-term result of continued muscle loss is frailty, loss of independence, and a big drop in the quality of your life.

## Muscle Mass: Your Anti-Aging Ally

The bottom line is "Use it or lose it!" Not surprisingly, inactivity—not age—is the biggest culprit in the loss of muscle mass. In a University of California study on master athletes, researchers found that these active adults had as much muscle mass as people ten to twenty years their junior. Fitness truly does keep you young!

What else erodes your muscle mass? There are several other factors, many of which are linked to the other aging culprits we've already discussed.

- *Insulin resistance.* Insulin stimulates the creation of muscle protein, but as insulin resistance increases with age and the onset of metabolic syndrome, it can undermine the rebuilding of your muscles.
- *Increased cortisol.* Running hand in hand with insulin resistance is a rise in cortisol, which breaks down muscle cells.
- *Too much inflammation.* A factor in insulin resistance, it also appears to speed the erosion of muscle tissue.
- *A decline in hormones.* The loss of growth hormone and testosterone as we age is strongly related to a drop in muscle mass.

The number one treatment for shrinking muscles is to exercise more often, especially with strength training. Studies have shown that with strength training, even elderly patients can restore the amount of muscle mass that would normally be lost in ten years with a short ten-to-twelve-week exercise program. The Age-Busting Fitness regimen in Chapter 6 includes the best muscle-building exercises and will help you work on twelve parts of your body two or three times a week to rebuild strength and muscle mass. You will also be able to reduce insulin resistance and inflammation by coupling the workout I recommend with the Ten Years Younger Diet for weight control.

## Your Brain

Most of us are more terrified of losing our memory than we are of cardiovascular disease or cancer. We dread being unable to care for ourselves or to function to our full capacity. One of my patients, Ken, had been an extremely successful businessman, having formed several thriving companies. Part of a loving family, he was active in his community and in philanthropy. But he came to me because his memory was slipping. He couldn't keep track of the details in the many business and charitable organizations in which he was involved. At the age of 60, he exercised vigorously every day, but kept himself going on coffee. In fact, the more coffee he drank, the more wired he felt. He seldom slept more than six or seven hours. Trying to be health conscious, he ate sushi every day for lunch.

While Ken's usual laboratory studies and exam were normal, I found that his memory speed was lower than predicted for his age, and his mental flexibility was quite low. Test results showed that his mercury, homocysteine, and cortisol levels were elevated. It also struck me that he was eating too many refined carbs. Fortunately, there was a great deal I could do to restore Ken's mental performance.

Several key processes are involved in the accelerated loss of your brain cells, including excess inflammation, metabolic syndrome and diabetes, mercury toxicity, chronic stress, and elevated homocysteine levels. Fortunately, the Ten Years Younger Program shows you how to manage these conditions to minimize loss in brain function.

As nationally recognized neurologist David Perlmutter explains, inflammation can set a brain on fire—that is, the brain cells are burned by inflammatory compounds. And sadly, unlike many other tissues in the body, nerve cells don't have the same potential to rebound after an injury. Significant brain damage can in fact result from long-term inflammation.

What causes this inflammation? Your diet plays a big role. As I explained previously, when you eat refined carbs (sugary sweets; bread, bagels, or pasta made with white flour; pretzels and chips) your proteins become sugarcoated. This is toxic to your brain cells and causes their rapid destruction. Unfortunately, the hippocampus, the area of your brain responsible for memory and advanced mental function, is the most sensitive to inflammatory damage from sugarcoated proteins, so memory loss occurs. Not surprisingly, then, metabolic syndrome and diabetes, which are very common health problems in the United States, are having a dreadful impact on cognitive performance on a grand scale. It's likely that millions of people are losing brain function at a time when the Ten Years Younger Program can prevent and even reverse some of this loss.

Toxins, and mercury in particular, also speed brain cell injury. Clinical laboratories note that mercury levels greater than 5 parts per million pose an elevated risk to our health. I measure mercury levels in my clinical practice routinely, and I see levels greater than 5 parts per million in red blood cells all the time, usually because people eat the wrong types of fish. Not surprisingly, research has shown that if you eat tuna (which can be higher in mercury than other fish) more than weekly, it slows your information processing. While scientists debate which specific harms are directly related to mercury exposure, the simple thing to do in the meantime is to limit your exposure as best you can. The information I present in Chapter 5 and Appendix D will help you identify seafood sources that are high in healthful omega-3 fats but still low in mercury.

Chronic stress and high cortisol levels are also related to the deterioration of the memory center. High cortisol levels are strongly associated with cell death, in particular in the hippocampus. Excess caffeine intake, chronic sleep deprivation, and chronic unmanaged stress all elevate cortisol levels. In contrast, getting adequate sleep and exercising regularly have been shown to lower cortisol levels and enhance cognitive performance, and are associated with a lower risk of Alzheimer's disease.

Finally, as I noted earlier, elevated homocysteine levels are associated not only with an increased risk for heart attacks and strokes but also with memory loss. Homocysteine is toxic to the energy-producing structures in your cells (the mitochondria), and it is especially damaging to the mitochondria in your brain cells. The higher your blood level of homocysteine, the higher your risk of Alzheimer's disease. Fortunately, adding foods and supplements that lower homocysteine levels is easy to do, safe, and effective.

Obviously, stress management and avoiding foods that hurt you are simple first steps to reversing the problems associated with memory loss. You can also add helpful foods, such as all those brightly colored fruits and vegetables emphasized in the Ten Years Younger Diet, as these pigments protect brain cells from damage from oxidative stress. In particular, resveratrol, a recently identified anti-aging compound discovered in red grapes and red wine, blocks inflammation and is associated with brain protection.

Omega-3 fats from seafood or fish oil are also particularly important in protecting brain function. First, omega-3 fats from seafood are very effective in blocking inflammation. They also enhance blood sugar control, decreasing brain cell damage from sugarcoated proteins. Finally, they help keep cell membranes flexible, enhancing and potentially increasing communication between brain cells. It is no surprise that people who eat more fats from seafood also have much lower rates of Alzheimer's disease.

## Your Bones

If you think of your body as a purely mechanical structure, you may judge it by its appeal to the human eye. Yet your bones and muscles also hold vast reserves of minerals and proteins that play a critical role in how your body functions. As you move and exercise, you stimulate your muscle and bone tissue to grow stronger. And building bone and muscle mass is like building a solid retirement fund. It gives you capital for your future.

I like to think of our bones as a retirement bank account. You store calcium and other minerals in your bones, just as you put money in the bank. The more calcium and minerals deposited there, the stronger and denser they become. One of your goals in becoming ten years younger is to increase your bone mass, providing you with a beautiful reserve of minerals that will promote vitality and longevity well into your golden years.

We are all born with enough calcium in our "bone account" to last throughout our childhood. From puberty until you reach the age of 21, the density of your bones increases quickly. It plateaus there until you're 30 and then gradually drops for the rest of your life. Most people don't realize that they need to build their lifetime calcium account between the ages of 13 and 21. Had they known this, they might have downed more calcium (e.g., more nonfat milk and fewer Cokes) and been a bit more active as a teenager!

## How Do We Lose Bone Mass?

Cells within your bones are continuously dissolving calcium (and other minerals such as magnesium, phosphorus, and boron) and releasing them into the bloodstream. In fact, every day your bone cells remove about 300 mg of calcium. At the same time, other cells redeposit these minerals into your bones. But unless you redeposit the full 300 mg of calcium you've lost, your bone mass will decrease, and your bones will lose their strength.

Your bone-recycling cells are under the direct influence of your hormonal and immune systems. Inflammation, too much cortisol, certain medications like high doses of steroids (used to treat asthma, arthritis, and autoimmune diseases, especially long-term), and insulin resistance also increase the rate at which calcium leaches from your bones. Other factors that deplete calcium include too little activity, too much salt, too much animal protein, too much cola, too much caffeine, and any tobacco.

When your bones weaken, they become brittle. Once you lose about 40 percent of your total bone mass, you are in a state of what I call bone poverty. This loss usually corresponds to a diagnosis of osteoporosis. Losing additional bone density puts you at an immediate increased risk for disabling fractures.

About 10 million Americans currently suffer from osteoporosis and another 20 to 25 million have mild bone loss (called osteopenia). More American women die from an osteoporosis-related hip fracture than from ovarian, uterine, and breast cancer combined. Though we rarely associate osteoporosis with males, a man of 50 or older is more likely to break a hip from osteoporosis than to get prostate cancer.

After age 30, the only way you can substantially increase your bone density is with prescription drugs that are used to treat advanced osteoporosis. Better would be to prevent loss in your bone account in the first place. Fortunately, with the Ten Years Younger Program you can slow and nearly stop the loss that normally occurs.

## Take Some Advice from NASA

Young and fit astronauts sent to man the International Space Station have lost substantial bone mass because of the severe inactivity associated with weightlessness. Some even developed osteoporosis within a couple of months. To combat this, NASA has spent about $10 million to ship special gym equipment to the space lab. In order to offset the lack of gravity, astronauts must spend several hours a day exercising on resistance machines so that they can maintain their bone density.

Here on earth, your activity level also plays an enormous role in maintaining your bone mass. Each step you take stimulates your bones to deposit calcium. Lie on the couch for a while and your bones release and lose calcium. The more active you are, the stronger your bones will be. Weight-bearing exercise is terrific for your bones—walking, jogging, or using an elliptical trainer. When you lift weights, you also stimulate bone tissue to strengthen and deposit calcium. Age-Busting Fitness is your first line of defense against bone loss.

Since calcium is the currency your bones use, increasing your calcium intake and limiting the calcium that is pulled unnecessarily from your bones will improve your long-term calcium retirement fund. Add calcium to your diet by eating green leafy veggies, nonfat dairy products, and calcium-fortified foods. Even soy beans and sardines are great sources of calcium. The Ten Years Younger Diet contains a wide range of calcium-rich foods and shows you how to start making smart lifestyle choices that will help you on this front.

At the same time, you also want to limit foods and drinks that deplete calcium from your bones. You should:

- Limit your salt (sodium) intake to less than 2,400 mg daily.
- Reduce animal protein (meat, poultry, and fish) to no more than 10 ounces a day.
- Avoid or limit colas, as they contain phosphoric acid, which increases the calcium you excrete.
- Drink no more than 1 to 2 cups of coffee a day. (In contrast, tea is good for your bones!)
- Steer clear of all tobacco products.

Depending on your age and physical condition, calcium supplements are also a wise choice. In Chapter 8, I'll help you identify how much calcium you need every day, especially as different people have different calcium intake requirements. The Common Calcium Sources chart in Appendix C will clarify how much you're currently getting from your diet. If you don't eat enough calcium to reach your needs, I'll explain the best way to get it through supplements in Chapter 10.

## Your Skin

Forty-six-year-old Sally came to see me because her skin had become blotchy. She'd spent most of her childhood in Boston, where she'd acquired severe sunburns two or three times each summer. For the last three years, Sally had lived in Florida—causing more sun troubles. She was recently divorced and had started dating again, and she hated having spots on her skin at this critical juncture in her life.

When I examined her, I saw that Sally had fair skin, yet her face, neck, and arms were dotted with many small brown sunspots. Her forehead, cheeks, and upper chest also showed irregular color. But the condition of her skin was worse than we could detect with the naked eye. When I shone an ultraviolet light over it, so that we could see the true extent of the sun damage, Sally started to cry.

I sat her down, listened to her concerns, and reassured her that I could make her skin look smoother, softer, and much younger if she would follow six easy steps. Ten weeks later, the blotches and discoloration were gone, and some of the fine wrinkles had disappeared, too.

The most common cause of accelerated skin aging is tanning and exposure to the sun. Compare the skin around your underarms to your forearms. The underarm skin is smoother, softer, and has more regular color. It seems plumper and less wrinkled. Now look in the mirror. The skin on the left side of your face may look older and blotchier than the skin on the right. That's because your left cheek is exposed to more sunlight while you're driving in the car!

Healthy skin is soft, smooth, and even. It has enough fat and collagen to give you a youthful contour and complexion with minimal wrinkling. But sunlight can increase the presence of free radicals inside skin cells, damaging DNA, collagen, and normal cell function. Tobacco smoke is equally harmful. The six-step plan that I'll share with you in Chapter 8 is the same as the one that worked for Sally and hundreds of other patients I've treated over the years. After ten weeks on my skincare regimen, Sally looked ten years younger. She was delighted about her new appearance and felt more confident as she re-entered the world of dating.

To understand how certain skin-care products can make your skin appear healthier, less wrinkled, and more radiant, you need to be aware of basic skin structure and cycling. Your skin is made up of three layers:

- *The epidermis.* This is the outer layer that you can see. It gives your skin its texture, color, and moisture. If your epidermis is rough or dry, your skin looks older.
- *The dermis.* This layer, just below the epidermis, is what gives your skin its thickness and shape.
- *The subcutaneous layer.* Below the epidermis and the dermis, this layer separates your skin from your muscles and body parts. It consists of fatty tissue, nerves, and blood vessels.

The outermost layer, the epidermis, is constantly recycling. New epidermis cells form at the border of the dermis and gradually migrate to the surface. As the cells move up, they become drier and rougher. In fact, the thicker your skin (the more layers of cells within the epidermis), the older it looks. It normally takes a cell twenty to forty days to make this journey. But as you age, the skin cell cycle slows down so your oldest skin cells show for a longer time. Happily, treatments that speed up the cycle reveal younger skin cells and make your skin look softer and smoother.

Fats in the epidermis layer also help to make your skin look moister and younger. Diet is a factor here. Ultra-low-fat diets can make your skin appear drier and older. But a diet with 20 to 30 percent of calories coming from healthy sources of fat (as recommended in the Ten Years Younger Diet) will improve your skin's appearance greatly.

Bingeing on sugar-rich foods, which are bad for you in so many other ways, also sugarcoats the collagen (a protein) in your skin and increases wrinkles. But the Ten Years Younger Program will help you reverse the damage and protect your collagen to prevent further wrinkles.

All in all, the Ten Years Younger Program aims to protect your circulation, metabolism, brain, bone and muscle mass, and skin from accelerated aging. While that might sound like a tall order, turning back the clock is what this program is all about. And now it's time to let the program start working for you. In Chapter 3, I'll show you how to assess your own physiological age, so that you too can measure your own progress as you begin taking off the years.

# How Old Are You Really?

YYou know what's written on your birth certificate, but as you're now well aware, your chronological age may not match your biological age. In other words, you may be older than you think. So, don't you want to know how old you *really* are?

In this chapter, I'm going to help you uncover this vital but often hidden piece of information. Not only will we solve the mystery of your real age, but the tests I'll be sharing with you will help you establish your baseline before you begin the Ten Years Younger Program. They'll also give you realistic goals to shoot for as you go through the program. Then, at the end of ten weeks, you'll repeat the same tests to show off your success.

There are five key things we can measure to give us a true sense of your biological aging:

1. Aerobic fitness
2. Strength
3. Body fat
4. Cholesterol
5. Brain function

In the pages that follow, you'll find several options to calculate each of these markers. While ideally you should test yourself with all five throughout the program, you can get a good read on your progress if you follow even two or three over the course of the next ten weeks. I'll also share other aging tests at the end of this chapter that you might want to have done at your doctor's office before you start.

## Understanding Your Ten Years Younger Goals

Since overall fitness levels normally decrease by 1 percent a year, in general your Ten Years Younger goal will be to increase your fitness by 10 percent over ten weeks. Many of the tests will give you a performance number that compares you with others your age. You can also use that score to measure yourself against people in other age groups and to determine where you'd really like to be in terms of your fitness level. For example, the maximum heart rate (pulse) you can reach with vigorous exercise is a predictor of your biological age. An easy way to estimate your appropriate maximum achievable heart rate with exercise is to subtract your actual age from the number 220.

Here's how it works. Linda is an average, relatively fit 50-year-old. When you push her into a flat-out run on the treadmill, she may reach a maximum heart rate of 170 beats per minute (220 − 50 = 170). This is fine, and appropriate for her age, but it could be even better. The good news for Linda is that if over the next ten weeks she eats well, exercises daily, noticeably improves her fitness level, and then repeats the treadmill test, it's likely that her maximum heart rate will be 180 beats per minute. She will now have the heart fitness of a healthy 40-year-old—ten years younger!

Someone who is less fit than Linda, such as her 50-year-old best friend, Marcia, may with vigorous exercise only reach 160 beats per minute. Biologically, this tells us that Marcia is ten years *older* than her birth certificate says. Her heart responds like a 60-year-old's—not a good thing! Marcia's goal in following the Ten Years Younger Program will be to actually achieve the average heart rate for her age. Though not as dazzling as Linda's accomplishment, this is still a great improvement for Marcia that will continue to yield health benefits for her in the long run.

And as her level of fitness increases, she may indeed begin to shave additional years off her biological age.

I've set up many of the tests so you can accomplish them on your own without too much trouble or expense. I also suggest more extensive testing available from your doctor or at the gym, if you're interested. And in each case, I offer healthy profiles, whether you're in your 20s or your 60s, so that you know what your assessment should look like. You'll also find tables in this chapter that show norms by gender and age (broken into decades), many of which have been established by the American College of Sports Medicine.

## Assessing Aerobic Fitness

Aerobic fitness is one of the keys to feeling and staying young, and it's absolutely essential for lowering your physiological age. Because fitness levels naturally decrease over time, measuring your aerobic fitness allows you to assess your overall health as well as your rate of aging. You'll find here several ways to do this, including your maximal achieved heart rate, one-minute heart rate recovery, MET level, and $VO_2max$. Bear in mind that a treadmill test can't always assess your true level of fitness. If you have leg, back, foot, or hip pain that limits your running, you won't be able to push yourself to your maximum potential.

### Test 1: Take Your Pulse

The simplest way to measure your aerobic fitness is to find the *maximum* heart rate you can reach while exercising. As a physician, I'd like first to clarify the risks and benefits of maximal exercise testing. If you push yourself to your highest effort during exercise, there's a very small risk (1 in 10,000) that you could have a cardiovascular accident (such as a fainting spell, heart attack, or, even more rarely, sudden death). The worse your health and fitness level, the higher your risk becomes. That tiny risk of having a significant cardiovascular event exists in my clinic, too. But in truth, if you were to encounter a problem during testing, what better place to have it than at your doctor's office with medical equipment and trained staff immediately available?

At best, I recommend that you perform this kind of exercise testing with your physician. If that doesn't work for you, I'd like to suggest working out at the gym with an exercise physiologist or trainer, or simply doing it at a gym with staff in the vicinity. Even if they're not supervising you directly, it's good to have someone present in the extremely unlikely case that you feel dizzy. Obviously, if you're young, healthy, and fit, you might choose to do this test without anyone observing. A good rule of thumb: The more out of shape you are, and the more significant medical problems you have, the more important it is that you do this test with a physician or with an exercise physiologist in a gym.

Having clarified the risks, there are enormous benefits to doing this exercise and defining your real maximal heart rate. This score will help you make the best use of your fitness program and derive the most benefit within a reasonable time. In Chapter 6, I'll explain how to use this heart rate number to develop your aerobic exercise program. But here's how you find the number in the first place.

**What You'll Need:** a treadmill, a wristwatch that shows seconds

1. *Find your pulse at rest (or wear a heart rate monitor).* Before you begin exercising, gently place your fingers over the radial artery on your inner wrist or use a pulse-measuring tool such as a chest band. Using your watch, count the number of heartbeats within a 15-second period. Multiplying by 4 gives you your pulse rate for one minute.

2. *Warm up.* Start off gradually on the treadmill, giving yourself a 3-minute warm-up at a brisk walking pace. Then gradually increase your pace.

3. *As your pace builds, find your maximum, comfortable exertion level.* This means pushing yourself to the point where you are breathing hard, puffing, and just barely able to talk in short sentences but clearly unable to sing. Your stride is still steady (you aren't stumbling), your color is good, and you could keep on going a few more seconds.

4. *Now check your pulse again.* Using your watch, count the number of heartbeats within a 15-second period, say 42. Multiply this by 4 (42 beats × 4 = 168 beats per minute). This is your maximal achieved heart rate. (Note: Be sure to do this the old-fashioned way. Treadmills and exercycles with hand measuring devices may not be accurate enough, as they usually record only a three-beat sequence and yield varying heart rates.)

5. *Compare your maximal achieved heart rate to the formula for determining the optimum rate for a person your age:* 220 – your age = normal maximal heart rate.

On average, a fairly fit 40-year-old can comfortably reach a maximum heart rate of 180. (That's 220 – 40 = 180.) If you're 40 and can reach a heart rate of 190, then you have the relative cardiac fitness of an average 30-year-old. At age 50, my own heart rate with maximum, comfortable exercise goes to 190. This reassures me of good cardiac fitness.

Write down the maximum heart rate you achieved, because you're going to use it to determine your exertion level for aerobic exercise in Chapter 6. Bear in mind that this equation won't work if you're taking blood pressure medications such as beta blockers that limit your heart rate. You might also get an inaccurately high pulse if you overuse stimulants such as caffeine and decongestant medications.

A better predictor of your heart's fitness, although not a measure of physiological age, is to track how quickly your heart rate decreases after peak exercise. You want to see a rapid drop to indicate good heart fitness; it means your heart is able to readily adjust to accommodate varying levels of physical stress. In a 2005 article in the *New England Journal of Medicine* that studied more than 5,000 people, French cardiologist Xavier Jouven and his colleagues found that a one-minute heart rate recovery is one of the most important measures for predicting your risk of sudden death.

To discover how quickly your heart rate drops after the pulse test, quickly reduce your exercise level to a very slow walk, say 1.5 miles per hour without incline. Walk in this way for 60 seconds and take your pulse again. I like to see a minimum 25-beat drop at one minute, and I'd prefer to see more than a 30-beat drop. At two minutes, your heart rate should have dropped by at least 42 beats. This indicates a good cardiac fitness level.

If your heart rate doesn't drop by at least 12 beats after one minute, your risk of a cardiovascular event (heart attack, stroke, or sudden death) in the near future would be quite high. In several studies across the country that measured whether exercise stress tests predict the risk of future cardiovascular events in people between the ages of 30 and 80, with or without heart disease, the one- or two-minute heart rate recovery was judged to be the best tool. Again, if you're taking blood pressure or other medications that modify your heart rate, you may be unable to measure your heart rate recovery accurately.

## Test 2: Measure Your METs

No, this is not the name of a New York baseball team! METs is a term that describes how much energy you use while performing a particular activity, as in met-abolic energy burning rate. The usual measurement for your overall exertion level is your "MET level achieved." One MET of energy is what you burn lying completely still in bed. If you're running

MET LEVELS FOR VARIOUS JOBS AND ACTIVITIES

| OCCUPATION | METS |
|---|---|
| Receptionist | 1.0–2.0 |
| Housekeeper | 1.5–4.0 |
| Farm worker | 3.5–7.5 |
| Construction worker | 4.0–8.5 |
| Miner | 4.0–9.0 |
| Mail carrier | 2.5–5.0 |
| Medical professional | 1.5–3.5 |
| Walking with a suitcase | 7 |
| Cleaning floors | 4 |
| Cooking | 3 |
| Gardening | 4 |
| Pushing a power mower | 5 |
| Sexual intercourse | 5 |
| Making your bed | 5–6 |

on a treadmill machine at a 14 percent elevation at 3.4 miles per hour, you will reach about 8.0 to 8.3 METs during the first minute.

Most people should comfortably achieve at least 10 METs on a standard treadmill fitness test. Many of my robust 80-year-olds still make at least 10 to 12 METs, and with time and training you should be able to reach this level, too. Twelve METs is a very good level of fitness, and 13.5 METs is excellent. My truly athletic participants from their 30s through their 60s may reach 15 to 18 METs.

Doing well on a MET assessment is not just a matter of pride; it has important implications for your life. For every one-MET increase in fitness, your risk of a heart attack, stroke, or sudden death drops by 12.5 percent. If you can increase your fitness level by two METs (from 8 to 10), you would decrease your risk by 25 percent!

How do you measure METs? Physicians worldwide use a standardized treadmill test to gauge cardiovascular function. The most common test is called the Bruce Protocol. How long you're able to continue on the treadmill indicates your MET level. The table below gives you an approximate MET score based on your speed and elevation, which are increased every three minutes. To calculate your score, read the number of METs achieved at the end of each minute you complete, and continue until you reach your maximal exertion level. Ideally, this should be done with a physician, but it could be performed with a skilled exercise physiologist, and in truth you could measure this on your own with most treadmills.

**What You'll Need:** a treadmill with timer and the capacity to increase incline

Start the machine at the speed of 1.7 miles per hour with a 10 percent elevation. (This should be an easy walking warm-up speed.) After three minutes, increase promptly to 2.5 miles per hour and a 12 percent elevation. Continue to increase the settings every three minutes. When you reach your maximal, comfortable exertion level (breathing hard and just barely able to talk in short sentences), note the time elapsed and the elevation, measure your maximal heart rate—check your pulse for fifteen seconds and multiply that number by 4—and then immediately decrease

| MINUTES COMPLETED | SPEED (MPH) | ELEVATION (% GRADE) | MET LEVEL MEN | MET LEVEL WOMEN |
|---|---|---|---|---|
| 1 | 1.7 | 10 | 3.2 | 3.1 |
| 2 | " | " | 4.0 | 3.9 |
| 3 | " | " | 4.9 | 4.7 |
| 4 | 2.5 | 12 | 5.7 | 5.4 |
| 5 | " | " | 6.6 | 6.2 |
| 6 | " | " | 7.4 | 7.0 |
| 7 | 3.4 | 14 | 8.3 | 8.0 |
| 8 | " | " | 9.1 | 8.6 |
| 9 | " | " | 10.0 | 9.4 |
| 10 | 4.2 | 16* | 10.7 | 10.1 |
| 11 | " | " | 11.6 | 10.9 |
| 12 | " | " | 12.5 | 11.7 |
| 13 | 5.0 | 18* | 13.3 | 12.5 |
| 14 | " | " | 14.1 | 13.2 |
| 15 | " | " | 15.0 | 14.1 |

*If your treadmill doesn't go beyond 15 percent elevation, at 10 minutes adjust the incline to 15 percent and increase your speed to 4.4 miles per hour and at 13 minutes maintain the 15 percent incline and increase the speed to 5.4 miles per hour.

the speed to 1.5 miles per hour with no elevation. For example, 45-year-old Michelle reaches her maximal exertion at 11 minutes and 15 seconds, and therefore reaches 10.9 METs. She is in good but not excellent physical shape.

While you're in the midst of the METs test, it might also be helpful for you to assess your *perceived* exertion level—how hard do you feel you're actually working? This will help you be mindful of the intensity of your workout while doing the aerobic exercises in the program. So while you're on the treadmill, note how hard you are pushing it. Give your exertion a number value on a scale of 1 to 20. A level of 20 would be near collapse—you'd be unable to speak in two-word sentences. That's too much! Ideally, you should strive to attain an exertion level of 12 to 15, which is somewhat hard. At this level you should be able to speak in short sentences but be too short of breath to sing. This is a great range for sustained exercise, and what you'd like to reach each day during your aerobic workouts. You might also want to push yourself to a 17 for short intervals, where you're sweating, you're nearly spent and puffing, but you're still able to run smoothly and talk in short but not long sentences.

## Test 3: Find Your VO$_2$max

The gold standard for aerobic fitness testing is measuring VO$_2$max. This computes the volume of oxygen you burn during peak exercise—a great measure of your total body fitness level. Because it accurately predicts how old you are on a cellular level, VO$_2$max is the best test for Accelerated Aging Syndrome.

Every single cell in your body has a tiny power plant that burns oxygen to produce energy, even when you're resting. These power plants are called mitochondria. The better the food you eat, and the more often you exercise and increase your heart rate, the larger your muscle mass will grow, the more of these little power plants you'll accumulate, and the better they'll function. Healthy mitochondria can burn more oxygen than those that are sickly. Measuring your VO$_2$max reveals the total capacity of your mitochondria—that is, your total energy-burning capacity.

Like other fitness markers, VO$_2$max usually decreases by 1 percent a year. But whether you're 30 or 70, almost everyone can improve their VO$_2$max. It's never too late. In fact, during my Ten Years Younger study, participants who exercised at least five days a week and added 30 grams of fiber daily to their diets increased their VO$_2$max by 29 percent! If after 10 weeks of healthier living, you were able to increase your VO$_2$max by only 10 percent, you still would have become ten years fitter. Happily, increasing your VO$_2$max is easy with strength and aerobic training coupled with my Ten Years Younger Diet.

Usually VO$_2$max is measured at the doctor's office. If you were being assessed at my clinic, I'd have you run on a treadmill or pedal a bike as fast as you comfortably could while wearing a mask that measures the volume of oxygen your mitochondria burn. Your VO$_2$max would be reported as the volume of oxygen burned per minute per kilogram of body weight.

The great news is that you don't actually have to test your VO$_2$max level at your doctor's office. If you want to forgo the time and expense (around $300 to $400, though your insurance may cover most of the cost of this test if you have heart disease, diabetes, or other cardiovascular problems), simply multiply your MET level by 3.5. That predicts your $VO_2$max fairly well. For instance, if we were to multiply Michelle's MET level of 10.9 by 3.5, we could predict that her $VO_2$max would be 38.2. At 45 years of age, that puts her in the 85th percentile for aerobic

## $VO_2$MAX TESTING FOR MEN
### AEROBIC CAPACITY (ML/KG/MIN)

| AGE | 20-29 | 30-39 | 40-49 | 50-59 | 60+ |
|---|---|---|---|---|---|
| PERCENTILE | | | | | |
| 90 | 51.4 | 50.4 | 48.2 | 45.3 | 42.5 |
| 80 | 48.2 | 46.8 | 44.1 | 41 | 38.1 |
| 70 | 46.8 | 44.6 | 41.8 | 38.5 | 35.3 |
| 60 | 44.2 | 42.4 | 41.8 | 38.5 | 35.3 |
| 50 | 42.5 | 41 | 38.1 | 35.2 | 31.8 |
| 40 | 41 | 38.9 | 36.7 | 33.8 | 30.2 |
| 30 | 39.5 | 37.4 | 35.1 | 32.3 | 28.7 |
| 20 | 37.1 | 35.4 | 33 | 30.2 | 26.5 |
| 10 | 34.5 | 32.5 | 30.9 | 28 | 23.1 |

## $VO_2$MAX TESTING FOR WOMEN
### AEROBIC CAPACITY (ML/KG/MIN)

| AGE | 20-29 | 30-39 | 40-49 | 50-59 | 60+ |
|---|---|---|---|---|---|
| PERCENTILE | | | | | |
| 90 | 44.2 | 41 | 39.5 | 35.2 | 35.2 |
| 80 | 41 | 38.6 | 36.3 | 32.3 | 31.2 |
| 70 | 38.1 | 36.7 | 33.8 | 30.9 | 29.4 |
| 60 | 36.7 | 24.6 | 32.3 | 29.4 | 27.2 |
| 50 | 35.2 | 33.8 | 30.9 | 28.2 | 25.8 |
| 40 | 33.8 | 32.3 | 29.5 | 26.9 | 24.5 |
| 30 | 32.3 | 30.5 | 28.3 | 25.5 | 23.8 |
| 20 | 30.6 | 28.7 | 26.5 | 24.3 | 22.8 |
| 10 | 28.4 | 26.5 | 25.1 | 22.3 | 20.8 |

Adapted with permission of the American College of Sports Medicine's *Guidelines for Exercise Testing and Prescription,* 6th Edition, 2000. Data provided by Institute for Aerobics Research, Dallas, TX.

fitness for her age. If you're in the 85th percentile, that means your performance is the top 15 percent for your age group and gender. The 10th percentile means only 10 percent of people in your age group performed worse than you did, and 90th percentile means that 90 percent of people in your age group turned in a worse performance than you did.

If you were to move from one age group column to the previous one (even if you remained in the 30th percentile), you would be ten years younger. For example, if a 45-year-old woman could reach a $VO_2$max of 28.3 now, and after 10 weeks of the program could reach a $VO_2$max of 30.5, she would have improved from the 30th percentile to the 50th percentile for her age group. Plus, this new $VO_2$max is enough to put her in the range of a woman in her 30s. She's gone from the 30th percentile for a 40-year-old to the 30th percentile for a 30-year-old; fitnesswise she would be 10 years younger.

Your 10-week goal is to increase your $VO_2$max by ten years. Thinking beyond the next ten weeks, my ambitious long-term goal for you is to reach the 70th percentile for the age group that is ten years younger than you are. Of course, I don't expect you to achieve this right away, but it is absolutely achievable over the long haul, and it will serve you well.

## Testing Strength

Given what you've just read about mitochondria, you can see why increasing your muscle mass by 10 percent would make it easier for you to become the equivalent of ten years younger. Muscles burn calories and keep you trim, so increasing your muscle mass means having a bigger motor to burn calories from sugar and fat. And not surprisingly, our body's natural loss in muscle mass as we get older often leads to weight gain and obesity. All too often, we're not even aware that we're losing muscle. Take one of my study participants, 53-year-old Jill. When she started the program, she'd been sitting behind a desk for the last five years, and although seemingly trim and fit, she'd begun to notice that her body was changing. "I'm a little wider in the hips, and I have a little belly," she confided. "I took seventeen years of dancing lessons, so I thought I was a fit person. But what surprised me once I started the Ten

Years Younger Program was how much strength I *didn't* have. I was totally amazed."

So how do you gauge muscle mass? For years, scientists would dunk people into large tanks of water to calculate their lean muscle mass, but the expense and the sheer hassle of having to jump into a tank of water have limited this sort of testing. Even today, special tests such as electrical impedance and DEXA can be used to measure your body composition, but there are many confusing limitations when it comes to using these methods. In the end, the easiest way to measure your muscles is still simply to test your strength.

## Test 4: Push-ups and Abdominal Crunches

Your ability to perform abdominal crunches and push-ups is an excellent indicator of your muscle strength and mass—the more you can do, the stronger you are and the bigger your muscles!

The American College of Sports Medicine has developed tables (which I've adapted below) that can help you determine your fitness level and your current strength in relation to the optimum level for your age. Compare your level to others in your age group or see how your numbers stack up against people who are younger or older. These charts also let you calculate how much you need to improve in order to increase your strength by ten years. For instance, if 45-year-old Ken can do 19 push-ups (in the 70th percentile for his age), he would need to perform 24 push-ups to improve his performance by ten years.

> **What You'll Need:** a floor mat, a metronome (optional), masking tape, and a tape measure or ruler

A few ground rules before you start doing push-ups:

- Women should perform push-ups with their knees on the floor, but men must do their push-ups on their toes.
- You must perform the push-ups consecutively without resting in between.
- Your chin but not your stomach must touch the floor.

PUSH-UPS

| AGE | 20-29 | | 30-39 | | 40-49 | | 50-59 | | 60-69 | |
|---|---|---|---|---|---|---|---|---|---|---|
| GENDER | M | F | M | F | M | F | M | F | M | F |
| PERCENTILE | | | | | | | | | | |
| 90th | 41 | 32 | 32 | 31 | 25 | 28 | 24 | 25 | 24 | 23 |
| 80th | 34 | 26 | 27 | 24 | 21 | 22 | 17 | 17 | 16 | 15 |
| 70th | 30 | 22 | 24 | 21 | 19 | 18 | 14 | 13 | 11 | 12 |
| 60th | 27 | 20 | 21 | 17 | 16 | 14 | 11 | 10 | 10 | 10 |
| 50th | 24 | 16 | 19 | 14 | 13 | 12 | 10 | 9 | 9 | 6 |
| 40th | 21 | 14 | 16 | 12 | 12 | 10 | 9 | 5 | 7 | 4 |
| 30th | 18 | 11 | 14 | 10 | 10 | 7 | 7 | 3 | 6 | 2 |
| 20th | 16 | 9 | 11 | 7 | 8 | 4 | 5 | 1 | 4 | 0 |
| 10th | 11 | 5 | 8 | 4 | 5 | 2 | 4 | 0 | 2 | 0 |

Adapted with the permission of the Canadian Fitness and Lifestyle Research Institute.

- Your back must stay straight and your movements must be clean—slow, smooth, and steady is the key.
- You must keep moving—if you stop to rest for one second, you're done.

If you're a 30-year-old woman who is only able to do 12 push-ups, your goal should be 14 or better. If you can do 14, why not work toward 22 to 32? That puts you in the 70th percentile of the age group that's ten years younger! Jill told me, "When I started the program, I could only do 2 push-ups. I had the strength of a 70-year-old. When I ended the program, I had the strength of a 40-year-old. Now that's really motivating!"

You can also use crunches to measure your muscle strength. To do this properly, use a metronome and set it for 40 beats per minute. You'll be doing one crunch with each beat—a little more than one per second. Or, you can simply count a quick "one one thousand, two one thousand" to keep the same pace.

Before you begin, lie on your back with your knees bent and your arms at your sides. Place a tape line where your fingers end. Then place a second tape line 3¼ inches down toward your feet if you're 45 or older and 4¾ inches away if you're less than 45. Now lie down again, your

ABDOMINAL CRUNCHES

| AGE | 20-29 | | 30-39 | | 40-49 | | 50-59 | | 60-69 | |
|---|---|---|---|---|---|---|---|---|---|---|
| GENDER | M | F | M | F | M | F | M | F | M | F |
| PERCENTILE | | | | | | | | | | |
| 90th | 76 | 70 | 75 | 55 | 75 | 50 | 74 | 50 | 53 | 50 |
| 80th | 76 | 45 | 75 | 43 | 69 | 42 | 60 | 30 | 33 | 30 |
| 70th | 66 | 37 | 61 | 34 | 57 | 33 | 45 | 23 | 26 | 24 |
| 60th | 51 | 29 | 49 | 27 | 36 | 27 | 35 | 20 | 19 | 19 |
| 50th | 39 | 25 | 31 | 21 | 27 | 21 | 27 | 19 | 16 | 13 |
| 40th | 26 | 22 | 24 | 21 | 23 | 17 | 21 | 15 | 9 | 9 |
| 30th | 26 | 17 | 20 | 12 | 19 | 14 | 19 | 10 | 6 | 3 |
| 20th | 13 | 12 | 13 | 10 | 11 | 5 | 11 | 0 | 0 | 0 |
| 10th | 10 | 5 | 10 | 0 | 3 | 0 | 0 | 0 | 0 | 0 |

Adapted with the permission of the Canadian Fitness and Lifestyle Research Institute.

arms extended at your sides, your fingertips touching the first tape line. The idea is to have your fingers touch the second tape line with each and every crunch; don't count it if you come short. You'll be measuring the maximum number of crunches you've performed without missing a beat. If you stop for even two seconds, you are finished.

Increasing your ability to do push-ups and crunches is an easy way to drop your physiological age by 10 years. It is also a terrific way to improve your shape and to prevent back problems. As always, shoot for the 70th percentile of the age group below you. But to become ten years younger and ensure that your total muscle mass—not just that in your arms and abs—has increased by at least 10 percent, your strength training routine should include at least twelve different exercises, not just these two. You'll learn all about these age-defying moves in Chapter 6.

## Measuring Body Fat

Normally your body fat increases by 1 percent a year after the age of 40, but with accelerated aging, you may be gaining 2 to 4 percent a year. To lower your age by ten years, you'll need to decrease your body fat by 10 to 20 percent, depending on your weight gain.

How does this work? Take John, a 200-pound man whose body fat has been increasing by 1 to 2 percent a year. Thirty percent of his weight is composed of fat. That means he's carrying around 60 pounds of fat on his frame (200 pounds × 30% = 60 pounds). To be ten years younger, John would have to shed 9 pounds of his fat mass in order to lose 15 percent (60 pounds × 15% = 9 pounds). This 9-pound decrease in fat mass is entirely realistic if he follows the ten-week program in this book. In fact, this was the average loss in fat mass noted during my Ten Years Younger study.

Our goal in my research was to have those participants who were overweight at the beginning lose 1 pound a week. Given all the claims made by fad diets these days, you might feel this is disappointingly small. But many studies have shown that the most successful weight loss rate over the long haul is one pound a week. Furthermore, you'll also be adding lean muscle—which weighs more than fat—so even if the number on the scale drops by only 10 pounds, you'll still be losing substantial amounts of body fat and the size of your clothes should shrink noticeably.

So how is body fat measured? Again, there are several approaches we can take.

## Test 5: Measure Your Waist and Hips

As discussed above, your Ten Years Younger weight loss goal shouldn't be calculated on your bathroom scale. Most scales can't tell the difference between fat and muscle. You *want* more muscle, since it makes you look trim and fit. So rather than stepping on the scale, pull out that old-fashioned tape measure. It's going to help you determine how much fat you're carrying around.

Slip the tape measure around your waist. Measure the smallest circumference between your lowest rib and the top of your hipbone along your side. Take a big breath, relax your tummy, and blow out. Measure while your lungs are empty and your tummy is relaxed.

Now measure your hips. Choose the largest horizontal hip circumference you can. Be careful not to let the tape ride up or down, as that will give you an inaccurate hip circumference.

## WAIST-TO-HIP CIRCUMFERENCE RATIO

### ADVERSE HEALTH RISK FOR WOMEN

| AGE | LOW | MODERATE | HIGH | VERY HIGH |
|---|---|---|---|---|
| 20-29 | Less than 0.71 | 0.71-0.77 | 0.78-0.82 | More than 0.82 |
| 30-39 | Less than 0.72 | 0.72-0.78 | 0.79-0.84 | More than 0.84 |
| 40-49 | Less than 0.73 | 0.73-0.79 | 0.80-0.87 | More than 0.87 |
| 50-59 | Less than 0.74 | 0.74-0.81 | 0.82-0.88 | More than 0.88 |
| 60 and up | Less than 0.76 | 0.76-0.83 | 0.84-0.90 | More than 0.90 |

## WAIST-TO-HIP CIRCUMFERENCE RATIO

### ADVERSE HEALTH RISK FOR MEN

| AGE | LOW | MODERATE | HIGH | VERY HIGH |
|---|---|---|---|---|
| 20-29 | Less than 0.83 | 0.83-0.88 | 0.89-0.94 | More than 0.94 |
| 30-39 | Less than 0.84 | 0.84-0.91 | 0.92-0.96 | More than 0.96 |
| 40-49 | Less than 0.88 | 0.88-0.95 | 0.96-1.00 | More than 1.00 |
| 50-59 | Less than 0.90 | 0.90-0.96 | 0.97-1.02 | More than 1.02 |
| 60 and up | Less than 0.91 | 0.91-0.98 | 0.99-1.03 | More than 1.03 |

Adapted with permission from Heyward, Applied Body Composition Assessment. Human Kinetics, 2004.

Next, calculate your waist-to-hip ratio. How to do that? Simply divide your waist measurement by your hip measurement. Thirty-three-year-old Alicia's waist was 26 inches and her hips were 35 inches. Twenty-six divided by 35 gave her the ratio of .74. According to the above chart, that number would put Alicia at a moderate risk for major health problems, such as diabetes and heart attacks, for a woman her age.

In contrast, 200-pound John's waist and hips were both 39 inches. At age 50, this 1.0 ratio puts him at high risk of major health problems.

Once you've done the calculation, use the applicable chart to determine your risk level for your age and gender.

Remember, however, that this ratio is helpful only up to a point. No matter what your hips measure, a waist larger than 35 inches for a woman and 40 inches for a man is one of the warning signs of metabolic syndrome (see Chapter 1).

## Test 6: Body Mass Index (BMI)

Tall and thin? Short and squat? A good way to determine your body composition is to compare your weight in relation to your height. To address this very issue, scientists have created a standard measure, popularly called the body mass index, or BMI. Overwhelming evidence shows that if your BMI goes above 25, your health is at risk. The risk increases linearly from a BMI of 25 to 30, but above 30 (the obesity mark) further weight gain increases your risk of death and serious disease exponentially.

Your BMI is your weight in kilograms divided by your height in meters squared (kg/m2). (If you prefer to calculate your BMI in pounds and inches, divide your weight in pounds by your height in inches, then divide that number by your height in inches again, and then multiply the whole shebang by 703.) If you don't feel like doing the math, the table below shows the most common BMIs for both men and women.

The good news here is that if your BMI is more than 30, even a modest weight loss can produce a big drop in risk. If your BMI is over 30, then at the very least your Ten Years Younger weight goal should be a BMI of less than 29.

However, you should take care to choose a realistic weight goal and strategy. If you have a BMI of 35, a major step toward better health is to aim for a weight that helps you reach a BMI just under 30. It's unrealistic for a 5-foot-6-inch person who weighs 210 pounds with a BMI of 35 to aspire to a weight of 150 and a BMI of 24 as a first step. A weight of 180 and a BMI of 29 still have enormous health benefits and are much more achievable. Once you've stabilized at this new weight for several months, you can assess what other long-term lifestyle changes you're willing to make for additional improvements.

You should also be aware that BMI doesn't show the ratio of muscle to fat. Twenty-nine-year-old Peter could be all flab and his old college roommate, Matt, could be all muscle. But if they're the same height and weight, they'd have the same BMI. That's why people like Arnold Schwarzenegger would be the exception to the BMI rule. He might be quite heavy for his height but have little fat to show for it.

## BODY MASS INDEX

HEIGHT IN INCHES

| WEIGHT IN POUNDS | 58 | 59 | 60 | 61 | 62 | 63 | 64 | 65 | 66 | 67 | 68 | 69 | 70 | 71 | 72 | 73 | 74 | 75 | 76 |
|---|---|---|---|---|---|---|---|---|---|---|---|---|---|---|---|---|---|---|---|
| 100 | 21 | 20 | 20 | 19 | 18 | 18 | 17 | 17 | 16 | 16 | 15 | 15 | 14 | 14 | 14 | 13 |  |  |  |
| 105 | 22 | 21 | 21 | 20 | 19 | 19 | 18 | 17 | 17 | 16 | 16 | 16 | 15 | 15 | 14 | 14 | 13 |  |  |
| 110 | 23 | 22 | 21 | 21 | 20 | 19 | 19 | 18 | 18 | 17 | 17 | 16 | 16 | 15 | 15 | 15 | 14 | 14 | 13 |
| 115 | 24 | 23 | 22 | 22 | 21 | 20 | 20 | 19 | 19 | 18 | 17 | 17 | 16 | 16 | 16 | 15 | 15 | 14 | 14 |
| 120 | 25 | 24 | 23 | 23 | 22 | 21 | 21 | 20 | 19 | 19 | 18 | 18 | 17 | 17 | 16 | 16 | 15 | 15 | 15 |
| 125 | 26 | 25 | 24 | 24 | 23 | 22 | 21 | 21 | 20 | 20 | 19 | 18 | 18 | 17 | 17 | 16 | 16 | 16 | 15 |
| 130 | 27 | 26 | 25 | 25 | 24 | 23 | 22 | 22 | 21 | 20 | 20 | 19 | 19 | 18 | 18 | 17 | 17 | 16 | 16 |
| 135 | 28 | 27 | 26 | 26 | 25 | 24 | 23 | 22 | 22 | 21 | 21 | 20 | 19 | 19 | 18 | 18 | 17 | 17 | 16 |
| 140 | 29 | 28 | 27 | 26 | 26 | 25 | 24 | 23 | 23 | 22 | 21 | 21 | 20 | 20 | 19 | 18 | 18 | 17 | 17 |
| 145 | 30 | 29 | 28 | 27 | 27 | 26 | 25 | 24 | 23 | 23 | 22 | 21 | 21 | 20 | 20 | 19 | 19 | 18 | 18 |
| 150 | 31 | 30 | 29 | 28 | 27 | 27 | 26 | 25 | 24 | 23 | 23 | 22 | 22 | 21 | 20 | 20 | 19 | 19 | 18 |
| 155 | 32 | 31 | 30 | 29 | 28 | 27 | 27 | 26 | 25 | 24 | 24 | 23 | 22 | 22 | 21 | 20 | 20 | 19 | 19 |
| 160 | 33 | 32 | 31 | 30 | 29 | 28 | 27 | 27 | 26 | 25 | 24 | 24 | 23 | 22 | 22 | 21 | 21 | 20 | 19 |
| 165 | 34 | 33 | 32 | 31 | 30 | 29 | 28 | 27 | 27 | 26 | 25 | 24 | 24 | 23 | 22 | 22 | 21 | 21 | 20 |
| 170 | 36 | 34 | 33 | 32 | 31 | 30 | 29 | 28 | 27 | 27 | 26 | 25 | 24 | 24 | 23 | 22 | 22 | 21 | 21 |
| 175 | 37 | 35 | 34 | 33 | 32 | 31 | 30 | 29 | 28 | 27 | 27 | 26 | 25 | 24 | 24 | 23 | 22 | 22 | 21 |
| 180 | 38 | 36 | 35 | 34 | 33 | 32 | 31 | 30 | 29 | 28 | 27 | 27 | 26 | 25 | 24 | 24 | 23 | 22 | 22 |
| 185 | 39 | 37 | 36 | 35 | 34 | 33 | 32 | 31 | 30 | 29 | 28 | 27 | 27 | 26 | 25 | 24 | 24 | 23 | 23 |
| 190 | 40 | 38 | 37 | 36 | 35 | 34 | 33 | 32 | 31 | 30 | 29 | 28 | 27 | 26 | 26 | 25 | 24 | 24 | 23 |

## BODY MASS INDEX

HEIGHT IN INCHES (top row) / WEIGHT IN POUNDS (left column)

| Weight in Pounds | 58 | 59 | 60 | 61 | 62 | 63 | 64 | 65 | 66 | 67 | 68 | 69 | 70 | 71 | 72 | 73 | 74 | 75 | 76 |
|---|---|---|---|---|---|---|---|---|---|---|---|---|---|---|---|---|---|---|---|
| 195 | 41 | 39 | 38 | 37 | 36 | 35 | 34 | 33 | 31 | 31 | 30 | 29 | 28 | 27 | 26 | 26 | 25 | 24 | 24 |
| 200 | 42 | 40 | 39 | 38 | 37 | 36 | 35 | 34 | 32 | 32 | 31 | 30 | 29 | 28 | 27 | 26 | 26 | 25 | 24 |
| 205 | 43 | 41 | 40 | 39 | 38 | 37 | 36 | 35 | 33 | 33 | 32 | 31 | 30 | 29 | 28 | 27 | 27 | 26 | 25 |
| 210 | 44 | 42 | 41 | 40 | 39 | 38 | 37 | 36 | 34 | 34 | 32 | 31 | 31 | 30 | 29 | 28 | 28 | 26 | 26 |
| 215 | 45 | 43 | 42 | 41 | 39 | 39 | 38 | 37 | 35 | 34 | 33 | 32 | 32 | 30 | 30 | 29 | 28 | 27 | 26 |
| 220 | 46 | 44 | 43 | 42 | 40 | 39 | 38 | 37 | 36 | 35 | 34 | 33 | 32 | 31 | 30 | 29 | 29 | 28 | 27 |
| 225 | 47 | 45 | 44 | 43 | 41 | 40 | 39 | 38 | 36 | 35 | 34 | 33 | 32 | 32 | 31 | 30 | 30 | 28 | 27 |
| 230 | 48 | 47 | 45 | 44 | 42 | 41 | 39 | 39 | 37 | 36 | 35 | 34 | 33 | 32 | 31 | 30 | 30 | 29 | 28 |
| 235 | 49 | 48 | 46 | 45 | 43 | 42 | 40 | 39 | 38 | 37 | 36 | 35 | 34 | 33 | 32 | 31 | 31 | 29 | 29 |
| 240 | 50 | 49 | 47 | 46 | 44 | 43 | 41 | 40 | 39 | 38 | 37 | 36 | 34 | 34 | 33 | 32 | 31 | 30 | 29 |
| 245 | 51 | 50 | 48 | 47 | 45 | 43 | 42 | 41 | 40 | 38 | 37 | 36 | 35 | 34 | 33 | 32 | 32 | 30 | 30 |
| 250 | 52 | 51 | 49 | 48 | 46 | 44 | 43 | 42 | 40 | 39 | 38 | 37 | 36 | 35 | 33 | 32 | 32 | 31 | 30 |
| 255 | 53 | 52 | 50 | 49 | 47 | 45 | 44 | 42 | 41 | 40 | 39 | 38 | 37 | 36 | 34 | 33 | 33 | 31 | 31 |
| 260 | 54 | 53 | 51 | 50 | 48 | 46 | 45 | 43 | 42 | 41 | 40 | 39 | 37 | 36 | 35 | 34 | 34 | 32 | 32 |
| 265 | 55 | 54 | 52 | 51 | 49 | 47 | 46 | 44 | 43 | 42 | 40 | 39 | 38 | 37 | 36 | 35 | 34 | 33 | 33 |
| 270 | 56 | 54 | 53 | 52 | 49 | 48 | 46 | 45 | 44 | 42 | 41 | 40 | 39 | 38 | 37 | 36 | 35 | 34 | 34 |
| 275 |  |  | 54 | 53 | 50 | 49 | 47 | 46 | 45 | 43 | 42 | 41 | 39 | 38 | 37 | 36 | 35 | 35 | 34 |
| 280 |  |  | 55 | 54 | 51 | 50 | 48 | 46 | 45 | 44 | 43 | 41 | 40 | 39 | 38 | 37 | 36 | 35 | 34 |

## Optional Test: Skin-Fold Thickness

You can also measure your body composition with a skin-fold thickness test. A technician uses calipers to gauge the thickness of your skin over the triceps arm muscle, just under the scapula on your back, and over your tummy. Many nutritionists, exercise physiologists, physical therapists, or trainers at the gym can perform this test. Although this technique is not precise, it does give a decent estimate of your percentage of body fat by measuring the thickness (fat content) of your skin, and can be used to follow changes in body fat over time.

## Optional Test: Bioelectrical Impedance

The new gold standard for measuring body composition and in particular for gauging fat mass has become electrical impedance. This test measures the strength and speed at which a mild electrical signal travels through your body. Fat tissue conducts this signal more slowly than lean muscle. I test body composition with bioelectrical impedance routinely on my patients. In addition to assessing body fat, it also measures lean mass

**BODY FAT PERCENTAGE RANGES AND HEALTH RISKS**

| ADULT MALE AGE RANGE | MODERATE RISK, UNDER-WEIGHT | DESIRED BODY FAT | MODERATE RISK, OVER-WEIGHT | HIGH RISK, OVER-WEIGHT | VERY HIGH RISK, OVER-WEIGHT |
|---|---|---|---|---|---|
| 18-39 | Less than 10% | 10-20% | 20-25% | 25-30% | More than 30% |
| 40-60 | Less than 10% | 10-22% | 22-27% | 27-34% | More than 33% |
| Over 60 | Less than 13% | 13-24% | 24-29% | 29-35% | More than 35% |
| ADULT FEMALE AGE RANGE | MODERATE RISK, UNDER-WEIGHT | DESIRED BODY FAT | MODERATE RISK, OVER-WEIGHT | HIGH RISK, OVER-WEIGHT | VERY HIGH RISK, OVER-WEIGHT |
| 18-39 | Less than 18% | 18-25% | 25-30% | 30-39% | More than 39% |
| 40-60 | Less than 20% | 20-26% | 26-33% | 33-40% | More than 40% |
| Over 60 | Less than 22% | 22-27% | 27-35% | 35-42% | More than 42% |

(the combination of bones, organs such as your kidneys, brain, and heart, water weight, and muscles) and calculates the ratio between the two.

Electrical impedance testing is rapidly becoming widespread in clinics, spas, and gyms. It usually costs from $20 to $30 in these venues, but many centers now do this for free as part of their normal assessment. Generally, the better machines are 98 percent accurate, which is excellent.

In the preceding tables, you'll find the recommended body fat percentages for men and women. Your Ten Years Younger goal is to reach your desired percent body fat range and stay there. My own personal goal has been to keep my body fat below 19 percent.

## Looking at Cholesterol

Cholesterol screening assesses your risk for cardiovascular disease, the number-one killer in the Western world if you combine strokes and heart attacks. Your cholesterol is determined by a quick blood test at your doctor's office, or you can even have blood drawn at a health fair. The cost for your complete cholesterol profile varies with laboratories, from free to between $15 and $40 per test, and the test is often covered by health insurance.

Nathan Pritikin, the founder of the Pritikin Program, taught that at best, your cholesterol level should be 100 plus your age. If you're 35 years old, your total cholesterol should be 135 or less. If you're 50, it should be 150. This gives you a nice goal to keep in mind with cholesterol screening. (Note this is the *optimal* level—the *average* level in the United States runs about 200!)

If your lifestyle remains unchanged, over your lifetime your cholesterol level generally increases by 1 mg/dl per year. So over ten years, you can anticipate that your cholesterol would jump from 150 to 160 mg/dl.

As I explained in Chapter 2, the ratio of your total cholesterol (TC) to high-density lipoproteins (HDL) is an excellent predictor of plaque formation in your arteries and of your risk of cardiovascular disease. But since total cholesterol and HDL are both important, your Ten Years Younger goal would be a 5 percent decrease in that ratio. Your total cholesterol should drop by 10 points, but your HDL cholesterol should stay the same. For example, Mary's total cholesterol is average at 200. Her HDL level is 40. That would give her a ratio of 5 (abnormally high). If she were to decrease her total cholesterol by 10 points (to 190) without changing her HDL, her overall ratio would improve to 4.75, which is a 5 percent drop.

While these reductions are great, they're not mind-boggling. Still, they do represent a reversal of ten years of age in relation to how your cholesterol increases. In the Ten Years Younger study, however, subjects with elevated cholesterol ratios saw a 12.8 percent decrease in TC/HDL ratios, and as I mentioned previously, we noted 29.5 and 33 percent decreases in earlier diabetic and adolescent studies. Truly outstanding! I'll teach you how to achieve similar results in Chapters 5 and 6.

## Assessing Brain Function

Of the five areas I suggest you measure, mental function or cognition is the most controversial and complicated. Nevertheless, I've included it here because I believe that maintaining your mental sharpness is critical to getting and staying ten years younger. *Cognition* refers to the act of knowing or thinking. If your cognition is functioning well, you are able to input information properly, process it, respond appropriately and in a timely manner, and remember the information for the future.

Why would you want to test your brainpower? Your ability to think improves from birth until age 20 to 30. Then, as with other body functions, it starts to decline. How quickly your mental function wanes is key. Early and subtle memory loss is difficult to assess with any sort of precision. Your ability to memorize typically starts to decline after the age of 40 but may remain well preserved into your 80s. And, in fact, many people sustain their attention span until they're quite old.

To assess whether you're experiencing a decline in cognitive function, ask yourself the following questions for your Brain Symptom Score:

- Do I lose things often (keys, pens, glasses)?
- Is it getting harder to find my car in a big parking area?

- Do I have trouble remembering a seven-digit phone number long enough to dial it?
- Do I find myself writing lists to help my memory more than I used to?
- Am I forgetting names of movie and sports stars I once knew well?
- Is it easier to remember an event from twenty years ago than two days ago?
- Do I have trouble dealing with math problems (balancing my checkbook, calculating percentages for tipping)?
- Am I challenged when I have to learn new things (software programs, instructions to put together a new barbecue)?
- Does my mind start drifting sooner than it used to during a detailed lecture or meeting?
- When working on a project, do I find it hard to get back into the groove after being interrupted by a phone call or office visitor?

Here's how to score yourself. If you've answered yes to:

- *None of these questions:* You're doing great!
- *1–2 questions:* You're fine, but you should watch for further cognitive loss.
- *3–4 questions:* This would cause some concern. Check with your doctor. (You might also find some helpful advice in Dr. David Perlmutter's *The Better Brain Book*.)
- *5 or more questions:* Further mental function testing might be necessary.

People whose brains operate at a high level may lose function dramatically without realizing it. While they might suspect they aren't as sharp as they used to be, the people around them usually don't notice until they've suffered a substantial decline in cognitive ability. Once this occurs, there's no guarantee it can be restored. Prevention is the best way to protect your mental performance. That means it's important to know your baseline.

Memory loss is difficult to quantify and predict. In contrast, mental speed or reaction time (your ability to respond quickly) and flexibility (your capacity to respond to rapidly changing situations and questions) drop steadily after age 30 and are frequent early signs of accelerated aging. This makes them good measures for your mental age. Since all of us lose some thinking power over time, it's important to identify these losses early so you can take steps to prevent or slow them. Many patients I see find that their thinking isn't as sharp as it used to be, that their reaction time has slowed, and that they're cognitively less flexible. But there are actions you can take. In fact, both reaction time and cognitive flexibility can rebound with healthy eating and regular exercise. This is often the first improvement participants note when following the Ten Years Younger Program—they feel sharper mentally. Subjects who did aerobic exercise at least five days a week in my Ten Years Younger study experienced a 9.1 percent increase in reaction time, a 24.6 percent jump in cognitive flexibility, and a 44.3 percent increase in attention span.

Pharmaceutical companies have long utilized computerized tests to measure cognition for their research studies. Today you can access these tests through the Internet. They're easy to take, and many people actually find them fun to do. You sit at a computer for about thirty minutes, watch the screen, and respond to prompting by using only a couple of keys on a keyboard. I prefer the tests that measure mental speed and flexibility, because they can tell you about your mental age. Bear in mind, however, that cognitive testing by itself can't be used to diagnose diseases, memory loss, or other problems. It's just one tool among many that a doctor would use to assess your brain function.

In my clinic, I've been using a test called CNS Vital Signs to determine cognitive function. You receive a report indicating memory, mental speed, reaction time, attention, and cognitive flexibility. If your own physician doesn't offer this type of testing, it's also available on my Web site, www. tenyearsyounger.net. The cost of the test varies from $50 to $70. Make sure you follow the instructions correctly and are not interrupted during the test, since that might affect your score. Ideally, as you go through the Ten Years Younger Program, you'd like to see your mental speed increase, your reaction time drop, and your cognitive flexibility rise.

Whether you follow your Brain Symptom Score or use a more objective test such as the CNS Vital Signs, I recommend that you continue

COGNITIVE TEST MEAN SCORES

| Age | 30s | 40s | 50s | 60s | 70s | 80s |
|---|---|---|---|---|---|---|
| Mental speed | 177 | 170 | 159 | 143 | 128 | 112 |
| Reaction time | 619 | 640 | 665 | 716 | 756 | 897 |
| Cognitive flexibility | 47 | 42 | 42 | 30 | 22 | 9 |

Adapted with permission from CNS Vital Signs

this type of testing yearly to make sure your cognitive function isn't waning without your having the opportunity to correct it.

# Other Biological Markers

In addition to the tests we've just discussed, there are others important to your long-term health. In particular, I'd like to mention several that measure your bone strength and future fracture risk, as well as assess your skin. You should take these tests regularly and monitor any changes.

## Your Bones

It's easy to measure the density of your bones. Density is an excellent yardstick of your bone strength and helps predict your risk for fractures. All women should have their bones scanned when they pass through menopause. (Most insurance companies will pay to check bone density in postmenopausal women once every two years.)

Some women, however, already have an elevated risk for osteoporosis. These special risk factors include:

- A history of fractures as an adult
- Fragility fracture (a broken bone without a serious injury) in a first-degree relative (parent or sibling)
- Weight below 127 pounds
- Smoking
- Use of oral corticosteroid therapy for more than three months
- Significant inactivity

- Very low calcium and/or vitamin D intake
- Poor diet with excessive salt, animal protein, and cola

Although you may have to pay out-of-pocket for this, women who have these risk factors should check their bone density at least once after turning 40. After all, the sooner you identify low bone density, the sooner you can prevent additional losses. Since men begin to fracture on average ten years after women, I suggest they check their bone density at least once sometime between ages 50 and 60.

DEXA testing is the method of choice; it's highly precise, and comparable to getting a bank statement in that it will tell you how much calcium you have in your bone account. Your report compares your bones to a 30-year-old of your gender and also to someone your age who has average bones. It gives you a specific score indicating the density of your spine, hip, and the neck of the femur, the area in the hip susceptible to breaking. Your doctor will usually tell you whether your bone density is good, borderline and needs watching, or diminished. In the last case, you might need medication.

You'll also want to ask for the total spine, total hip, and femoral neck mineral density number, in $g/cm^2$. A good bone density number is easy to remember: $1.0$ $g/cm^2$. When your bone density drops below $0.6$ $g/cm^2$, that would be worrisome for a future fracture. My hope is that you would live to be 100 and still have a bone density number above $0.65$ $g/cm^2$. That would give you reserve bone mass for your future. I'll tell you more about how to prevent bone loss in Chapters 4, 5, and 6.

## Your Skin

You're never too young to visit your primary care physician or dermatologist to assess the condition of your skin. He or she will look at your skin carefully and identify any possibly precancerous or cancerous lesions.

Shining ultraviolet light at facial and forearm skin in a darkened room can help you and your doctor determine whether you have any sun damage. Skin that has been damaged and may develop sun spots and uneven pigmentation in the future will show blotching and irregular coloration under ultraviolet light. Many people are unaware of how much the sun has hurt their skin, and they're shocked to see the results.

In Chapter 9, I'll focus on how to make your skin look ten years younger.

By now, you should have a fairly clear picture of exactly how your body is aging. Once you've established your baseline, you can work on improving your performance with realistic lifestyle changes over time. The whole idea behind these tests is that they're practical and can be easily repeated to monitor your progress. So use them regularly to see just how far you've come! And if you're feeling discouraged by your initial results, don't worry—it's never too late to be ten years younger. In Part II, I'll show you how to do it.

# TURNING BACK THE CLOCK

# CHAPTER 4

# The Sweet Sixteen Vitality Foods

I magine a buffet displayed in front of you. It features hearty servings of grilled salmon, sole, trout, and shrimp as well as chicken and turkey breast along with platters of steamed crab, mussels, oysters, and lobster from pristine waters.

There are fresh, colorful vegetables and an array of green salads in abundance. To the left sit bowls of blueberries, raspberries, peaches, plums, and cherries along with slices of melon, papaya, and avocado. To the right are plates laden with luscious red ripe tomatoes and plump steamed artichokes. Farther on is a tray with almonds, hazelnuts, pecans, and walnuts and a platter with herb-seasoned wild rice.

You see another bowl wafting a heavenly aroma—whole-grain pasta covered with fresh tomato sauce made with garlic and basil. A golden omelet sprinkled with herbs and sautéed onions decorates yet another plate. And for dessert, you spy strawberries dipped in dark chocolate, a delicious chocolate mousse, and mango smoothies. Lined up to drink with this feast are pitchers of iced green tea, elegant red wine, hot cocoa, and pure refreshing water.

Sounds fantastic? Too good to be true? Not at all.

Welcome to the Ten Years Younger Diet.

You probably noticed that four of the seven Aging Accelerators I discussed in Chapter 1 involve changes in body shape and metabolism. It goes without saying, then, that food plays a compelling role in your health and longevity, and that nutrition itself can be a potent anti-aging ally. For example, depending upon your initial status, it is possible to drop your cholesterol level and your TC/HDL ratio by 10 to 25 percent with the right kind of eating. By the same token, some foods, like refined carbohydrates (white bread, white rice, and table sugar), can raise your blood sugar and insulin levels and lower your healthy HDL levels substantially. These foods set you up for metabolic syndrome and ultimately prevent your HDL from doing its job.

A key requirement of the Ten Years Younger Diet is your consistent commitment to transforming yourself from supersize to just-right size. There is no doubt that losing excess weight and building lean muscle mass can lengthen and even save your life. But the diet in this book goes much further than simple weight control. I stand by the principle that adding healthy foods to your diet is more important than cutting out unhealthy ones. For this reason, you'll likely find that this diet is relatively painless when compared to others. And no starvation is required! If you're going to live longer, I want you to feel great—and taking pleasure in food is part of that.

The truth of the matter is that, as we saw in Chapter 2, one delicious meal—maybe a slice of grilled wild salmon perched on fresh field greens with tomatoes, with a side of black beans and wild rice seasoned with fragrant herbs and sliced almonds—can deliver powerful anti-aging nutrients to your cells, leave your arteries squeaky clean, and promote blood circulation and energy. It can fight metabolic syndrome, diabetes, cancer, osteoporosis, and heart disease and revitalize your skin. A different lunch (say, a cheeseburger and fries with a shake on the side) leaves you sluggish as it clogs your arteries with plaque and constricts your circulation. It makes you vulnerable to the same array of maladies that the Ten Years Younger lunch averts. Starting right now, you're going to be choosing the first kind of meal whenever you eat, and the recipes and meal plans in Part III will help you do this. And now it's time to introduce the cornerstone of the Ten Years Younger Diet: the sixteen Vitality Foods.

# The Sweet Sixteen Vitality Foods

As I said earlier, one of the main ideas behind the Ten Years Younger Diet is that adding the right foods is more important than cutting out unhealthy choices. But which foods do you add?

There are sixteen types of food that are especially good for your heart and your circulation, and work actively to fight metabolic syndrome and support your bones and skin. On my Web site, www.tenyearsyounger. net, you'll find a complete list of one hundred anti-aging Vitality Foods that appear in the recipes in Part III. But for now, meet my "sweet sixteen"—the easy list of Vitality Foods that when added regularly to your diet will begin turning back your clock on a cellular level.

1. *Green Leafy Vegetables.* For every serving (1 cup) of green leafy vegetables you add to your daily diet, you cut your risk of a cardiovascular event by 25 percent. That means just 2 more cups daily of green leafy vegetables should slash your risk for a stroke or heart attack nearly in half. That's a powerful change with very little effort. Greens are also loaded with calcium, fiber, and folic acid, as well as a host of cancer-preventing plant pigments. Spinach, dark green lettuce, broccoli, collard greens, bok choy, and kale are just a few of the greens you can choose from. You should aim to enjoy at least 2 cups of green leafy veggies every day.

2. *Lean, not mean, protein.* Seafood, chicken and turkey breast, beans and soy, and nonfat dairy products are excellent lean protein sources. While chicken and turkey may not contain many anti-aging compounds, eating more of them does suppress hunger and makes it easier to feel satisfied on fewer calories. If you include healthy protein with each meal, you'll minimize surges in blood sugar levels, too. For weight control, I encourage you to enjoy 20 to 30 percent of your calories from healthy, lean protein sources.

   By contrast, mean proteins include fatty dairy products (such as 2 percent milk, with 35 percent of calories from fat), most red meats, sausage, and dark meat poultry, which are loaded with artery-clogging saturated fat.

3.  *Seafood.* Studies show that there are many anti-aging benefits from eating seafood. In fact, fish consumption can actually lower risk of death, as well as reduce irregular heartbeat, blood stickiness, and triglycerides. Seafood consumption can also improve blood sugar regulation, boost brain function, and decrease inflammation in people with inflammatory bowel disease or rheumatoid arthritis. In Chapter 5, I'll help you discover seafood choices that are rich in healthy omega-3 fats and low in mercury, helping you select the best catch. Pass the fish, please!

4.  *Beans and legumes.* One-half to 1 cup of beans daily lowers bad cholesterol (LDL) by 5 percent while raising your healthy cholesterol (HDL) 2 to 3 percent. Beans also suppress hunger and help to stabilize blood sugar levels, and are loaded with cancer-fighting compounds. Yes, they're known as the "musical fruit," but studies have shown that if you eat beans daily for a month, gas production drops. It is best to begin by consuming them in small quantities every day (say ¼ cup) and gradually increase portions over time. There are dozens of different types, and you can enjoy them as a side dish or add them to soups, salads, rice, and pasta dishes. If you don't have the time to soak and cook dry beans, canned beans will make your life easier; just rinse them well before eating, to wash away any extra salt and sugar that might be packed in the can.

5.  *Soy.* Soy products used to be limited to tofu, but today it's easy to enjoy a serving of soy a day. Most groceries carry soy-based veggie burgers, soy hot dogs and sausage, and calcium-fortified soy milk. These products lower cholesterol and blood sugar levels and are packed with cancer-fighting compounds—fiber, antioxidants, calcium, and many anti-aging nutrients. Edamame (fresh soybeans out of the pod) make a terrific snack, and they're so easy to prepare—just pop them into the microwave or boil them in water for a few minutes. (Try my edamame recipe on page 293.)

    I recommend trying several brands of soy products because you may like some more than others. Years ago, when I first decided to try soy milk, I bought six brands at once, poured a glass of each, and taste-tested them until I found the one I liked best. A few were awful! None tasted like milk, and it took me some time to adjust to this fact. Then I tried my favorite brand with cereal, coffee, tea, and cocoa, until I was sure I'd found a combination I could enjoy daily. Now I drink a cup of soy milk every day. Even chocolate soy milk is a good choice, and although it has a few more calories than plain soy milk, it's a worthy dessert.

6. *Whole grains.* Whole grains such as barley, buckwheat, wild rice, quinoa, and oats are actually tastier than refined, processed grains, they're more natural, and they help prevent weight gain, metabolic syndrome, and diabetes. When you follow the Ten Years Younger Diet, the fiber in whole grains (especially barley) blocks the blood sugar and insulin surge after a meal, so you'll stay satisfied for longer, too—even though you've eaten fewer calories.

7. *Cruciferous vegetables.* Toxins—poisonous foreign chemicals (such as heavy metals, industrial chemicals, pesticides, drugs, and various pollutants)—enter your body through your skin and the air you breathe, but especially through your intestines. You also produce toxins in the form of free radicals when you metabolize hormones and drugs and burn calories for energy. As we've seen, these toxins accumulate in your body and can cause diseases, including cancer.

   Fiber-rich cruciferous vegetables—cabbage, bok choy, broccoli, kale, cauliflower, and Brussels spouts—are high in chemicals that detoxify and remove cancer-causing compounds from your body. They're also great sources of vitamin C and calcium. You can eat these vegetables raw, steamed, or lightly sautéed, but be careful not to overcook them or they'll lose their valuable properties.

8. *Berries.* Blueberries, blackberries, raspberries, strawberries, cranberries, and bilberries, are among the brightly colored fruits and vegetables that have so many antioxidant benefits. They're also packed with fiber. Not only does sprinkling them over a salad or cereal make your meal visually more beautiful, but the colorful

pigments found in berries are some of the most powerful anti-aging compounds known to science. Berry pigments seem especially important for protecting brain cells and the cells lining your arteries from free radical damage and consequential aging.

9. *Nuts.* Nuts are packed with protein, nutrients, anti-aging compounds, and fiber. They'll help you feel full, and while they do contain fats, they are mostly healthy fats that will lower your cholesterol. Recent research published in *The Journal of Obesity Related Metabolic Disorders* found that people who eat up to 3 ounces (2 to 3 handfuls) of almonds daily lose more weight than those who eat other complex carbohydrates. Nuts appear to benefit both your heart and your waistline—every study to date has shown that eating nuts regularly decreases your risk of heart attacks, strokes, and death.

10. *Flaxseed.* Ground flaxseed is an excellent source of omega-3 fats (one of the key elements of the Ten Years Younger Diet). Omega-3 fats are good for everyone, but they are especially important for women with perimenopausal and menopausal symptoms. One tablespoon of ground flaxseed daily is an excellent nutritional supplement. (Flaxseed oil lacks fiber and can go rancid quickly and become packed with free radicals, so it's a poor choice, and whole flaxseed passes through your intestinal tract without being absorbed.) You can use a coffee mill to grind it, or buy it freshly ground. I keep the ground seed in an airtight container in the refrigerator so it's handy to sprinkle on my oatmeal, smoothies, or salads; it has a pleasant nutty flavor. If you eat eggs, then consider buying omega-3-enriched eggs commonly sold in grocery stores; the hens have usually been fed flaxseed. Though more expensive than ordinary eggs, they have half the saturated fat and a healthy dose (up to 300 mg) of omega-3 fats into the bargain.

11. *Fresh garlic.* Believe it or not, fresh garlic lowers your total cholesterol about 7 to 9 percent, raises HDL slightly, decreases clotting, lowers blood pressure, and boosts your immune function. But do stick to the real thing! Deodorized garlic (in pills) doesn't reduce cholesterol effectively because allicin, the chemical that gives garlic

its aroma, is also what gives it its cholesterol-lowering punch. To maximize allicin, smash the cloves with a wooden spoon or the flat side of a chef's knife. Let the juices in the garlic sit for a few minutes. At home, I serve 1 to 2 cloves of garlic per person every day. Throw it into your salad dressing, stir-fry dishes, soups, and rice dishes. Just about any meal goes well with garlic. It is a staple in Mexican, Chinese, Indian, French, Spanish, Greek, and Italian cuisines and appears often in the recipes you'll find in Part III.

But do be careful. While completing my chef internship at the Four Seasons restaurant in Seattle, I discovered that if you overcook garlic until it turns brown, it becomes bitter, and this also ruins its medicinal properties. So add crushed or finely chopped garlic during the last one or two minutes of cooking to give your meals the richest flavor and maximize their cholesterol-lowering benefits.

12. *Fresh herbs and spices.* Have you ever wondered why herbs smell so great? Think of that pasta sauce simmering on the stove. One whiff and you're salivating. Like a bee drawn to the scent of flowers, we're biochemically attracted to herbs. And by weight, they're the most densely packed anti-aging foods you can find. I encourage you to splurge on a minimum of 1 teaspoon of dried or 1 to 2 tablespoons of fresh herbs daily. Thyme, rosemary, oregano, sage, basil, cumin, mint, chives, dill, turmeric, and cilantro are all wonderful, heart-healthy choices. Not only do they make your food look, smell, and taste great, they're terrific for your health, too.

Also, don't be stingy with ginger. It adds a zesty, citrus-like tang and goes well with Indian curries, Asian stir-fries, desserts, and marmalades. It's also quite good for you. Two thousand years ago, the Chinese made ginger a staple in their diets, and we've recently learned that there is good reason for this. Ginger contains several potent antioxidants and, like garlic, it helps decrease blood stickiness, which prevents unwanted clots. Used regularly over weeks, it acts as an anti-inflammatory to relieve joint pain and arthritis without increasing the risk of stomach ulcers. (In fact, people use ginger to *treat* stomach ulcers.)

The simplest way to enjoy ginger with your meals is to grate fresh ginger directly into your food while it is cooking—it's particularly fabulous when grated over stir-fries. It grates easily, and don't worry about the skin (although you may prefer removing it for aesthetic reasons).

13. *Green tea.* Green tea, a staple in the Asian diet, is loaded with antioxidants, and drinking green tea regularly has been associated with reduced cancer rates. Black tea, though good for you, doesn't quite measure up to its green cousin. It has only 20 to 50 percent of the flavonoids (antioxidant compounds found in many foods) of green tea. To make the latter, growers chop, roll, and quickly heat tea leaves. Heating traps the antioxidants, giving green tea its healthful properties.

Green tea is also rich in L-theonine, a chemical compound that enhances mental function and learning while heightening concentration (independently of caffeine). Studies have demonstrated that L-theonine also increases alpha brain waves, which provide a sense of calm while reducing some of the jitteriness caffeine can produce. Similarly, the catechins in green tea are chemical compounds that decrease cancer risk and enhance your metabolism, helping to prevent weight regain after weight loss. Quite a healthy punch from a little tea bag!

Green tea has a pleasant although slightly bitter flavor that I've learned to enjoy. Make a weak cup at first to appreciate the subtle flavor. If it still seems bitter, either make it weaker still, or add one packet of Splenda or ¼ to ½ teaspoon of honey. I aim to drink a cup of green tea each afternoon. I also enjoy drinking a glass of iced decaffeinated green tea in the evening. And sometimes I add decaffeinated green tea to my dessert smoothies.

14. *Nonfat yogurt.* Nonfat yogurt is the healthiest dairy food—it's loaded with lactobacilli, healthy bacteria that normally live within your intestinal tract. Lactobacilli protect you from harmful bacteria, lower your cholesterol, and nourish your intestinal tract. For women, eating yogurt packed with lactobacilli is also associated with decreasing the risk of vaginal yeast infections. Eating yogurt

has been shown to enhance your immune system, prevent intestinal infections, and possibly even help fight cancer. Plus nonfat yogurt is loaded with protein and calcium—without the saturated fat of regular yogurt.

Nonfat yogurt is great in dips and sauces. Mix it with lemon juice, mustard, or soy sauce for a great veggie dip. Add it to curries at the last minute and use it in place of sour cream. Just don't cook it or it will curdle.

15. *Red wine.* Far from an indulgence, one 5-ounce serving of red wine a day helps keep you young. It raises your HDL, decreases your risk of clotting, lowers overall oxidation, and cuts your risk for dementia. It also improves insulin sensitivity—helping with blood sugar regulation. The key is stopping at one glass, and definitely not drinking more than two. The risks from drinking more than two servings of alcohol daily are substantial and include devastating strokes, obesity, and cancer.

When choosing between types of alcohol, red wine is the richest source of antioxidants of all. But if you avoid red wine, I'd suggest white wine over beer, and beer over hard liquor. Of all the alcoholic choices, hard liquor is the most irritating to your liver.

While 100 percent red grape juice does provide many of the antioxidants found in red wine, grape juice can raise blood sugar levels, potentially lowering HDL cholesterol levels. In contrast, one serving of red wine a day raises HDL levels nicely. If you can't limit your red wine consumption to 1 to 2 servings daily, or if you just don't like the effects of alcohol, and you have good blood sugar control, 8 ounces of red grape juice daily with a meal would be a good alternative.

16. *Cocoa and chocolate.* Good news for chocolate lovers everywhere! A serving of cocoa decreases clotting and the oxidation of LDL into plaque. Pure cocoa also helps dilate your arteries—improving their function, your blood pressure, and reducing the risk of clotting. Cocoa is rich in magnesium and packed with anti-aging and stress-relieving compounds. I find a cup of nonfat cow's milk or calcium-fortified low-fat soy milk mixed with cocoa to be a great

dessert and surprisingly satisfying for my sweet tooth. (See cocoa recipe on p. 240.)

Real chocolate is a winner too. Like cocoa, dark semi-sweet chocolate is packed with anti-aging and stress-relieving compounds. It also decreases LDL oxidation. But again, pay attention and always read the ingredients label. Most "chocolate" is not chocolate at all but a mixture of sugar, milk, butter, and palm oil, with only a trace of cocoa. The milk in milk chocolate negates the benefits of eating dark chocolate. The first ingredient should be cocoa, the second cocoa butter, and the third sugar. Vanilla (or vanillin) and lecithin are acceptable too and make chocolate taste terrific. But if you see palm oil, milk products, or butter, search for another brand.

Chocolate is high in calories, so you can't eat a whole bar regularly if you want to lose weight. But in small amounts, real dark semi-sweet chocolate is wonderful. The Mayans of Central America were right to treat it like currency, and it's no wonder it took Europe by storm. So, *if* you can reasonably limit your chocolate habit to one to two squares a day for dessert, go for it. And savor every bite.


All of these terrific foods will optimize your ability to lower your cholesterol, stabilize your blood sugar level, improve your metabolism, suppress your hunger—all part of fighting your aging enemies. What's even better, they'll make your meals taste great! So now that you're familiar with some of the essential ingredients in the Ten Years Younger Diet, let's move on to Chapter 5, where you'll learn the principles that make the diet work.

# The Ten Years Younger Diet

How can you integrate the Sweet Sixteen Vitality Foods into your everyday eating habits? The Ten Years Younger Diet and daily food plans listed in Part III will help you. We'll get into those in a minute, but before we do, let's focus on the diet itself and exactly how it works to help you reverse the aging process.

The diet is built around ten simple principles:

1. Eat at least 30 grams of fiber a day.
2. Consume 4 to 5 cups of colorful fruits and vegetables daily.
3. Reduce saturated fat and shun trans fats.
4. Choose healthy omega-3 fats (from seafood, nuts, and soy).
5. Substitute whole grains for highly processed, refined foods.
6. Seek out foods rich in calcium and magnesium.
7. Hydrate.
8. Save room for dessert.
9. Watch your portion sizes.
10. Select healthy snacks.

In this chapter we'll explore these principles and their anti-aging benefits. But remember that even though they are distinct, they impact and overlap with one another in very helpful ways. For instance, as you increase your portions of colorful fruits and vegetables and whole grains, you'll naturally move toward your goal of 30 grams of fiber, you'll increase your intake of calcium and magnesium, you'll benefit from the water contained in fruits and vegetables, and you'll eat healthy snacks too. It's all so much easier than you think—and best of all, it's delicious.

## Principle #1: Eat at Least 30 Grams of Fiber a Day

Fiber, also called roughage, is the portion of plant food that isn't digested. Scientists have divided fiber into two categories, soluble and insoluble, based upon which types of fiber dissolve in a laboratory setting. (These categories are not clearly related to what happens in your intestinal tract, though.) Soluble fiber is best at lowering cholesterol and blood sugar levels. Insoluble fiber feeds the healthy bacteria in your intestinal tract and helps to keep you regular by providing bulk to your large intestine. You don't have to worry about which foods have soluble and insoluble fiber; all you need to do is enjoy a mixture of fiber-rich foods including fruits, vegetables, beans, soy products, nuts, and whole grains and you've got it covered.

How does fiber help to make you ten years younger?

- It lowers your cholesterol levels by blocking the absorption of cholesterol from your gut into your bloodstream.
- It lowers blood sugar levels by slowing the release of sugars from your stomach to your intestines and decreasing the absorption of sugars into your bloodstream.
- It delivers a whopping dose of antioxidants—most of the anti-aging compounds that come from grains are in the fiber-rich outer layer.
- It binds to bad chemicals in your intestinal tract, carrying them out of the body with other waste and helping to detoxify your system.

Fiber-rich foods are also often an excellent source of minerals—such as selenium and magnesium—that help to protect you from cancer. Best of all, the more fiber you eat, the fuller you'll feel, and the less room you'll have for unhealthful foods and snacks. Why is this so? Fiber makes you feel full because it swells with fluid in your intestinal tract. It also makes you feel full on account of something called calorie density—a key part of understanding which foods keep us healthy and why.

## Calorie Density

Answer the following question: If every night you ate a pound of raspberries or a pound of Oreo cookies, which would result in your gaining weight? The cookies, of course, and to make matters worse, they'd provide no nutritional value. But since you're eating the same amount of each food—a pound—you'll feel similarly satisfied or full from either one. Why is this true?

The short answer is calorie density, which is a fancy way of saying calories per pound of food. While I was the medical director at the Pritikin Longevity Center, Robert Pritikin focused many of his lectures on this concept. Simply put, your stomach feels full when you eat foods that are heavy. Part of feeling full has to do with the weight of food in your stomach. Two foods with the same weight but different numbers of calories per pound will give you about the same sense of fullness. Obviously, if you want to lose weight, you'll choose the lower-calorie-density foods over high-calorie foods. Thus you'd choose raspberries over Oreos.

Take pasta and broccoli. Eating a pound of broccoli (128 calories) or a pound of cooked pasta (500 calories) will make you feel similarly full. But the pasta has more than three times the calories—it has a higher calorie density. If you cut the amount of pasta in your dish in half and replace it with an equal amount of broccoli, you'll drop your calorie intake from 500 to 314 calories per pound and you'll feel just as satisfied. A big improvement.

Generally, the higher the fiber and water content in foods, the lower the calorie density. Fiber provides weight but isn't absorbed in the gut. Water also provides weight and, as you know, doesn't have any calories. So the more fiber and water in your diet, the fuller you'll feel without consuming more calories. Not surprisingly, then, eating more fiber-rich foods results in weight loss and a slimmer waistline. For instance, the fiber and water in a large green leafy salad eaten before dinner would be filling but would have fewer calories per pound (lower calorie density) than most main-course dinner choices. So with the salad as a first course, you end up feeling satisfied even if you've eaten a smaller entrée. Studies have actually shown that adding a low-calorie-density salad before your entrée will decrease the total calories you consume over the course of dinner by 10 percent.

So on the Ten Years Younger Program, you're going to be choosing foods that have both high fiber and low calorie density. That's your winning combination. The chart below provides the calorie/fiber ratio for many common foods. You'll see that broccoli is clearly the standout choice! For a more detailed list and to determine how much fiber you're actually eating every day, see the fiber table in Appendix B.

The one clear exception to the low-calorie-density rule is nuts. Yes, they're high in calories and fat, but as I mentioned in Chapter 4, they are one of the Sweet Sixteen Vitality Foods and have many age-busting benefits: They're packed with fiber, calcium, and heart-protecting fats, and most are low in saturated fat, too. In fact, nuts are so important to your health that I question the wisdom of any diet program that restricts fat to less than 20 percent of calories, as such severe control would prevent you from enjoying adequate amounts of nuts. If a program allows for generous amounts of seafood, tofu, and other soy products (all of which contain healthy fats), you'd be hard-pressed to follow its guidelines and still get all the incredible health benefits that come from simply eating 1 to 2 handfuls of delicious nuts daily. The best choices are raw or dry-roasted nuts without salt.

One caveat: The average American fiber intake is pretty low—about 10 to 12 grams daily. If your fiber consumption falls into this range, be sure to increase your fiber intake slowly, by 5 to 10 grams a week. At this rate, it should take the average person two to four weeks to reach the goal of 30 grams a day. Increasing your fiber too quickly (jumping from less than 10 grams a day to more than 40) may overwhelm your intestines and cause you to become gassy, to feel distended, or to have

| FOODS AS COMMONLY EATEN | CALORIES PER POUND | FIBER IN GRAMS PER POUND |
|---|---|---|
| Broccoli | 128 | 12 |
| Strawberries | 137 | 12 |
| Green beans | 161 | 9 |
| Carrots | 195 | 15 |
| Orange | 211 | 13 |
| Apple | 266 | 10 |
| Oatmeal | 300 | 6 |
| Tofu | 344 | 6 |
| Crab | 393 | 0 |
| Bananas | 418 | 7 |
| Shrimp | 452 | 0 |
| Cod | 480 | 0 |
| Pasta (whole-wheat) | 500 | 20 |
| Pasta (white) | 627 | 5 |
| Rice (brown) | 504 | 10 |
| Rice (white) | 558 | 4 |
| Lentils | 533 | 18 |
| Black beans | 599 | 19 |
| Chicken breast | 688 | 0 |
| Rainbow trout | 698 | 0 |
| Parmesan cheese | 720 | 0 |
| Salmon | 841 | 0 |
| Prime rib | 1,029 | 0 |
| Ice cream | 1,065 | 0 |
| Cheesecake | 1,373 | 0 |
| Blue cheese | 1,600 | 0 |
| M&M's | 2,180 | 0 |
| Granola bar | 2,368 | 1 |
| Chocolate chips | 2,917 | 1 |

abdominal cramping. The meal plans in Part III and the fiber table in Appendix B will help you to add fiber to your diet comfortably and safely. In fact, the people participating in the Ten Years Younger study told me that the fiber table made it easy for them to add fiber—they simply needed to find either recipes rich in fiber from the meal plans or foods in the fiber table they liked and eat them more often. Ideally, you should drink at least eight glasses of water or other hydrating fluid daily to support your intestines' ability to handle this new regimen.

### Choosing Fiber-Friendly Snacks

Periodic snacks with fiber are a great way to get your desired 30 grams and also cut down on your daily calorie intake. I often enjoy soup in the late afternoon—vegetable soup with beans, veggies, and spices in a clear broth has very few calories, tastes great, and leaves me satisfied. After that, I'm not starving when I get home, and I eat less at the dinner table. Apples are another perfect afternoon snack. Their fiber and water will make you feel full, and for only about 60 to 80 calories! Combine an apple, pear, or orange with half a handful of nuts and you've got a cure for the late-afternoon munchies.

As I said before, nuts are a particularly healthy high-fiber snack. But I do want to caution you to be sensible. If you snack on nuts by the *jarful*, you can quickly run up your calorie count. I could easily down four handfuls watching a ballgame. But that exceeds 1,000 calories. It isn't easy to achieve weight control if you have 1,000-calorie snacks every day. So limit yourself to enjoying 1 to 2 ounces of nuts daily. That's roughly one or two handfuls.

## Principle #2: Consume 4 to 5 Cups of Colorful Fruits and Vegetables Daily

"Four to 5 cups?" you say. "I'll never be able to do that!" That's exactly what my research participant Jill said when she joined the Ten Years Younger Study. "When I was told to eat 4 to 5 cups of vegetables and fruit," she recalls, "I thought, 'Oh my gosh, I can't eat that many veggies!' But it's amazing how easily you can do it if you take an apple and an orange to work with you and have raspberries or blueberries on your cereal in the morning—already you've got at least 1½ cups of your fruit down. If you eat a big salad with different vegetables on it along with your choice of protein for lunch, you just added another 3 cups. Add a cup of broccoli, zucchini, or green beans with dinner and you're done for the day. If you missed a salad with lunch, then have one with dinner. If you didn't have a piece of fruit with lunch, then enjoy some fruit with dessert. It's not as difficult as it seems in the beginning."

## Carotenoids

Why are brightly colored fruits and vegetables so good for you? First of all, nobody is going to eat too much broccoli or romaine. You'll stay full by eating these high-fiber and low-calorie-density foods, so following Principle #2 will help you follow Principle #1. But more important, colorful fruits and vegetables are loaded with potent antioxidants and cancer-fighting compounds. The source of these antioxidants has to do with plant physiology. Plants use energy from sunlight to grow, a process that, like any other energy-producing process, generates a great deal of free radicals. To protect themselves from these free radicals (along with sun damage and disease), plants produce over 600 types of antioxidants in the form of pigments or colors, which are called carotenoids. When we eat the plants, we absorb the carotenoids and their anti-aging compounds. During the summer, when the plant is actively growing, the predominant pigment you'll see is chlorophyll, which gives plants their greenish hue. As the growth phase drops in the fall, chlorophyll production stops and the green disappears. Now the yellow, orange, and red pigments become visible, but they've really been there all along.

Berries, pomegranates, tomatoes, green leafy vegetables, and other brightly colored produce all contribute to making you ten years younger, as their carotenoid-rich pigments protect your cholesterol from oxidation and extinguish the free radicals that attack your DNA. Here are some of the most commonly studied carotenoids, all potent anti-aging allies.

- *Lycopene.* Lycopene is found in the red-orange pigment in tomatoes, watermelon, and pink grapefruit. When you eat tomatoes or tomato sauce, the lycopene is absorbed just like other nutrients and carried through the blood, where it helps prevent your cholesterol from being oxidized and converted to plaque. But it's also delivered to your skin, where it helps shield your cells from ultraviolet damage, commonly called sunburn. You'll actually burn more slowly after a meal rich in tomato sauce! Does that mean you can drink tomato juice and lie on the beach all day in Florida without any sunblock? Of course not—you'll still burn. But it does mean that these plant pigments slow damage to your skin. Yes, a diet rich in tomatoes will actually give you younger-looking skin.

You can increase your absorption of lycopene by cooking tomatoes, as the heat breaks down the cell walls inside the tomato, releasing more lycopene to be absorbed. Tomato sauce cooked with olive oil increases the absorption even further, as lycopene needs fat to be well absorbed. A marinara sauce made of tomato paste provides wonderful nutrients to your diet, which explains why you'll see these ingredients in so many of my recipes.

- *Beta-carotene.* The plant pigment beta-carotene is found in orange fruits such as apricots, mangoes, papayas, peaches, and cantaloupes; orange vegetables such as carrots, yams, and squash; and green leafy vegetables. Beta-carotene protects your cells from free radical damage, and in nonsmokers it likely decreases cancer risk by protecting cell membranes and DNA from damage. Beta carotene is also converted into vitamin A, which prevents certain types of blindness and decreases cancer risk.

  A word of caution about taking vitamin A or beta-carotene supplements in pill form. While many multivitamins contain beta-carotene, too much of it blocks the absorption of other carotenoids, including lutein and lycopene. Also, the hundreds of toxic chemicals in tobacco products convert beta-carotene into a harmful carcinogen, making beta-carotene supplements likely harmful to smokers.

  Vitamin A supplements can also be harmful in excess. Rest assured, though, that your body is smart enough to convert beta-carotene into vitamin A from food only when it needs it. No toxicity from plant-based vitamin A (derived from beta-carotene) has ever been reported in a medical journal. So in this case, you are better off forgoing supplements altogether and getting your carotenoids from a diet rich in colorful fruits and vegetables.

- *Astaxanthin.* Astaxanthin originates in algae but then moves up the food chain into small shellfish and other seafood. While it's really a plant-based carotenoid, it becomes useful to us humans as a potent antioxidant in certain seafood. It shows up as the orange-red pigment in wild Alaskan salmon, shrimp, trout, lobsters, and crab, all of which are packed with this healthy carotenoid. Astaxanthins block LDL oxidation into plaque and provide an excellent nutrient source.

In shellfish, the astaxanthin is bound to a blue pigment, rendering the color of raw shellfish a dull purple to brown. When you cook shellfish, the bond holding the blue and orange-red pigments is broken, and the true astaxanthin color can be seen.

- *Lutein and Zeaxanthin.* The best sources of lutein and zeaxanthin are dark green vegetables. These blue-green pigments protect the vision center in your eyes, the macula, from damage called macular degeneration—one of the leading causes of blindness in Americans today. You'll see that by Phase Three of the Ten Years Younger Program, I'd like you to eat at least 2 to 3 cups of dark greens such as salad daily.

## Flavonoids

Plants not only produce carotenoids to protect themselves but also produce a second class of chemical compounds called flavonoids that act as potent antioxidants. In addition to fighting oxidation, flavonoids also have cancer-fighting and clot-busting properties. The most studied flavonoids are the anthocyanins, resveratrol, and quercetin.

- *Anthocyanins.* Foods containing the red and blue pigments known as anthocyanins—such as blueberries, raspberries, plums, and cherries—are especially effective in fighting aging. These pigments have been shown to block LDL cholesterol from being oxidized into plaque more powerfully than almost any other food. Blueberries, pomegranates, and red and black beans are claimed to be the best foods you can eat to prevent LDL from clogging your arteries. Anthocyanin pigments also protect brain cells from free radical damage. And as an added bonus, these foods are full of fiber.

- *Resveratrol.* Researchers have recently found that resveratrol, a chemical found in red grape skins (and which is concentrated in red wine), appears to activate a gene that slows aging. Resveratrol is also a highly potent antioxidant that is especially adept at extinguishing free radicals, and it has both anti-inflammatory and clot-blocking powers that decrease the risk of stroke and heart attack. Resveratrol has been shown to block the progression of early cancer cells; in laboratory settings, it encourages certain cancer cells to commit suicide through a process known as apoptosis, or cell death.

- *Quercetin.* Quercetin, found in tea, apples, and onions, is yet another flavonoid with potent antioxidant powers, protecting DNA from free radical damage that can cause mutations in cells that lead to cancer, and preventing cholesterol from being oxidized into plaque.

One of my biggest beefs with low-carb diets is their lack of adequate fruits and vegetables and the resulting loss of all the carotenoids and flavonoids they contain. Your mother was right, and the low-carb promoters got it wrong—you *should* eat your carrots!

## Principle #3: Eat Less Saturated Fat and Shun Trans Fats

In the past, doctors told their patients that in order to avoid a heart attack they should avoid foods high in cholesterol. But recently we've found that cutting out saturated and hydrogenated fats is much more effective in lowering dangerous LDL than watching your cholesterol intake. Saturated fat speeds the formation of arterial plaque, especially in people with metabolic syndrome and diabetes. Worst of all, saturated fat actually stimulates your liver to *create* cholesterol—and your liver can produce up to 4,000 to 5,000 mg of cholesterol daily! It has a much greater impact on your LDL and HDL levels than simply eating an extra 100 mg of cholesterol. Foods that are overloaded with saturated fat include fatty dairy products (cheese, butter, and high-fat milk—2 percent milk and whole milk) and fatty meats (red meat, sausage, and bacon).

Cutting saturated fats will improve your cholesterol profile and your health. The American Heart Association recommends a diet limiting saturated fat to not more than 7 percent of your total calories. So if you stick to the National Cholesterol Education Program recommendations, you could have about 16 grams daily. But studies of heart patients who closely followed these recommendations found that plaque still grew in their arteries over time. While these recommendations are a terrific improvement for average Americans, as far as I'm concerned, keeping saturated fats to 3 to 5 percent of your total calories (about 12 to 16 grams daily) would be ideal.

Let's look at the saturated fat table to see what this means in terms of daily food servings. (You'll find an even more detailed list in Appendix A.) If every day you drank 1 cup of skim milk, ate 1 or 2 organic omega-3 enriched eggs, whisked 1 teaspoon of extra-virgin olive oil into your salad dressing, and snacked on 1 to 2 ounces of almonds, and if each week you had a generous 6-ounce portion of salmon, sole, and shrimp, you'd be eating only 6 to 8 grams of saturated fat daily. Add an ample chicken breast to two or three meals a week and an extra tablespoon of extra-virgin olive oil to your salad, and you reach 11.5 grams, still decent. But go a step further and add a typical store-bought muffin, a hunk of cheese, a plate of cookies, and a big slice of pie and you leap into the unacceptable zone. So if you want to keep your circulatory system and arteries in the best possible shape, you really can't afford to splurge on saturated fats too often.

Note that while people have avoided shrimp because of its cholesterol content, it is low in saturated fat, rich in astaxanthins, and has omega-3 fats. Plus, studies have shown that shrimp lowers triglyceride and total cholesterol/HDL levels. That's why you'll see shrimp in my recipes often.

Worse than the harm caused by saturated fat, however, is that caused by trans fats or hydrogenated fats (found in solid shortening, margarine, and many processed foods and packaged baked goods as well as most fried fast foods). These nasty fats worsen cholesterol (raising your LDL cholesterol while dropping your healthy HDL levels) while also increasing

## SATURATED FAT CONTENT

| FOOD ITEM (SERVING SIZE) | SATURATED FAT (GRAMS) |
|---|---|
| Fruits and vegetables (1 cup) | 0.0 |
| Canola oil (1 tsp) | 0.3 |
| Skim milk (1 cup) | 0.3 |
| Bread, whole-wheat, 1 slice | 0.3 |
| Shrimp | 0.4 |
| Bagel, 1 medium | 0.5 |
| Sole (6 ounces cooked) | 0.6 |
| Olive oil (1 tsp) | 0.6 |
| Egg (1 from flaxseed-fed hen) | 1.0 |
| Peanut butter (1 tbsp) | 1.5 |
| 1% milk (1 cup) | 1.5 |
| Egg (one, regular) | 2.0 |
| Chicken breast (broiled, 6 ounces) | 2.0 |
| Bacon (2 strips) | 2.2 |
| 2% milk (1 cup) | 2.4 |
| Butter (1 tsp) | 2.4 |
| Salmon (coho, wild, 6 ounces cooked) | 2.7 |
| Almonds (3 ounces) | 3.0 |
| Oreo cookies, 3 ounces | 3.7 |
| Ice cream (½ cup) | 4.5 |
| Whole milk (1 cup) | 4.5 |
| Croissant | 6.6 |
| Mrs. Field's muffin (4 ounces) | 7.0 |
| Cheese (Swiss, 1.5 ounces) | 7.5 |
| Ground beef (extra lean, 6 ounces cooked) | 8.0 |
| Cheese (cheddar, 1.5 ounces) | 9.0 |
| Hostess Fruit Pie | 10.0 |
| Steak, sirloin (6 ounces) | 12.3 |
| Ground beef (regular, 6 ounces cooked) | 15.0 |

your risk of heart attacks and cancer and aggravating your insulin resistance and risk for diabetes. If in doubt, always read the label. If it lists "partially hydrogenated" *anything*, skip that item altogether. In a restaurant, ask if they use hydrogenated fats in the foods they serve, and insist upon choices that are free of these harmful products.

## Principle #4: Eat Healthy Omega-3 Fats

While the Ten Years Younger Diet steers you away from saturated and trans fats, I wholeheartedly believe that other, healthful fats are some of your most potent anti-aging allies. Chief among those are the omega-3 fats. There are actually two types of omega-3 fats, and both are beneficial to your health. Long-chain omega-3 fats come from cold water seafood, and excellent sources include salmon, trout, sole, sardines, herring, mussels, and oysters. These foods decrease inflammation, clotting within blood vessels, and abnormal heart rhythms, and lower cholesterol. Omega-3s help with blood sugar regulation by increasing insulin sensitivity, which makes them extremely important for people with metabolic syndrome and diabetes. They also have brain benefits, especially in cutting the risk of developing Alzheimer's disease, depression, and memory loss, by improving brain cell membrane flexibility, and by decreasing brain inflammation. In fact, at least 50 percent of your brain is made of omega-3 fats. They also appear to rejuvenate your skin by enhancing skin cell membrane flexibility and minimizing skin inflammation.

Healthy plant sources of omega-3 fats (also called medium-chain omega-3 fats or *alpha linolenic acid*) are found in soy, organic expeller-pressed canola oil, green leafy vegetables, flaxseed, and many nuts. These plant-based omega-3 fats lower cholesterol, are loaded with fiber, contain plant hormones that minimize menopausal and perimenopausal symptoms, and are a good source of lignans (fibrous compounds that decrease cancer risk). Unlike seafood sources of omega-3 fats, plant-based omega-3 fats don't have the ability to reduce clotting, heart rhythm irregularities, or inflammation.

Seafood, nuts, avocados, extra-virgin olive oil, and organic expeller-pressed canola oil are my favorite healthy sources of fat. Either they are rich in the omega-3 fats mentioned above or they contain monounsaturated fats (found especially in avocados and olive oil), which are associated with other benefits, including lowering your cholesterol, enhancing immune function, and protecting your cholesterol from being oxidized into artery-clogging plaque. To me, a combination of food sources rich in monounsaturated fat and omega-3 fats optimizes your health.

However, in addition to omega-3 fats, there are also omega-6 fats, and here's where the healthy fats issue gets complicated. While omega-3-rich foods block inflammation, omega-6 foods (including grain oils like corn and sunflower oil) actually increase inflammation and clotting. Some omega-6 fat is compatible with good health, as long as you ingest adequate amounts of the healthy omega-3s to counterbalance it.

In choosing seafood as a source for omega-3 fats, keep in mind how the food chain works. Tiny shrimp and other shellfish eat omega-3-rich algae. Small fish eat these shrimp and shellfish. Bigger fish eat the small fish. So as you go up the food chain, the levels of omega-3 fat increase. Mussels and oysters filter lots of omega-3-rich algae too, so they are also rich in omega-3 fats.

When choosing among oils you'd use for cooking, baking, and making salad dressing, I'd stick mostly with organic expeller-pressed canola oil and extra-virgin olive oil. If you can't find this kind of canola oil, stick to olive oil. For desserts and salad dressings, nut oils are also healthy and delicious. On occasion for flavoring special dishes, you could also use modest amounts of sesame and peanut oils—about ½ to 1 teaspoon per serving.

## The Mercury Dilemma

Just as omega-3 fat levels increase as you move up the food chain, unfortunately so do levels of toxic metals such as mercury. Seafood with high mercury content may reverse some of the benefits you derive from adding omega-3 fats to your diet. Where does the mercury come from? Human activity. Coal-burning plants, industry, and even batteries all release this toxic chemical, polluting our air, rivers, and groundwater. Eventually, the mercury makes its way to the sea, where levels have increased fifteen- to twenty-fold in the past thirty years. And as mercury levels rise in the sea, they build up in the algae and tiny organisms living there. The fish we eat consume the algae and smaller organisms, so as we move up the food chain, the levels of mercury increase as well. Usually, the bigger the mouth, the higher on the food chain; the higher on the food chain, the greater the mercury content. Shellfish and smallmouth fish are generally low in mercury and other heavy metals; fish at the top of the food chain, such as swordfish and shark, are the worst.

As a starting point, excellent choices of seafood high in omega-3 fats and low in mercury are wild salmon, sardines, herring, mussels, oysters, and low-mercury-area trout. Those that have moderate omega-3 fats but are still low in mercury include most shellfish (crab, shrimp, clams, Caribbean lobster, and squid), sole, flounder, small halibut, small mahi-mahi, perch, cod, and similar smallmouth fish. Other choices that have moderate mercury levels that you could eat one to three times a month include albacore tuna (the white- rather than red-flesh tuna), grouper, bass, Maine lobster, and snapper. I'd also suggest you limit sushi tuna (bluefin, with red flesh) to not more than once a month. If you eat these often, you should have your doctor test your mercury level to ensure that it isn't elevated. As for fish to avoid completely, there are four: swordfish, shark, tilefish, and barracuda.

If you have an allergy to seafood or really don't enjoy it but are eager to reap the benefits of omega-3 fats, you should consider taking an omega-3 supplement. I'll review these in Chapter 10.

## Principle #5: Substitute Whole Grains for Highly Refined, Processed Foods

The one area that low-carb promoters (Atkins, the Zone, Sugar Busters, South Beach Diet), high-carb promoters (Pritikin, Ornish, and Barnard), Andrew Weil, Nicholas Perricone, and myself all have in common is that we all preach the evils of refined carbohydrates such as white bread, white rice, processed fruit juices, table sugar, chips, and popular cereals like Cocoa Puffs.

Not only are these "foods" empty of all nutrients and full of sugar, but they lack fiber and vital anti-aging compounds. They don't even satisfy your appetite. In fact, most people experience a quick rise in blood sugar (or "sugar rush") and then feel hungry an hour later. As a result, highly processed and refined foods greatly contribute to accelerated aging, as they promote rising insulin levels and insulin resistance, which are associated with an expanding waistline and fat being deposited in your arteries and liver.

## Why Are Refined Carbs Bad for You?

If a whole grain such as a wheat berry is ground into white flour, most of its beneficial bran coating is removed. Similarly, brown rice is made into white rice by removing the outer bran covering during processing. Bran

### Glycemic Index and Glycemic Load

Glycemic index is a measure of how high your blood sugar levels rise after eating carb-rich foods. Sudden rises in blood-sugar levels worsen hunger, weight gain, inflammation, and both cholesterol and blood sugar levels. To measure a food's glycemic index, researchers test blood-sugar levels in people after feeding them a specific quantity of various carb-rich foods. The higher a food causes your blood-sugar level to rise, the higher its glycemic index. But glycemic index is not a perfect measure of how a food will impact your body and your weight, and many diet authors have erred in overemphasizing this concept. It would be far better to look at *glycemic load* because it starts where glycemic index leaves off.

Once nutritionists know a food's glycemic index, they look at how much carbohydrate is in the food itself. Take carrots, with a moderately high glycemic index of 47 (a rating that banishes them from low-carb diets). Since their carb content per pound is low (only 6 grams for ⅓ cup serving), their glycemic load is actually quite low at 3. That means, if you eat a serving of carrots, your blood sugar wouldn't rise all that much. And this Vitality Food is packed with anti-aging compounds, fiber, and nutrients. Avoiding carrots because of their glycemic index would be a mistake.

By choosing low glycemic load carbs, you minimize spikes in blood sugar, reduce insulin surges, and suppress hunger. This is why I emphasize low glycemic load foods for the Ten Years Younger Diet. So enjoy healthy carbohydrates, in particular those listed in Chapter 4, the Sweet Sixteen Vitality Foods, as they are generally low in glycemic load and also rich in nutrients, antioxidants, and fiber. For more information on glycemic load, visit my Web site, www.tenyearsyounger.net.

contains multiple anti-aging and antioxidant compounds that protect the grain from damage and disease. In fact, a grain wrapped in its fibrous bran coating can last thousands of years in a tomb in Egypt, Thailand, or Mexico, and often will still germinate if planted today. The anti-aging benefits of the bran layer in whole grains are incredible. But remove the bran and you remove many of the grain's anti-aging benefits.

Moreover, when you eat something made from refined white flour, you digest and absorb the sugars much more quickly than you would if the wheat had remained in its original form. This creates an immediate surge in your blood sugar, which in turn stimulates your pancreas to make insulin, which then causes your sugar levels to drop. As they do, your body senses the drop in blood sugar and stimulates your appetite— so you eat again. This cycle of eating refined carbs, rapid blood sugar rise, blood sugar storage as fat, blood sugar level drop, and repeated hunger is one factor behind the recent spike in obesity rates.

Elevated insulin levels in the bloodstream also slow your metabolism, and over time you will reach insulin resistance, the first step toward diabetes and accelerated aging, which we discussed in Chapters 1 and 2. This is why the Ten Years Younger Diet substitutes whole grains for white flour, white pasta, and white rice, which are highly processed, diabetes-inducing foods. Not only do you add fiber when you choose whole grains, but you also minimize surges in blood sugar levels.

## Principle #6: Seek Out Foods Rich in Calcium and Magnesium

Your diet can either build or deplete your bones, and it goes without saying that you want to improve your bone health. Calcium, magnesium, and healthy sources of protein combined with exercise support excellent bone health. Adequate calcium is also associated with better weight control and weight loss. Studies have shown that people who take in 1,000 to 1,500 mg of calcium daily lose more weight than those on a low-calcium diet. So if you think it's just about your bones, think again—calcium has broader anti-aging benefits. So how much calcium do you need? That depends on your lifestyle.

Let's look at two extremes. A person who is a true "couch potato," who eats salt and animal protein in great excess, drinks more than 4 cups of coffee and colas a day, and smokes cigarettes is likely to lose bone density even with an intake of 1,500 mg of calcium daily. (See Chapter 2.) In contrast, someone who exercises an hour a day (with weight-bearing and strength-training activities), who avoids coffee and colas, limits salt and excessive animal protein, and doesn't smoke could maintain his or her bone density with only 700 to 800 mg of calcium a day. More typical are those who try to eat well and exercise but are only doing about 75 percent of what they should. If this is your profile, you should give yourself an added cushion and be sure to consume 1,200 mg of calcium a day. If you already have osteopenia or osteoporosis, I would recommend 1,500 mg.

You can of course take calcium supplements, but you should endeavor to get as much calcium directly from foods as you can. Most green leafy vegetables and beans contain about 100 mg of calcium per cup, and whole grains have about 20 mg per cup or serving. All calcium-fortified drinks such as soy milk, rice milk, and calcium-fortified orange juice seem to have the same calcium content as cow's milk—about 300 mg per cup.

Unlike calcium, which we hear about regularly, magnesium is an oft-overlooked mineral. It improves bone health, but it also improves blood sugar control, blood pressure control, and bowel function; it lowers your risk for heart attacks and strokes; and it enhances many anti-aging enzyme reactions.

Magnesium is found in whole grains, green leafy vegetables, and legumes. Most of us are magnesium deficient, and we would benefit in many ways by adding extra magnesium to our regimen. The recipes in the Ten Years Younger Diet will help you do so with ease, and you'll also find suggestions for magnesium supplements in Chapter 10 and on my Web site, www.tenyearsyounger.net.

## Principle # 7: Hydrate!

Your body is 80 percent water—you need fluid to survive. But many of us fail to drink enough of the right kinds of liquids each day. We need 8 cups of fluid, but beware of caffeinated coffee, tea, and colas, as well as alcohol. Alcohol and caffeine are diuretics—they actually cause your body to filter water out of your system through urination, so despite the fact that you're drinking all these liquids, you won't actually get hydrated! In fact, if this is all you drink during a day you may feel tired and constipated all the time. Water, on the other hand, is the ultimate hydrating drink. It's cheaper than soda and better for you too. Next time you feel like your energy is waning, try a tall cool glass of water—either still or sparkling—instead.

Drinking the wrong kinds of fluids can also tack on extra calories. A 12-ounce can of cola typically has 140 calories. If you drink one can a day for a whole year, you've added an extra 51,100 calories to your body fat stores in the form of 14 pounds. If you normally drink one soda daily, skip it, or switch to diet soda or water, and you should lose 14 pounds of fat over the next year.

This is not to say, however, that only water is permissible as a beverage. Fiber- and protein-rich drinks (such as a smoothie made with frozen berries, ground flaxseed, and soy milk) shouldn't be lumped in with drinks that provide nothing but empty calories. Furthermore, unlike soda and wine and even water, they contain fiber, which will help you feel full—allowing you to cut calories in other areas as you take off the years. If you don't have problems with weight control, then fruit juices such as orange juice can provide healthy vitamins and nutrients.

## Principle #8: Don't Forget to Save Room for Dessert

The worst snacking time for most people is between dinner and bedtime, so plan to serve yourself something healthy and tasty during this danger zone. Many wonderful desserts can be made with anti-aging ingredients. Frozen berries whirled in a blender with nonfat soy milk, skim milk, or nonfat yogurt makes a great smoothie. I usually add 1 or 2 teaspoons of ground flaxseed per serving, just to up the omega-3 and fiber content.

Cocoa, as we've seen, is heart healthy, so enjoy a cup of nonfat, no-sugar-added cocoa with soy milk or skim milk daily. Small amounts of real chocolate are beneficial too—just watch out for the calories. For an occasional treat, try my wife's wonderful Chocolate Mousse with Grand Marnier on page 239. It's fabulous and healthy at just 200 calories. Or combine fruit with some tapioca and sprinkle some low-fat, nutty granola on top and pop it in the oven. It makes a terrific dessert. (See the Peach and Raspberry Crumble recipe on page 295.) You'll find plenty of dessert recipes to help you with this principle in Part III.

## Principle #9: Watch Your Portion Sizes

Studies have shown that portion sizes in our society have increased substantially since the late seventies. To no one's surprise, fast food has seen the largest jump. Hence familiar slogans like "Supersize me!"

Generally, the more leafy vegetables you eat, the fuller you'll feel and the less room you'll have for less healthful foods. The foods that need portion control are the ones high in calorie density. Very-high-fat foods such as cheese, peanut butter, and oils, for instance, should be limited to only 1 to 2 teaspoons per meal. And you should restrict serving sizes of potatoes with the skin and even whole grains such as brown rice and whole-wheat pasta to ½ to 1 cup at any given meal.

At the annual meeting of the North American Association for the Study of Obesity in October 2003, researchers at Penn State University presented data showing that if people are served larger portions, they eat them. But serve yourself a smaller portion, and you'll eat less! It's as simple as that. Even eating off smaller plates will lower how many calories you eat. Offer someone one cookie, and they'll eat one cookie; give them a plate, and they probably won't stop at just one.

If you're working for better weight control, don't bring platters full of food to the dinner table, family style. Try plating the meal in the kitchen, putting the extra food away for lunch or dinner another day, and serving a smaller portion. You should find that you eat less without feeling hungry. If you need more volume, add extra vegetables to your dinner plate—they'll help fill you up!

## Ten Years Younger Portion Recommendations

- For whole grains (brown rice, whole-wheat pasta, whole-grain cereal, and other grains), 1 cup per meal. (For weight loss and blood sugar control, limit to 3 to 4 cups maximum daily.)
- For potatoes eaten with the skin, up to ¾ cup. Mashed or baked without the skin, not more than ½ cup per serving.
- For oils (extra-virgin olive oil and organic expeller-pressed canola oil), ½ to 1 teaspoon per meal. Better yet, use a spray can for 1 to 2 seconds.
- With nuts, 1 to 2 ounces or 1 to 2 handfuls a day.
- 6 ounces a day of high-fat seafood such as salmon, sardines, and trout (4 ounces is about the size of your palm).
- 6 to 8 ounces daily of low-fat seafood such as shellfish, sole, and cod (about the size of your hand).
- Limit serving size of lean poultry to 4 to 6 ounces per meal.
- For soy products (edamame, soy milk, tofu), no more than 2 to 3 cups daily.
- People who have problems with blood sugar regulation should limit their fruit intake to not more than three servings daily (a serving is an apple or a cup of grapes). For those who have no blood sugar problems, no restrictions.
- No limit for salads, vegetables, and beans.

# Principle #10: Select Healthy Snacks

I encourage healthy snacks with the Ten Years Younger Diet. While you should plan on three meals a day plus a tasty yet healthy dessert, eating a modest snack before a meal takes the edge off your appetite, helping you with portion control. And the afternoon snack is critical for many people. The key is eating the right kind of snacks in the right proportions.

Midmorning snacks are optional. Some people will find the act of eating breakfast in itself to be a big change. If this is you, asking you to eat a midmorning snack would be unrealistic. But for those who are terribly hungry around 10:30 or 11 A.M., a serving of yogurt, an omega-3 enriched, free-range, organic hard-boiled egg, or a piece of fruit will make a big difference in controlling your hunger all day.

The Rescue Snacks listed in the meal plans in Part III are intended for moments when you need to be saved from an attack of the munchies. When you feel like bingeing on a bag of chips, cookies, or candies, consider something hearty and satisfying instead. Nuts, sardines or smoked oysters with rye crispbread, and soy meats (such as soy sausage) are chewy and satisfying, and they leave you feeling full. The protein adds some weight to your stomach, and these foods are also low in the refined carbs that trigger binge eating. When you're feeling tempted, the worst snacks would have low fiber and protein and high glycemic load, such as chips, cookies, breads, candies, and other sweets. These refined snacks are *not* filling and, as your blood sugar spikes up and down, often trigger continuous eating. No wonder they say, "Bet you can't eat just one." You truly can't!

## Before You Begin the Diet

Just as with the other aspects of your health that you measured in Chapter 3, the first step with the Ten Years Younger Diet is to assess your current eating habits. I want you to track your diet over three days, choosing one weekend day and two weekdays. The most helpful things to track are:

- Total fiber intake
- Omega-3 fat intake
- Saturated fat intake
- Total intake of colorful fruits and vegetables

Tables in Appendixes A, B, and D will help you to calculate your average intake, even without filling out food questionnaires or seeing a nutritionist. Optimally, once you begin the ten-week program, you would then reassess every two to four weeks how much fiber, saturated fat, and fruits and vegetables you're eating. While it might seem tedious to calculate these quantities, many research studies have shown that if you write down what you eat, it empowers you to make substantial changes in your eating patterns.

**Based on the ten principles, here's what you're shooting for:**

- More than 30 grams of fiber daily
- 5 cups of colorful fruits and vegetables daily
- At least 2 to 3 grams daily of omega-3 fats (with at least 1 of those grams from seafood sources)
- About 12 to 16 grams of saturated fat daily
- 1,200 mg of calcium a day
- 8 cups of fluid a day
- Whole grains rather than refined carbs

Follow these guidelines and you'll achieve a high nutrition score for longevity and vitality!

Many of the Vitality Foods I've recommended on these pages have multiple benefits. But none of these foods is as effective if you eat it in isolation. The aging process within us works in a delicate balance, much like an orchestra playing a Mozart symphony, in which each instrument has a critical role—simply adding more horns and clarinets will not improve the performance. It's the same with antioxidants: You need the whole team of age blockers if you're going to be ten years younger.

In the same vein, I've often heard people—even some of my co-workers—complain about recipes that have more than four ingredients. I find this tragic, because the truth is that, much like music, nutrition, and taste depend on harmonies and synergies. Think back to that Mozart symphony. Now, shrink the sound down to just three instruments. It just won't resonate as deeply, and it won't have the complexity that makes it your favorite piece.

Nutrition and taste are the same. Combining anti-aging ingredients such as ginger, garlic, chili, lemon juice, and oregano with soybeans and plant pigments plus adequate fiber, lean protein, and healthy fats creates a powerful anti-aging meal. Together, these agents protect your cell membranes and DNA vastly more effectively than any one of them could alone. It is the combination that is essential. If you want your food to taste great while you maximize your anti-aging capacity, you'll seek out and prepare meals that have multiple ingredients!

We all have five essential taste centers: sweet, sour, bitter, salty, and pungent (as with mushrooms). Unfortunately, the average American diet overstimulates just two of these centers: sweet and salty. In fact, many of us are so used to eating bland food made from butter, white flour, salt, and sugar that our palates explode when we taste something flavorful; we can't handle the zing. In Part III, you'll find recipes that keep you younger while they literally sing with flavor. The Ten Years Younger Diet taps into all five taste centers, delivering a nutritional yet tasty punch that harmonizes flavor and health.

And now let's move on to the second pillar of the Ten Years Younger Program: exercise.

# CHAPTER 6

# Age-Busting Fitness

When Rick started the Ten Years Younger research study, he'd grown increasingly out of shape because he'd stopped exercising. "I'm 47," he told me. "Up until four or five years ago, I did a lot of running to keep fit—thirty miles a week or so. I ran a lot of road races and occasionally 5K and 10K races. I even did triathlons for a while. But I had a problem with a lower disk injury. When I'd go on the triathlons, I used to think it was muscle spasms, but I found out after having an MRI that I actually had a herniated disk in my back. The mileage of training, the pounding on it, constantly irritated it. So I stopped running when I was 43. But that's when I ballooned up 25 or 30 pounds or more, which made me less active in other areas of my life—not just with running."

The Ten Years Younger fitness regimen did Rick a world of good. He had visible results soon after starting the program, which kept him motivated. "You really do see the change," he told me. "I didn't weigh myself, but I could tell by the notches on my belt that I was losing weight and getting in shape. I lost 17 pounds during the 10 weeks, and 4 inches off my waistline!"

Better yet, Rick was able to resume activities he'd believed were lost to him forever. He now plays basketball and tennis with his seventeen-year-old son. "I have a lot more endurance and strength than I did prior to participating in the program. I'm looking forward to going snowboarding this winter in Colorado. This is the best shape I've ever been in. I think that the weight loss combined with building strength and stretching has helped me tremendously."

Best of all, Rick has enjoyed a surge in confidence. "The program has made a big difference in my life. I feel better about myself; I feel healthier. My energy level is up, my clothes fit better—all of those things get your self-esteem back up." And the fact that he can play sports with his son again is a change that truly makes life worth living.

## The Anti-Aging Benefits of Exercise

As we've seen, regular exercise is one of your key allies in turning back the clock, and one of the three pillars of the Ten Years Younger Program. Studies have shown that you can actually restore 75 percent of the muscle mass lost over 10 years with a short 12-week exercise program. Exercise fights the seven Aging Accelerators in many ways: It boosts your energy, builds muscle and strengthens your bones, perks up your metabolism and helps control blood sugar, lowers inflammation and free radical levels, supports your immune system, enhances your circulation by increasing your blood vessels' ability to dilate, and increases your HDL, the "good" cholesterol that prevents arterial blockage.

Exercise is not only good for your body's physical function, it also helps your mind. Your mental efficiency increases by about 15 percent when you follow an exercise program. In my Ten Years Younger study, we saw a 10 to 29 percent increase in various aspects of brainpower in people who exercised 5 days a week. If it normally takes you 10 hours to complete all your tasks at work, then you should be done in 9 hours or less.

Finally, whereas most of the other parts of the Ten Years Younger Program tackle the inside—the parts of your body invisible to the eye—exercise is one component that will make you younger on the *outside*. You will look firm and toned, and have curves from muscle definition, rather than excess pounds. Your clothes will fit better, and you'll be able to reclaim those smaller sizes you long thought were lost to you. Your svelte new physique will be a great sign that your muscle mass has increased while your fat has diminished. And maintaining a regular aerobic exercise regimen is the best way to keep the extra weight off. Think of it this way: If you ate one 200-calorie candy bar every day for a year on top of your normal eating habits without increasing your activity, you would gain roughly 20 pounds. On the other hand, if you added an activity that burns 100 calories every day, such as walking a mile, you'd lose 10 pounds over one year without changing your other eating habits or activities. Which would you choose?

To top it off, exercise leaves you feeling terrific—much more energized and alive. That's yet another reason why it's such an integral part of my anti-aging program. As Doris explained after her ten weeks in the program, "I have a lot more energy. On the weekends, I used to need naps on both days. But now I don't feel so tired anymore. I can keep going, and in the end I can get a lot more accomplished." Fifty-three-year-old Sherilyn had the same experience. "I feel great!" she said. "In fact, I used to come home from work and be pretty sedentary and not do much. Now I have more energy, and I'm a lot less tired."

## The Age-Busting Fitness Program

Age-busting fitness has three key elements: aerobic exercise, strength training, and stretching. In the Ten Years Younger Program, your aerobic workout involves raising your heart rate, preferably to 70 to 80 percent of your maximum rate, and keeping it in this range for 30 to 60 minutes five to six days a week. When focusing on the aerobic element, you'll walk, jog, swim, or bike daily to burn calories and boost your resting metabolic rate. And you'll improve quickly, progressing from 20 to 25 minutes of aerobic exercise five days a week to 40 to 60 minutes of aerobic activity six days a week.

As you know by now, muscles not only impact your metabolism and rate of calorie burn, but they also provide proteins in the form of amino acids to repair tissues, fight infections, and create anti-aging compounds essential to life. Toned, well-maintained muscles are one of your biggest anti-aging weapons, so muscle-building exercise—or strength training—is the second piece of your exercise regimen. You'll engage in strength training twice a week during Phase One, but by Phase Three, you'll have advanced to three times a week.

Which muscles will you focus on? While you have hundreds, you're going to aim at building an even dozen: those around your knees, hips, spine, shoulders, elbows, and ankles. For the knees, hips, shoulders, and elbows I'll emphasize extension and flexion activities that build the big power muscles in your body: hamstrings, quads, calves, back, abs, glutes, deltoids, biceps, and triceps. While you may not know where all these muscles are just yet, they are the power plants that move you through space and burn the most calories during exercise and at rest. If you want the biggest bang for your exercise buck, you'll focus on these major hitters. Not only do they burn fat, they also provide muscle definition and sex appeal—a real plus!

In addition, I'll focus on muscle groups that are essential for independence as we grow older. Those most commonly associated with disability include the muscles that stabilize the shoulder joint, back, knees, and pelvic floor. The last of these are critical for sexual function and urinary and bowel control, so you certainly don't want to neglect them. I'll also add an exercise for your shoulder's rotator cuff that will stabilize your shoulder movements, and some trunk-twisting stretches to help support your spine. And for safety's sake, I'll also ask you to stretch every day after your workout, keeping your muscles flexible and supple as well as strong. Stretching—the third element of the Ten Years Younger fitness program—helps prevent the kinds of injuries that would undermine your progress.

The exercises are organized in an even and balanced way. You'll work on your quadriceps, the large muscles in the front of your thighs, but also your hamstrings, the muscles at the back of your thighs. You'll strengthen your chest muscles for a firm, lifted look but also work on the opposing muscles in your upper back, to ensure good posture.

The program is designed to help even the most deconditioned participants start rebuilding their lean muscle mass in a way that's gradual enough not to cause injury but yields remarkable results. It's never too late!

Even though five days may seem like a lot, it's gentle consistency that does the trick. Weekend warriors who push themselves to complete exhaustion once or twice a week deplete their antioxidant defense systems, and consequently they get sick more often—not a Ten Years Younger goal! And if you exercise above 85 percent of your maximum heart rate, you will actually generate more free radicals than your antioxidant system can handle. Yes, you are burning more calories, but at the risk of aging yourself in the process. It's just not worth it. As always, I recommend that you work with a medical provider to ensure that your goals are realistic and safe.

## Aerobic Exercise: It Keeps You Young at Heart

Researchers have shown that regular physical activity actually slows the aging process. In one study conducted on a group of aging runners, those who maintained their lean body mass through aerobic exercise lived longer and better. Why should this be so? Maintaining a healthy weight is one reason, but there are also chemical reasons for engaging in aerobic exercise. One of the answers involves C-reactive protein (CRP), a substance your liver creates in response to bodywide production of inflammatory compounds (see Chapter 1). Regular exercise lowers CRP levels, and it decreases your risk of a heart attack or stroke by up to 40 percent.

Indeed, of all the options for preventing and treating cardiovascular disease in both men and women, the single most effective choice is not medication but aerobic exercise! Simply walking every day would likely cut the risk of all cardiovascular events by 33 percent. And when you increase your exertion to a brisk walk, a hike in the hills, or jogging and get your heart rate up, you'll experience even greater benefits, including greater energy, vitality, and weight loss.

### Walking Away the Pounds

As we've seen, something as basic as walking—if you do it consistently—can yield tremendous weight loss results. Generally, those who succeed with long-term weight loss walk at least 3 to 4 miles a day or use exercise machines to burn at least 2,000 to 2,500 calories every week. And people who exercise at least 5 but often 6 to 7 days a week have the best results.

With this in mind, the Ten Years Younger Program recommends:

- Forty to 60 minutes of aerobic exercise 5 to 6 days a week (burning about 2,500 calories per week) for weight *loss*
- Thirty to 40 minutes of aerobic activity 5 to 6 days a week (burning about 2,000 calories per week) for weight *maintenance*

That may sound like a lot, but here's how you can manage this exercise schedule efficiently. Most of us burn roughly 100 calories walking one mile. Therefore, to lose one pound (about 3,500 calories) you'd need to walk 35 miles. For most people this is impossible in a single day, and for many even 5 miles a day for a week would be difficult at best. However, it might be possible to walk 21 miles a week—that's 3 miles a day. In one day alone you'd burn 300 calories, and over one year you could burn 109,500 calories. If your eating habits remained unchanged, you'd lose 31 pounds. That's the power of consistency!

If during that walk you increased your heart rate to 70 to 80 percent of your maximum, you would burn 10 to 15 percent calories more *after* exercising due to the rise in your metabolic rate. That takes off an *extra* 3 to 5 pounds in the short run and over the long haul will help prevent weight regain.

Walking also helps to prevent and reverse metabolic syndrome. One of the first steps toward defeating insulin resistance and gaining insulin control is activity, which will improve your blood sugar levels by depleting the energy your muscle cells have stored as glycogen. You want your muscles to be building and depleting energy every day; this process will help restore muscle cell sensitivity to insulin. If you've become insulin resistant, the first week on the Ten Years Younger Program may show mixed results, as your blood sugar levels may tend to bounce around. But by the second week, you should notice clear improvements in blood sugar control and blood pressure. Walking has also been called the best prevention and treatment for diabetes.

If you are in good health and are used to some form of activity, you might want to exceed my minimal recommendation of walking at least 3 miles a day. During your exercise time, your heart rate should reach 70 to 80 percent of your maximum achieved heart rate (see Chapter 3). This gives you a nice metabolic calorie burn. With your health provider's permission, spend at least 40 minutes daily in this heart rate zone to prevent metabolic syndrome, and 45 to 60 minutes in this zone daily to reverse it. Not everyone can reach this level of exercise all at once. Depending on

## YOUR AEROBIC WORKOUT

Your aerobic activities can include bicycling, jogging, swimming, brisk walking or hiking, an aerobics class at the gym (low-impact, step, spinning), or working out on a treadmill, a stationary bike, or an elliptical machine. You should plan on working out aerobically 30 to 60 minutes a day, five to six days a week. Here's what the aerobic portion of your daily workout should look like:

- Start with an aerobic warm-up at 50 to 60 percent of your maximum heart rate for 3 minutes. Focus on nice smooth steps with good form. You don't need to spend time stretching before you work out unless there's a specific injury you're coping with. Better than stretching is to be sure you warm up slowly.
- Next, reach aerobic activity at 70 to 85 percent of your maximum heart rate for 30 to 60 minutes. This is your *aerobic zone*—an important concept for your exercise routine. If your initial fitness level is too low to tolerate 30 minutes in your aerobic zone, alternate 5 minutes in your warm-up zone with 5 minutes in your aerobic zone until you can sustain your aerobic-zone level.
- Cool down for 2 to 3 minutes. Stopping suddenly can leave you dizzy; it's much better to go back to 50 to 60 percent of your maximum heart rate for a couple of minutes.
- Now stretch for 5 to 10 minutes. Stretching decreases injuries, thereby ensuring that you exercise regularly without taking weeks off because you've hurt yourself. (See below for my stretching recommendations.)

your condition, you might have to start with a twenty-minute walk daily and gradually increase your activity week by week.

### Interval Training

Interval training is your ticket to maximizing your aerobic performance. As you advance to Phases Two and Three of the Age-Busting Fitness Program, you will be adding interval training once or twice a week. Here's how it works: At the midpoint of your aerobic workout, take your pulse or use a pulse meter to track your heart rate. Then push yourself to 85 to 90 percent of your maximum rate (you determined your rate in Chapter 3) and keep your heart pumping at that rate for one minute. Then slow the pace and let your heart drop to 65 to 70 percent of your maximum rate for one minute. Then do it again! Pick up the pace to 85 percent of your maximum and hold it for one minute. Repeat this cycle of one minute high and one minute low five times.

After you've engaged in interval training for a while, your maximum predicted heart rate will increase. In fact, after a while, the interval training will begin to feel easy. That's when you'll have to retest your maximum achievable heart rate because your heart will be responding as if you were ten years younger!

## Strength Training: The Secret to Shaping Up

We all want to feel good in our clothes and look great, and strength training can slim you down and bring back the muscle tone of younger years—probably two of your most important Ten Years Younger goals. How? Because muscles burn calories. In fact, one pound of muscle burns about 35 to 40 calories a day! That means one extra pound of muscle could burn an extra 1,000 calories a month, or 12,000 additional calories a year. And over the course of that year, that single pound of muscle would burn 3½ pounds of fat! So if you were to add 5 pounds of muscle to your frame—a realistic goal after several months of strength training—you'd lose 17½ pounds of extra fat a year. Imagine! That's more than the volume of four footballs.

While you might believe that strength training is something only bodybuilders do, in fact, it's one of the most important ways to become ten years younger. Women, in particular, benefit from the effects of weight lifting and strength training, mostly because they usually have much less muscle mass than men. (And no, you won't end up looking like Arnold Schwarzenegger!)

I've known many women who run on a treadmill for 30 to 45 minutes every day but still complain that they can't lose weight. When I measure their body composition, I usually discover that even though they are aerobically fit, their muscle mass is grossly depleted. Once they build up a decent muscle mass, they find it much easier to burn calories. In fact, I've known many women who needed to *gain* a few pounds of muscle before they finally succeeded in losing weight.

If you're completely out of shape, you too may need to build your muscles before you can successfully lose weight with an exercise program. No matter how old you are, it's possible. Even frail 90-year-olds have been able to markedly increase their muscle mass with strength training! By engaging in proper strength training three times a week, you will actually shift your body's composition and increase your total calorie burn by about 15 percent. That comes close to burning an extra 120 calories a day.

My program recommends strength or weight training three times a week for optimum results. But beware! You can't just build the muscle and then quit. Your muscles will simply shrink back to their old selves, and your fat will return. To maintain the beautiful new body you're creating, you'll need to work out at least once or twice a week. Remember, the Ten Years Younger Program is not a one-shot deal—it's a lifestyle change that requires ongoing attention for the best results.

## Elements of Strength Training

When you work with fixed-weight machines, you flex and extend your muscles. But in real life that's not enough. You have to stabilize your joints, not just flex and extend them. You need to keep them from twisting and falling from side to side. You need to build the stabilizing muscles in your trunk and core as well as those big power-hitting muscles. That is why Age-Busting Fitness encourages you to work with free weights rather than machines, and why many of the exercises I recommend require you to stand on the floor or incorporate the help of an exercise ball. Lifting free weights and doing your exercises on a ball will force you to use the little muscles that provide balance and joint stability. I've also thrown in some twisting moves to ensure that your trunk is strong, so you can accommodate all the activities that are essential to functioning optimally on a busy day.

You don't need to join a gym to do strength training, but you'll need some free weights in the form of various sizes of dumbbells so that you can work the twelve body parts mentioned earlier. Different parts of your body usually require different weights for optimum exertion. And as you'll see, an exercise ball is a wonderful strength-training tool, so I highly recommend you buy one if you aren't going to use a gym. Make sure to purchase a ball that suits your height. If it's the right size, you should be able to sit on it with your feet placed in front of you on the floor and your knees bent at a 90-degree angle. An exercise bench can also come in handy, but if you don't have one, don't worry. I've provided optional moves that don't require one.

However, if you're new to strength training, one big advantage of a gym is that it has all the equipment you'll need, making it easier to get started. Once you get the hang of strength training—and a four-week membership might be all you need to get in the groove—it is much easier to continue at home on your own.

One of the first steps is to identify how heavy a dumbbell you need for each movement. This varies from person to person. In general, you should be able to lift the weight smoothly at least 10 to 12 times. If you can't do 10 or 12 reps, it is too heavy; if you're able to lift it more than 16 times, the dumbbell is too light and you won't be adding enough stress to build muscle mass adequately. This varies greatly. One person might need to start with 3 pounds, while another might need to start with 30. I've noted an average starting weight for many of the exercises below, but the sensible thing to do is experiment to find the ideal weight for you.

Most people tend to envision their arms and legs doing all the work when it comes to strength training, but I want you to focus on your trunk or torso, too. Trunk strength is essential to preventing back pain, maintaining good posture, and gaining balance. You'll find that I've provided several options for some muscle groups such as your abs or your chest, and the exercises become progressively harder as you advance in your program. So you should begin working your abdominal muscles with simple crunches but then move on to crunches on the ball, which are more challenging and much more fun!

Here are your Ten Years Younger strength training guidelines at a glance. Aim to work out two or three days a week.

## YOUR STRENGTH TRAINING WORKOUT

- Work at least 10 to 14 body parts during each session (I pick an even dozen), but make sure to balance your workout. If you strengthen your biceps (elbow flexor), you'll also want to work out your triceps (your elbow extender). Similarly, if you do lots of crunches, make sure you also balance them out with back extension exercises. (See the exercise instructions below.)
- Lift your weight 12 to 15 times. If you can't manage at least 10 reps, the dumbbell is too heavy. But if you can lift it more than 16 times, the weight is too light. Try to use counts for up-and-down motions—such as "one one thousand" for up and "two one thousand" for down.
- Lift the weight smoothly and lower it slowly. (If you can't do that, return to a lighter weight.) Aim to feel a gentle burn as you lower the weight. Avoid jerky movements, as they cause injuries.
- While trainers may have you do 2 or 3 sets of each exercise (which can be good for teaching form), studies have shown that most of the benefit comes from performing just the first set. So if time is an issue for you, one set of 12 to 15 reps should give you more than 90 percent of your benefit, as long as you can just barely make the last couple of lifts. By Phase Three, I'll have you doing two sets of each strength training activity at least once a week to ensure that you are pushing yourself adequately to build the strength, tone, and shape you deserve for the time you've invested.

- With leg exercises, do *not* lock your knees. With arm exercises, do *not* lock your elbows. Again, this will help you avoid injuries.
- Exhale through your mouth on the upward motion (the most strenuous part of an exercise) and inhale through your nose on the down motion. And don't forget to breathe on each movement!
- Stretch after exercising, and hold each stretch for at least ten and preferably twenty seconds. (See below for instructions on stretching.)

# The Anti-Aging Moves

So what are the best muscle-building activities that you can undertake at home or at the gym? You'll learn the moves here. There are generally two kinds of strength training: machine training and functional training. Machine training isolates a specific muscle group and is effective for people aiming to beef up specific muscles. Functional training, on the other hand, reflects activities performed in daily life and helps build trunk muscles along with overall balance and strength. It has advantages over machine training in that it emphasizes strength and mobility for everyday activities (as opposed to lifting a 20-pound dumbbell). It also carries a lower risk of injury than machine training, which is why I stress it here.

Pick twelve activities below and repeat them two to three times a week.

## Functional Strength-Training Activities

### Abdominal Crunches

Everyone should be able to easily perform 75 crunches daily. If you can't do that yet, then you have a terrific opportunity to strengthen these core muscles. But be advised that old-fashioned sit-ups (which I performed in high school), where you touch your elbows to your knees, are now out of favor, as they can strain your back. Stick to crunches instead.

*Benefits:* Crunches build abdominal muscles and provide critical support for your spine. Strengthening those muscles is one of the best ways to prevent lower back pain. It's also a great way to firm up your tummy, and when combined with proper weight control, it can give you that sexy six-pack look.

*What you'll need:* A floor mat or other comfortable surface.

- Lie on your back with your feet flat on the floor and your knees bent at an angle of 30 to 45 degrees. Your arms are folded across your chest, one hand on each shoulder.
- Flex your pelvis, pushing your lower back into the floor and tilting your pelvis up; this protects your back during crunches.
- Now raise your upper back and head off the floor, lifting your shoulder blades about 1 to 2 inches from the ground. Hold for one second, and then lower down slowly. Repeat until you feel your abdominal muscles strain. Then take a break for 5 to 10 seconds and perform at least 10 more crunches.

*Tip:* Once you can easily reach 75 crunches, try this exercise with your feet lifted gently off the ground, keeping your pelvis flexed. This works your lower abs. Also, be sure your pelvis remains flexed with your back firmly pressed against the floor throughout your routine.

### Abdominal Crunches on the Ball

Once you're proficient at abdominal crunches on the floor, you can advance to the ball. It has the advantage of forcing you to use your whole trunk, subtly working your oblique stomach muscles as you balance yourself. This makes the exercises harder but also much more effective, as you are building the balance and strength you need every day to lift and carry objects.

*Benefits:* These are wonderful for people with back problems, and they give you a firm tummy. As with the regular crunches, these will help to give you that sexy six-pack look when combined with proper weight control.

*What you'll need:* An exercise ball.

- Sit on the ball with your feet on the ground and your arms folded across your chest. Now walk your feet forward and lean backward until your lower and mid-back are against the ball and your feet are a foot or two apart in front of you on the floor.
- With your pelvis flexed, curl up and lift your chest and head toward the ceiling until only your lower back pushes against the ball and you feel a strain in your abdominal muscles. Hold the up position for 3 to 5 seconds, then slowly lean back. Continue until your abdominal muscles tremble.

*Tip:* As these get easier, bring your feet closer together, until they are side by side, forcing you to recruit more trunk-twisting muscles for balance.

### Oblique Crunches on the Ball

This exercise works different muscles than the first two kinds of crunches.

*Benefits:* These are great for building the oblique muscles along the sides of your abdomen, which help you to twist your trunk. This exercise will tone your sides and, with proper weight control, help to form a shapely waist.

*What you'll need:* An exercise ball.

- Lie on the ball in the neutral position as if you were about to perform a crunch. Your feet are a foot or two apart on the floor; your lower and mid-back are lying against the ball.
- Now sit up and twist to the right, pointing your left elbow and shoulder toward your right knee. Be sure to keep your pelvis flexed throughout the twisting motion and your head aligned with your spine.
- Now lean back slowly into the neutral position, maintaining balance on the ball. Alternate sides, repeating 12 to 16 oblique crunches on each side.

## Back Extensions

This exercise balances the muscle groups used when performing crunches.

*Benefits:* Back extensions build the lower and upper back muscles, stabilizing your spine and preventing back pain. Doing back extensions on an exercise ball also helps to build your trunk's twisting muscles, as you are forced to balance. Back exercises should also help with your posture and give your back a sculpted look.

*What you'll need:* An exercise ball. If you are more advanced, you'll also need some small free weights.

- Lying facedown over the ball, brace your toes against the wall or another object. Your feet should be at least hip width apart, if not a bit wider. (The wider your feet are placed, the easier it is to perform this exercise. With time, you can bring your feet closer together.) Your hands are placed gently on the floor, and your abdomen is bent over the ball at about a 30-degree angle.
- Now lift your arms so they are extended out in front of you as if you were Superman flying. Your trunk and arms are in a straight line, with only your mid-tummy touching the ball. Be careful not to overextend or arch your back into a V. Hold for 1 to 2 seconds.
- Slowly and smoothly lower your arms and allow your stomach to bend so that your hands again touch the floor. Your feet should remain against the wall during the whole exercise.
- Repeat 12 to 16 times.

*Tips:* If you can't achieve 10 to 12 smooth extension lifts, make the exercise easier by holding your arms behind your back over your buttocks or along your sides. Lean forward until you are bent over the ball, then extend so that your trunk is straight, again keeping your toes against the wall. Once you've easily reached 16 back extensions, add a 2- or 3-pound weight to each hand. Continue to add weight as needed over time.

If you have back problems, avoid extending your back beyond the straightened neutral position.

## Chest Press

You can choose this exercise, or as you advance, do the chest press on the ball or push-ups. They all work the same muscle groups—your triceps, deltoids, and pectoral muscles.

*Benefits:* This builds your chest muscles and is also good for your triceps and shoulders. For women, the chest press helps to tone up the muscles under the breast, adding firmness, lift, and shape to the breast area. For men, it builds pec muscles that help you look great with or without a shirt on.

*What you'll need:* A bench (or as noted below, you can also perform this on the ball or on the floor) and two free weights that you can lift 12 to 16 times with smooth, even movements.

- Lie on your back on a bench with your knees bent and your feet resting on the end of the bench. Your legs should be bent at an angle of 30 to 45 degrees.
- Press your lower back into the bench, flexing your pelvis.
- Hold the weights next to your chest at breast level with your palms facing toward your knees. Your elbows are pointing down toward the floor.
- Now straighten your arms up into the air so they are perpendicular to your body. Don't let the weights touch at the top of the motion; this keeps your muscles working. Don't lock your elbows. Keep your body and wrists steady and pelvis flexed.
- Raise and lower the weights with smooth motions, counting "one one thousand" up and "two one thousand" down. You should just barely be able to lift the correct weight 12 to 16 times smoothly without jerking your arms or trunk.

## Chest Press on the Ball

You can also perform the chest press on the ball. It forces you to use your whole trunk to balance yourself, making the exercise harder but also much more beneficial.

*Benefits:* This builds your chest muscles, triceps, and shoulders and also works your obliques (or trunk twisters). You'll see the same appearance benefits as the chest press on the bench, along with extra firmness along your waistline.

*What you'll need:* An exercise ball and two free weights (most likely these will be 5 to 10 pounds lighter than the ones you used for the chest press on the bench or floor, because you'll need part of your strength to stabilize your trunk).

- Lie on your back against the ball. Your neck should be supported by the ball as well. Your legs are bent at an angle of 90 degrees with your feet flat on the floor, shoulder width apart. As you gain strength, bring your feet closer together, building additional trunk twister strength and balance.
- Hold the weights next to your chest at breast level with your palms facing toward your knees. Your elbows are pointing down toward the floor.
- Now straighten your arms up into the air so they are perpendicular to your body. Don't let the weights touch at the top of the motion, as they should remain shoulder width apart; this keeps your muscles working. Don't lock your elbows. Keep your body and wrists steady and pelvis flexed.
- Now slowly lower the weight to the start position.
- Repeat with smooth motions, counting "one one thousand" up and "two one thousand" down. You should just barely be able to lift the correct weight 12 to16 times smoothly without jerking your arms or trunk.

### Push-ups

You can perform either this exercise or the chest press.

*Benefits:* This is an excellent exercise to build triceps and pectorals (chest) muscles. It helps create firm and shapely chest, shoulder, and upper arm muscles, similar to the chest press.

*What you'll need:* A smooth, clean floor surface.

- Lie facedown with your palms on the floor, directly below your shoulders. (Beginners can start by doing the push-ups on your knees. As you build strength, you can perform the push-ups with your weight on your toes.)
- Inhale and straighten your arms, keeping your back straight, and pushing your trunk up and away from the floor.
- Now, slowly exhale and lower yourself back down until your chin just touches the floor. Your back remains straight at all times. (If your tummy or chest touches the floor before your chin, despite keeping your back straight, be sure you drop low enough that your elbows are bent to at least 90 degrees in the down position.)
- Continue raising and lowering yourself until you break form. Rest a few seconds, and then perform at least a few more.

### One-Arm Row

This exercise balances the muscles used in the push-ups and chest press exercises.

*Benefits:* Builds upper back and rhomboid muscles. This exercise provides you with a shapely upper back and helps your posture by pulling your shoulders back.

*What you'll need:* One free weight (average starting weight 10 pounds) and a bench or chair.

- Place your right knee on the bench or chair and rest your right hand on the bench in front of your knee.
- Hold the weight in your left hand.
- Lean forward so that your trunk is parallel to the floor and your left arm dangles toward the floor, your palm facing your standing leg.
- Inhale and pull your left elbow as high as you can, pointing toward the ceiling without shifting or rotating your trunk. Keep your arm close to your body.
- Exhale and slowly lower your left arm to the starting position.
- Repeat 12 to 16 times.
- Change sides and repeat, holding the weight in your right hand and placing your left knee and hand on the bench or chair.

## Biceps Curls

*Benefits:* Builds the biceps and the brachioradialis (upper forearm), giving you nice, shapely arms.

*What you'll need:* Two free weights (average starting weight 8 to 10 pounds).

- Stand with your knees slightly flexed and hold a free weight in each hand, your palms facing your legs.
- Keeping your upper arms stable and your elbows at your sides, raise your forearms upward, until your hands nearly reach your shoulders. Your palm rotates as you lift your arm so that it is facing your chest at the end of this motion.
- Lower your hands smoothly to the starting position. Repeat 12 to 16 times.
- Keep your trunk stable during your movements—your pelvis flexed and your abs tight—to protect your lower back.

## Triceps Extensions

This exercise balances the muscles used in the biceps curl.

*Benefits:* Good for building triceps muscles, and helps to create shapely arms.

*What you'll need:* One free weight (average starting weight 10 pounds).

- Hold a dumbbell vertically by one of its knobs with both hands behind your head, making sure your elbows are pointed forward and up.
- Now straighten your arms and extend your hands above your head, keeping your elbows close to your ears. Do not lock your elbows.
- Count "one one thousand" on the up motion, then slowly lower your hands behind your head and count "two one thousand" as you drop the weight to the down position. Repeat 12 to 16 times.

*Tip:* Watch to make sure your head is clear of the dumbbell. Keep your neck aligned with your spine.

## Overhead Press

*Benefits:* This builds your deltoids and trapezius muscles (shoulder and neck muscles) and triceps. It also gives you a shapely neck and shoulders.

*What you'll need:* Two dumbbells (average starting weight 5 to 10 pounds).

- Stand erect with your pelvis flexed. (If you find you are arching your back, perform this lift sitting instead to avoid back strain.) Hold a weight in each hand at shoulder height with your palms facing forward and your elbows out to your sides. To prevent shoulder strain, make sure your elbows don't bend more than 90 degrees.

- Now slowly press the weight up until your arms are nearly straight directly above your shoulders, without locking your elbows. Do not allow the weights to touch.
- Keeping your trunk still, lower the weight slowly.
- Perform 12 to 16 reps.

*Tip:* If you note pain or popping in your shoulder, stop immediately.

### Ball Squats

These are easy to do. As you get stronger you can progress to lunges (see below), which work the same muscle groups but require more strength and balance.

*Benefits:* These are great for shaping and firming your quads (thighs) and gluteal (buttocks) muscles.

*What you'll need:* An exercise ball and an unobstructed wall.

- Stand with your back to the wall, your feet about shoulder width apart.
- Place the exercise ball between the wall and your lower back and upper gluteal muscles.
- Flex your pelvis forward to protect your back throughout the movement.
- Lean back against the ball and walk your feet forward several steps. Walk far enough away so that your knees don't go over your toes when you squat.
- Now bend your knees until they're at an angle of 90 degrees and lower your body so the ball rolls down the wall. If you feel you want an extra push and you don't have a history of knee problems, bend your knees to 120 degrees, but no further.
- Make sure your weight is in your heels as you squat.
- Straighten back up to standing, squeezing your glutes as you stand.

## Lunges

This exercise works your quads (thighs) and glutes (buttocks) and also adds some work for your hamstrings.

*Benefits:* Lunges help build your quads and gluteals. They also enhance your balance. This is an excellent exercise for building shape, tone, and firmness.

*What you'll need:* Two free weights (average starting weight up to 5 pounds).

* Be sure to perform lunges with your pelvis flexed forward. If you extend your back and pelvis, you can irritate your lower back and spine.
* Stand with feet shoulder width apart.
* Holding one weight in each hand (you can also begin without weights), take a big step forward on your right foot, bending your right knee and lowering your left knee toward the floor. Stop when your left knee is just above the floor, and make sure your right knee doesn't extend beyond your toes. Your right knee should be bent at about a 90-degree angle when your left knee is close to the floor. Keep your weight in your front (right) heel. You want to feel a smooth dropping motion.
* Next, push back smoothly to your standing initial position.
* Repeat with your left foot, lunging forward while slowly dropping your right knee.

*Tip:* Once you can perform 20 to 25 lunges with each leg comfortably, add an extra five-pound weight to each hand. Gradually increase the weight so that reaching 15 to 20 lunges with each foot produces some moderate strain.

## Hamstring Bridge

This counterbalances the quad-enhancing exercises above, the squat and the lunge.

*Benefits:* You're working your buttocks and hamstrings to achieve well-toned and shapely thighs.

*What you'll need:* A chair or an exercise ball and an unobstructed floor surface.

- Lie on the floor with your back flat.
- Place your hands on the floor next to your hips.
- Place your heels either on the ball or on a chair.
- Lift your pelvis and buttocks off the floor as high as you can, pushing with the backs of your heels against the ball or chair. Feel the pull in your hamstring as you go up.
- Hold the position for two seconds, then lower your buttocks slowly back toward the floor.
- Lift again without resting your buttocks on the floor, keeping your muscles contracted between repetitions.
- Repeat 12 to 16 times.

## Calf Presses

*Benefits:* This builds your calf muscles and develops nice, shapely calves.

*What you'll need:* Two free weights (average starting weight 10 to 20 pounds).

- Stand erect holding free weights in each hand with your feet pointing forward, shoulder width apart.
- Slowly rise up on your toes, holding for half a second, and then slowly lower back down. Repeat 12 to 15 times.

## Shoulder Rotator Cuff Lifts

*Benefits:* This strengthens the small muscles beneath the larger deltoid muscles of the shoulder, which are critical for maintaining healthy shoulder function. This exercise won't make your shoulders look shapelier, but it will protect them so you can use them into your golden years.

*What you'll need:* Two small free weights (average starting weight 2 to 4 pounds).

- While standing with your pelvis flexed, hold a small weight in each hand with your thumbs pointed directly down toward the floor and your palms resting beside your thighs.
- Slowly lift your arms up in front of you with your hands a little more than shoulder width apart and your thumbs pointing to the floor, until they're shoulder height and parallel to the floor. Don't raise your arms above shoulder height; doing so can pinch tendons inside the shoulder.
- Now slowly lower your arms. Repeat 12 to 15 times.

### Kegel Exercises

Your bonus for a great sex life!

*Benefits:* These exercises are excellent for strengthening the pelvic floor muscles, enhancing sexual function for both men and women. In particular, these exercises can improve bladder control for women, especially after childbirth and through menopause.

*What you'll need:* Nothing!

- The easiest way to learn this exercise is to sit on the toilet, let your urine flow start, and then stop it. The muscles you use to stop the flow are your pelvic floor muscles. Contracting those muscles is called a pelvic lift.
- With time, you can learn to perform pelvic lifts during everyday activities, even when stopped at a red light, or when on hold on the phone. Nobody will notice that you're doing them.
- Perform 10 sets of 10 lifts daily, holding the lift for one second, or one set of 10 superlifts, holding the pelvic lifts for 10 seconds each.

## Stretching

Stretching after exercise decreases your risk for injuries and will improve your overall performance, making workouts more fun. The most common injuries are to the back, and people with tight hamstrings, in particular, run an increased risk for lower back pain and other injuries. So

I'd like to share with you my favorite stretches that increase flexibility from your heel to the back of your head. You can perform these four simple stretches in just a few minutes.

## Hamstring Stretch

- Sit on the floor with your legs extended out in front of you. Slowly lean forward and reach toward one foot at a time, feeling the stretch in your hamstring muscle, which runs from just below the back of your knee to your buttock.
- Hold your toes, one foot at a time, if you are able, and then feel the pull as you take deep breaths in and out. If you can't reach this far yet, just hold your ankle. With each exhale, bend deeper into the stretch, and with each inhale, note an added pull.
- Don't bounce. Maintain a steady stretch for at least ten and preferably twenty seconds.

## Calf Stretch

- Stand facing a wall with your arms extended out in front of you, touching the wall. Your palms lie flat against its surface.
- Now step backward about 1 to 2 feet with one foot, keeping the other foot in place, the knee slightly bent.
- Feel a pull in your calf muscles as you press the heel of your extended leg into the floor. Hold it steady for 10 to 20 seconds.
- Now bring the extended leg back to center and switch, stretching the back of the other leg.
- After completing the calf stretch on both legs, step back with one foot at a time into the same position, but this time keep the leg extended back slightly bent. This will help you feel a different stretch, lower on your calf. Repeat for both legs for 10 to 20 seconds.

## Lower Back Stretch

This stretch can be useful whenever you feel tightness in your lower back.

- Lie on your back.
- With your knees bent, pull your legs toward your chest with your hands behind your knees. Feel a gentle pull in your lower back as you hold this stretch for 20 seconds.

### Hip, Ileo-Tibial (IT) Band, and Lower Back Stretch

The ileo-tibial band is connective tissue extending from the hip to the outside of your knee along the outside of your thigh.

- Lie on your back with your arms out to your sides, perpendicular to your body.
- Pull your knees up and let them fall to one side. You should be able to touch your knees to the floor on your right without lifting your left shoulder off the floor, feeling a stretch along your lateral left hip down to the knee. Feel the stretch for 10 seconds.
- Now roll your knees over to the left, keeping your right shoulder on the floor, feeling the stretch over your lateral right hip down to the other knee. Hold it for 10 seconds. Repeat both sides.

In addition to stretching after exercise, one prolonged stretching session per week does wonders for tight muscles. Consider a 20-to-30 minute stretch session or a weekly yoga class.

## Avoiding Injuries

Injuries are the bane of all exercise programs. As soon as you're hurt, you stop the activity . . . and then you get out of the habit of exercising, lose momentum, and end up back where you started. Definitely unproductive! So the wise thing to do is avoid injuries in the first place. In fact, the reason for the gradual buildup in activities during the three phases of the Ten Years Younger fitness program is to help you sidestep this problem. Here are my recommendations:

- Never start out full blast. Always begin with a warm-up.

- Don't exceed 85 percent of your maximum heart rate. As noted previously, doing so increases your risk of accelerated aging.
- Cross-training during the week helps prevent injuries associated with overuse. By working on different aerobic exercise machines, or by alternating swimming, bicycling, walking, and running, you can decrease your risk of injury.
- Wear good-quality exercise shoes. If you are flat-footed (have fallen arches or pronate in excess), get rigid arch supports for your shoes. You can obtain custom-made orthotics from an orthopedist or standard ones from medical supply or sports shops.
- When it comes to strength training, if you're quite deconditioned, even doing 10 reps with 5-pound weights may be a challenge. Start slow if you have to—either with 3-pound weights, or by simply doing 6 or 8 reps until you feel more confident.
- Most strength-training injuries occur when using weight machines. If you're using machines, make sure the settings are correct for your size. (A trainer can help you set them up properly.) Lifting free weights, though it requires more skill, is much more functional and safer. It's also less likely to hurt you.
- If you have knee problems, don't squat more than 90 degrees, especially when carrying heavy objects.
- If you've never done strength training before, or if you have a history of injuries, consider working with a trainer to get started. But you don't need to do this every workout; that can become quite costly. Meeting once weekly, even if only for the first month, can ensure that your technique is safe and effective. It is also a good way to guarantee that you are pushing yourself hard enough to keep improving but not so hard that you hurt yourself.

When used in conjunction with the Ten Years Younger Diet, these exercises and safety precautions will not only help you look better, feel stronger, and walk sexier, but you'll be much healthier over the long haul. And that's the surest way to fight encroaching Aging Accelerators and both look and feel ten years younger.

# CHAPTER 7

# The Relaxation Routine

When Jennifer first came to see me, she was at the end of her wits. At 43, she was juggling being the mother of two lovely children, ages 9 and 11, with a busy real estate business in Clearwater, Florida. She was fed up with her husband, who was never home. For more than a decade she'd been the primary parent in charge of homework, dinners, running the household, and shopping. If the toilet overflowed, it was her job to fix it.

Despite a relatively healthy diet and trips to the gym several times a week, Jennifer was frustrated by her rising weight and, in particular, her expanding waistline. She could no longer fit into her favorite outfits, including the smartly tailored suits she wore to work. She was beginning to feel depressed and angry and found herself snacking on ice cream and cookies as consolation. In the last year alone, she had begun to look older than she really was.

What's more, as exhausted as she was, Jennifer slept only six hours a night. She drank too much coffee during the day and too much alcohol at night. She'd started skipping her workouts at the gym, and the increasing strain within her marriage had put a halt to any sort of romance or sex life.

"I'm stressed out of my mind," she admitted to me, "and I know it's impinging on everything. But I just can't figure out how to take back control."

From listening to Jennifer's story, it seemed to me that stress-related anxiety and depression were likely at the root of many of her problems. I knew that in order to overcome these issues, she needed to find a way to restore some peace and balance in her life. So I started off her treatment by sharing my Relaxation Routine—a simple, easy way to reduce high stress levels and all the negative side effects that will accelerate the aging process.

Jennifer went back to the gym and began working out every day. She cut back on caffeine and wine and practiced meditation for twenty minutes a day. She also made the commitment to me that she would sleep seven hours a night for a month. These steps helped her find the first inklings of peace and calm she'd felt in years. And these personal changes rippled out into other areas of her life.

Once in a better frame of mind, she sought counseling with her husband, and he became involved in the family again, which brought romance and intimacy back into their lives. The next time I saw Jennifer, she felt immensely better—and she looked better too!

As I explained in Chapter 1, stress is a potent Aging Accelerator. It increases oxidative stress by boosting your levels of cortisol and adrenaline and promoting weight gain (thereby irritating your arteries and triggering plaque formation), keeping your pulse and blood pressure high, and heightening your risk of stroke and heart attack. High levels of cortisol and adrenaline erode your bones and muscles, injure your brain cells, and cause insulin resistance, emotional fatigue, and depression. Too much long-term stress also disables your white blood cells, depleting your immune system and limiting your ability to fight intruding microbes and emerging cancer cells.

Not only is excessive stress physically harmful, it is also self-reinforcing. If you're stressed like Jennifer, you may not eat or sleep well. Often a downward spiral kicks in: The more stressed you feel, the less you exercise and the worse you eat. But the more weight you put on, the more stressed you become. Quickly your appearance, health, and lifestyle all spiral downward.

Your goal should be to reverse the downward spiral. If you commit to eating, sleeping, and exercising better, you'll begin to feel better, too. As your stress levels drop, it will become easier to continue to eat and sleep well and work out regularly. Your cortisol and adrenaline levels will drop, slowing the aging process. The Relaxation Routine outlined in this chapter will help you minimize the negative effects of stress in your own life.

On any given day, most of us have certain tasks or challenges that have the potential to cause us stress and worry, and when we think through our day in advance, we often see these challenges on the horizon. I like to envision my day as if I were sailing: I know that parts of the trip will be calm and fun, but I also know that rounding a particular rocky point will be difficult. The water will be choppy, the boat will pitch from side to side, and if I'm not careful, I might easily fret over this upcoming encounter all day, missing the more enjoyable parts of the sail.

However, I do have choices as to how I'll handle this patch of rough water. One option is to sail far around the coast, taking lots of extra time but avoiding the dangerous currents and waves. Another is to prepare the cabin below, batten down the hatches, and forge ahead with speed and determination. And both options call for planning—the worst strategy of all would be to get caught unprepared and be bashed against the rocky shore.

Dealing with stressful situations in your day isn't much different. You can't always predict the encounters you'll face, but you do get to choose how to deal with them and the stress they generate. Finding dedicated moments of peace and calm during the day is much like discovering a protected harbor when at sea.

Your goal on the Ten Years Younger Program is to find at least ten to thirty minutes of inner peace every day—time when you feel tranquil, loved, and relaxed. In truth, creating peace and calm requires more organization than it does time. The challenge—or perhaps the fun—is finding activities that suit you and making the time to do them. These precious moments should help you feel refreshed, and your mind should function with greater ease and clarity.

How you spend your time is up to you; there's no single right way to go about it. Deep breathing, yoga, and various forms of massage are effective relaxation techniques. One person might opt for quiet meditation or a long soak in a hot bathtub by the light of a fragrant candle. Another might choose to do a crossword puzzle or read a bedtime story to a child. A third might enjoy curling up with a great novel. You might simply enjoy playing gentle music or watching a sunset or gardening—anything that lets you take the time to appreciate the beauty in each day. Sometimes making time for peace and calm in your life requires the support of the critical people in your life. Involve loved ones in your relaxation goals. Their participation will not only provide support but also ensure that you really do take the time to recharge your batteries each day.

So, how can you plan for thirty minutes of soul-calming activity every day? There are many different ways to bring relief to both body and mind, but there are a few specific techniques that I prescribe to all my patients.

## Sleep: The Ultimate Relaxation

Sleep is incredibly important to looking and feeling ten years younger. You need rest to start fresh each day, but for many, a good night's sleep is elusive. Our worries over our jobs, bills, families, and relationships conspire to make us suffer from lack of and/or poor-quality sleep. But without adequate sleep your brain will act like a computer with too many programs open—sluggish and occasionally stalled. Shut down the computer, restart, and it runs quicker.

If you're feeling like your memory or recall abilities just aren't what they used to be, more sleep should be at the top of your agenda. Sleep actually increases melatonin and human growth hormone levels—both essential for brain function and health—while exhaustion increases cortisol levels, which, as I noted previously, results in damage to the hippocampus, the memory center of the brain. The bottom line is that most people need at least seven to eight hours of sleep a night to function optimally, and anything less than seven hours is inadequate for most people's best mental performance. So how can you make sleep your anti-aging ally? Here are a few rules:

- *Minimize or stop using stimulants.* It takes about seven hours for your body to eliminate half the caffeine in one cup of coffee. Drink four cups in the morning starting at 8 A.M., and by midnight you'll still have the caffeine equivalent of more than one cup of coffee floating through your bloodstream. If you are stressed, that stimulation may keep you from falling asleep. If you are exhausted, you might fall asleep, but once the exhaustion disappears, the slightest noise might wake you, and you won't get back to sleep. The caffeine impacts the quality of your sleep as well, limiting the deep sleep that is the most restorative.

- *Avoid alcohol before bedtime, since it, too, interferes with sleep.* It takes an hour to eliminate one serving and another hour before your blood sugar and metabolism return to a steady state. Have two drinks between 9 and 10 P.M., and four hours later you may startle awake as your blood sugar levels take a dive. If you enjoy a glass of wine with dinner, drink it at least two hours before going to bed.

- *Shun refined, processed carbs, such as ice cream, candies, and other sweets, at bedtime, because they create a cascade of hormonal reactions that will keep you awake.* After you eat sweets, your blood sugar level quickly rises, and a couple of hours later the resulting surge in insulin will cause your blood sugar level to dive just as precipitously, resulting in an arousal response. Indeed, your rapidly dropping blood sugar creates a spike in stress hormones (like adrenaline) and appetite, in an effort to protect your ever-active brain from the risk of dangerous low blood sugar levels.

- *Daily exercise improves your ability to fall and stay asleep.* But avoid working out within two hours of bedtime, as it increases your metabolism, raises your body temperature, and inhibits deep sleep.

- *Establish a good sleep routine.* Go to bed and wake up at about the same time (within thirty minutes) every day.

- *Identify a temperature that allows you to sleep comfortably.* You'll sleep better in a cooler room.

- *Avoid using sleeping pills with regularity.* Not only can they become habit-forming, but they disrupt normal sleep architecture and make it harder and harder to find a good night's sleep without sedation.

- *Talk to your medical provider about valerian.* This herbal remedy is derived from the common valerian plant, which grows in gardens across America. At least in the short term, studies have shown that 300 to 600 mg of valerian extract in pill form at bedtime can improve the quality and duration of sleep. But it isn't intended for long-term use.
- *Don't work in your bedroom.* Save it for sleep and romance.
- *If you can't sleep, don't fight it.* Don't yell at the clock. Don't be mad at yourself. Just get up, go to another room, and read until you feel sleepy. Then go back to bed.

## Exercise: Burn Away the Stress

Thirty minutes of aerobic exercise doesn't just burn away calories, it also helps melt away feelings of stress. After a decent workout, your muscles feel looser, you're calmer, and problems that seemed overwhelming may appear more manageable.

Daily exercise is also incredibly important in managing depression. Aerobic exercise releases endorphins, powerful brain chemicals that help with relaxation and pain control. Part of the buzz you'll feel after a workout comes from a natural endorphin high. The Age-Busting Fitness regimen in Chapter 6 will make a big difference in managing your stress.

## Limit Caffeine and Alcohol

If you're tired and stressed, it seems natural to turn to caffeine to pull you through the day. The problem with this strategy, however, is that while you do feel more awake, the caffeinated drink will also make you feel more wired and anxious. Excessive caffeine actually worsens your stress.

Aim to limit caffeine-containing beverages to no more than three servings a day. While a cup of coffee or maybe two is tolerable, more won't help you deal with the real problem. Consider a cup of green tea in the afternoon instead. Compounds in green tea heighten your alertness without caffeine and without that over-stimulated feeling.

If you drink too much caffeine during the day, you may feel you need alcohol to calm you in the evening. Not only is alcohol a depressant, it also disrupts your sleep (see above). An important step in managing excessive stress is to limit your daily intake to one serving each of caffeine and alcohol.

## Massage

Massage is a terrific way to loosen muscles and decrease tension, so you'll be enjoying a massage every two to four weeks while on the Ten Years Younger Program. Massage is also commonly believed to have detoxifying benefits—helping to release toxins from tissues by pushing chemicals from your lymphatic tissues and muscles into the bloodstream (though there is a lack of medical research to support this belief). Nonetheless, I recommend drinking at least one to two glasses of water immediately after a massage to help flush out any toxins that might have been released. If nothing else, massage feels great, and it's a great way to relieve the tension, aches, and pains that come with a stressful, busy life.

## Meditation: The Most Effective Stress Reliever

If you're able and willing, meditation is a tremendously effective way to reduce stress. It also lowers your blood pressure, decreases your heart rate, relaxes your muscles, and is effective for calming chronic pain. It provides rest and restores energy. In fact, for some, twenty to thirty minutes of focused meditation or deep prayer provides as much restoring rest as several hours of sleep. I feel terrific after I meditate. I'm calmer, I think more clearly, and I get more done after I've had a chance to clear my mind.

Meditation is not simply relaxation, however. It requires you to focus on your body and the moment, on letting go of your thoughts, and on paying attention to your breath. It teaches you to become present in the now.

You can discover how to meditate in a class or by yourself. Many meditation tapes are available in bookstores, natural food stores, and houses of worship. Try to listen to the first few minutes of the tape in the store before you buy it to make sure that the voice and setting will be soothing (if you hate the beach, for example, the sound of waves and seagulls on some of these tapes may not be all that comforting). You can now even find alarm clocks that play meditation music for 15 to 30 minutes once you get into bed.

## Share Love and Intimacy

Unlike muscle mass and fitness levels, there is no easy, objective measure for intimacy. But loving relationships are critical to a long and healthy life. In fact, intimacy plays an important role in your survival. In the Harvard Study of Adult Development, having a stable marriage and an adaptive coping style were two of the six most important predictors of aging well.

To be loved, you must love. Loving is an act of the will—to share kindness, consideration, and compassion. You don't have to "be in love" to share love. You can still act toward others with kindness, consideration, and compassion even if you're not intimately involved with them. Intimacy, by nature, requires companionship. Even a pet will do. We humans are social animals. Touch, for instance, is an essential need.

Keep in mind, however, that romance and sex are not the same thing. Romance soothes the soul rather than the body, and romantic acts linger and nourish us emotionally for days and sometimes weeks thereafter. In contrast, sex provides satisfaction, but only for a quick release—more like a photo flash than a soothing glow. A mixture of sex and romance can be terrific, but romance by itself can be more fulfilling in the long term.

## Choosing a Positive Attitude

When you start your day, you have a great deal of control over your attitude. You can be cheerful or glum. You can share a smile or a frown.

You also choose with whom you spend time during your day. If you're feeling down in the dumps or stressed, limit how much time you spend with irritable or bitter people—their state of mind can be contagious and will only reinforce your negative feelings. Instead, seek out those who are enjoying their lives. And avoid watching the news or reading the paper if they're packed with tension and distress. Read the comics, watch a comedy, or partake in activities that lighten your spirit.

## Outside Support and Counseling

Counseling isn't limited to people who suffer from more severe emotional and psychological problems. It can be very useful if you're having a hard time getting a handle on your stress. Counseling provides important insight into why we act, think, and feel the way we do, and this can help you through the rough spots. So don't be afraid to reach out for extra help if you need it. Once you know what the obstacles are—and sometimes it's easier to identify them with the help of an objective observer—you will be able to manage better.

The Relaxation Routine doesn't mean you can't or shouldn't have some stress in your life. In fact, I enjoy certain stressors because their challenges give me purpose. The key is managing the stress so that you can still find peace and happiness every day. Long-term stress management will also help you follow your Age-Busting Fitness plan and the Ten Years Younger Diet and remain focused on your own optimal health. In the next chapter, we'll learn how to manage another kind of stressor: toxins.

# CHAPTER 8

# Detoxification

I didn't pay much attention to the idea of detoxification during my first years as a physician. My office was packed with activity, and I spent the bulk of my time immunizing children, performing physicals and women's health exams, treating infections, and refilling medications for chronic diseases, in particular diabetes, arthritis, and high blood pressure.

But as my interest in nutrition, fitness, and aging grew, so did my frustration with health care's powerlessness to reverse many chronic illnesses, and I turned my attention to environmental toxins and the role they play in aging and disease. I found that in some cases, taking in too much toxic material (pesticides, alcohol, and cigarettes) seemed to play a substantial role in patients' chronic health problems. In other cases, patients' inability to neutralize the toxins they encountered seemed to be making them old before their time.

Toxins increase oxidative stress and free radical production, and over the years I have found that poor detoxification can speed aging and cause a drop in vitality. The brain, spinal cord, and nerves are especially sensitive to toxins, which can build up in these areas. Abnormal detoxification can also damage the mitochondria—those tiny energy power plants within each cell—as well as weaken your immune system, causing a system imbalance that can lead to excessive inflammation and tissue injury. This imbalance may also leave you open to more frequent infections and an increased cancer risk. Not surprisingly, since toxins increase inflammation and tax your overall energy production, the most common symptoms associated with poor detoxification are persistent body aches and fatigue. That's why detoxifying your system and avoiding toxins altogether are important parts of the Ten Years Younger Program.

## What Are Toxins?

Free radicals, heavy metals (such as mercury, lead, and cadmium), industrial chemicals, pesticides, drugs, and various other pollutants can accumulate in your body and cause disease. All of us have been exposed to an increasing number of toxic compounds through the air we breathe, the water we drink, and the food we eat. The EPA estimates that over 2 billion pounds of toxic chemicals are released into the environment in the United States yearly. Up to 25 percent of the U.S. population has suffered some degree of heavy metal poisoning.

Foreign chemicals can enter your body through your skin and lungs, but they enter primarily through the intestinal tract. Spread out your intestines, smoothing all the folds, and they would cover about one football field. The walls of this enormous organ allow nutrients, both large and small, to pass into your bloodstream. With all that is being absorbed into the body, it is extremely difficult to keep out toxins, although some are filtered out in this way.

In addition to these external sources of pollution, you also generate your own toxins as you metabolize a vast array of compounds, including hormones and the free radicals you make through energy production. These must be detoxified and removed from circulation. If poorly metabolized, for instance, estrogen can be converted into forms that increase your risk of breast cancer. Fortunately, you can change how you detoxify and metabolize estrogen by eating more soy, cruciferous vegetables, turmeric, and garlic. These simple additions to your diet can improve the type of estrogen metabolite your body produces.

# What Is Detoxification?

In order to stay healthy, your body must convert toxins into products you can safely eliminate. You rid yourself of these agents through the natural process called detoxification, which usually occurs in two steps: Toxic compounds in the bloodstream are converted into other compounds that can then be flushed out in the urine and feces. The first step is tricky, as it may actually render the original compound even more toxic than it was to begin with. But this chemical activity prepares the toxins for step 2 elimination. If the transformation is quick (in tiny fractions of a second), step 2 completes the process and safely converts the former toxin into a stable, nontoxic compound ready for excretion. Since detoxification removes toxins and wastes from your body, it slows biological aging and decreases your cancer risk.

However, some lifestyle factors can increase the step 1 reaction without boosting step 2. This is dangerous because step 1 products can be harmful. For instance, chemicals produced in charbroiling or barbecuing meats (*polycyclic hydrocarbons*) speed the production of free radicals in step 1. When meat juices drip onto an open flame, the heat transforms the protein into polycyclic hydrocarbons. As these modified hydrocarbons splatter back onto the meat, they create the crunchy texture that makes barbecued meats so popular. Unfortunately, this texture is very rich in heterocyclic amines (other potential carcinogens), which also increase your cancer risk.

Thus, by eating barbecued meat, you are flooding your system with cancer-causing compounds. And because these compounds also accelerate step 1 detoxification, you are increasing the production of other toxic compounds without speeding their removal. Worse, you could drink an excessive amount of alcohol or take antacid medications such as cimetidine along with the barbecued meat, which would slow the step 2 elimination process and give the toxins produced in step 1 even more time to damage your cells and organs before they are converted into stable compounds.

Alcohol in excess plays havoc with detoxification, as it acts like a VIP, demanding that your liver detoxify it first. This puts other toxins on a waiting list to be removed from your system. As they remain in your body longer, they have more time to cause damage. This is yet another reason why I recommend you limit your alcohol intake to preferably one and not more than two servings daily.

Fortunately, you can also choose to eat foods that improve step 2 detoxification, enhancing the elimination of cancer-causing compounds from your system. These include cruciferous vegetables (cabbage, bok choy, broccoli, kale, cauliflower, and Brussels sprouts), turmeric (often found in curry powder), garlic, rosemary, and soy products, all part of the Ten Years Younger Diet.

Surprisingly, grapefruit also impacts detoxification. It's rich in a chemical compound called naringenin, a blocker of certain metabolic pathways. A single glass of grapefruit juice can decrease metabolism of particular drugs like statin medications (cholesterol-reducing drugs) by up to 30 percent. Because of this property, I usually recommend that people taking statins avoid drinking grapefruit juice. But since it usually takes about two grapefruits to make a glass of juice, eating half a grapefruit every other day would have only a minimal impact. If, however, you were already taking the maximum dosage of a statin and your liver function tests were borderline or you were on other medications that might impact drug metabolism, I would avoid grapefruit altogether.

## The Leaky Gut Syndrome

While your liver performs most of the detoxification that goes on in your body (that's one of its primary roles, after all), it depends on your intestinal tract to prevent too many toxins from leaking into your blood supply in the first place. But if you have what's known as a leaky gut, your intestine will allow large, undigested molecules to pass into your bloodstream. This is a big load for your liver to handle and may overwhelm its ability to detoxify all these compounds.

There are many causes of a leaky gut. One is the use of anti-inflammatory medications that can put holes in your intestinal tract. Even the newer (COX-2 inhibitor) anti-inflammatory drugs, such as Celebrex, Mobic, and Bextra, can still cause significant intestinal leaking. These newer agents cause 40 percent less bleeding than ibuprofen, naprosyn, and the other older anti-inflammatory medications, but that doesn't mean they're free of adverse effects, as we know from recent research showing a very rare but real link with heart attacks.

Food allergies increase both oxidative stress and inflammation to a significant degree. They can also cause marked irritation to your intestinal tract, injuring your intestines' protective lining, accelerating a leaky gut, and thus allowing large loads of material to float freely from your intestinal tract into your bloodstream. The most common causes of food allergies are dairy products and gluten (commonly found in wheat, oats, rye, and barley). Although serious food allergies in people who are completely healthy seem fairly rare, in those individuals with intestinal complaints and unexplained health problems, food intolerances are quite common. More and more people seem to suffer from vague, poorly defined problems related to fatigue, aches and pains, and intestinal ills—all of which can be exacerbated by food allergies and food intolerances. If you have these types of concerns, always start with a visit to your medical provider. But if your symptoms persist, I strongly recommend at least a trial of a dairy- and gluten-free diet for three weeks to see if your symptoms resolve.

Another frequent cause of a leaky gut is an unhealthy balance of bacteria. Your intestinal tract contains more bacteria than there are cells in your body—over 400 species! The term "intestinal ecology" refers to the balance among the cells lining the intestinal tract, the microbes growing there, and immune cell activity. The first step to ensure a healthy balance is to eat at least 30 grams of fiber daily, which is a cornerstone of the Ten Years Younger Diet Plan. Without healthy fiber, good bacteria dwindle in numbers and bad bacteria flourish. Abnormal intestinal bacteria increase inflammation, irritating and injuring the intestinal wall, and leading to a leaky gut. They can even trigger systemwide autoimmune diseases such as inflammatory bowel disease.

Restoring normal intestinal ecology, therefore, can decrease inflammation and a leaky gut and strengthen normal detoxification. This means encouraging the presence of healthy intestinal bacteria (in particular, species of bifidobacteria and lactobacilli). You can take probiotic supplements containing billions of bifidobacteria and lactobacilli, but it may take several months for your system to become balanced. Eating more healthy fiber, as provided in the Ten Years Younger Diet, is the easiest and best way to maintain healthy intestinal ecology, as fiber provides the nourishment for healthy bacteria to thrive. Regularly eating yogurt with live cultures is another way to enhance intestinal ecology.

Antibiotics can also wreak havoc on intestinal ecology. They fight bacteria that can cause infections, but they also kill the good bacteria in the process. A typical course on antibiotics can decimate millions of healthy bacteria in your digestive tract. Far too often physicians will write a prescription for antibiotics not because they think their patients need them but because they believe their patients want them. Always be clear with your doctor that you will take a course of antibiotics, but only if obviously indicated, such as when you have bacterial pneumonia. Also, consider using probiotic supplements (such as live-culture yogurt or bifidobacteria and lactobacilli pills) to restore healthy bacterial numbers after the antibiotic treatment is completed. Maintaining a healthy intestinal ecology will minimize intestinal gut leaking and maximize your body's ability to detoxify.

Finally, optimal liver function is essential for normal detoxification. Too much alcohol can impair your liver and increase intestinal permeability, worsening detoxification overall. When your liver can't metabolize toxins, they're absorbed by other tissues, in particular fat. Since your brain and nervous tissue are rich in fat, toxins commonly accumulate in the nervous system, accounting for the increased rate of Parkinson's and Alzheimer's disease that we see with chronic toxin exposure. Furthermore, toxins that accumulate in body fat can be released back into the body further down the line. Unfortunately, fat releases toxins most often during times of severe stress, compounding the strain your system is under.

## Detox Testing

People who are at high risk for toxicity problems include those who have a:

- Family history of Parkinson's disease or Alzheimer's disease
- Strong family history of cancer

- High sensitivity to odors (perfumes, other fragrances)
- History of fibromyalgia with other signs of chronic inflammation
- High sensitivity or paradoxical responses to medications
- High exposure to chemicals or pesticides in the workplace

If you find yourself on this list, you may want to seek out specialized testing. Women with a strong family history of breast cancer may discover with testing that they produce the more dangerous metabolite of estrogen, increasing their risk. The dietary recommendations I made above can be helpful in reducing that danger. Many medical providers work with laboratories that can assess and measure specific aspects of detoxification.

## How You Can Enhance Your Own Detox Process

There are a variety of things you can do to maximize your body's ability to rid itself of toxins as well as decrease your contact with them.

- *Limit your exposure.* Do all you can to purify your environment. Avoid harmful chemicals, such as pesticides, solvents, and harsh cleansers (spray-on oven cleaners, lye, bleach). At the very least, wear protective clothing such as gloves, a face mask, and goggles when you come in contact with these chemicals and other toxic materials, and ensure adequate ventilation whenever recommended.
- *Avoid all tobacco products and even passive, secondhand smoke.* Only thirty minutes of passive exposure to tobacco smoke a week causes documented harm and increases your risk of a heart attack by 20 percent.
- *Drink plenty of purified water.* Adequate hydration flushes toxins out of your body. I've installed reverse osmosis systems (tap water is pumped through a membrane to remove even the smallest chemical compounds and improve the taste) in my home to ensure clean drinking water. Distilled water is even better, but it comes at an added cost. Simple filters (like the one on your refrigerator) may

improve flavor, but they may be inadequate to remove tiny chemicals from your drinking water.

- *Buy organically produced food whenever possible.* It isn't realistic to buy 100 percent organic, but the more you buy, the better for you and the environment.

- *Always rinse produce in the sink to minimize pesticides.* Studies have shown that submerging fruits and vegetables in water with a few drops of dishwashing soap can remove nearly 90 percent of pesticide residues; just be sure to rinse off the soap, too. Waxed fruit, such as apples and cucumbers, doesn't respond to rinsing, so it is best to either buy organic or unwaxed choices or peel nonorganic waxed fruit—of course, most of the powerful anti-aging nutrients are in the peel.

- *When grilling meat, poultry, and fish, to minimize the formation of carcinogens don't exceed 400° F.* Marinating with vinegar, lemon juice, or other acidic solutions and vinaigrettes markedly reduces carcinogen production.

- *Eat an abundance of fiber to enhance your intestinal ecology.* A healthy intestinal tract fed fiber will leak fewer toxins. In the same regard, avoid antibiotics and anti-inflammatory medications when possible to maintain a healthy intestinal ecology and to minimize a leaky gut.

- *Don't microwave with plastic plates or wrap.* When heated, plastic can release many harmful chemicals. Use glass or ceramic plates when microwaving and cover your food with waxed paper or a paper towel.

- *Avoid all processed sandwich meats.* They contain many chemicals, including nitrites.

- *Avoid excessive alcohol intake.* It decreases your liver's ability to remove toxic compounds.

- *Eat foods that improve detoxification.* Enjoy a cup of cruciferous vegetables daily. Enjoy garlic, rosemary, and turmeric on foods frequently. Aim to eat 1 to 2 servings of soy daily.

- *Maintain a healthy weight.* Excess body fat will store extra toxins.

- *If you have allergy problems, consider allergy testing.* If indicated, pull up carpeting from bedrooms and preferably the entire home. Consider using a HEPA filter to remove allergens and pollens from the air. If you have dust mite allergies, be sure to use special pillow and mattress covers and remove the carpeting in your home in favor of wood or ceramic flooring—starting with your bedroom.
- *Be careful with dry cleaning.* It can leave solvent residues. Talk to your dry cleaner about your options in limiting your chemical exposure. Consider leaving your newly cleaned clothing in the garage for a day to ventilate before placing it in your closet or on your body.
- *Enjoy plants in your home and work area.* Spider plants and philo-dendrons are especially helpful in removing airborne toxins.
- *Limit your exposure to paint, solvents, lacquers, nail polish, and nail polish removers.* Either ensure adequate ventilation or wear a breathing mask.
- *Practice organic gardening.* If you do use pesticides, always cover your skin with gloves, long-sleeved shirts, and pants. Wear goggles and use a mask. Don't spray pesticides on a windy day.
- *Limit your mercury exposure.* Mercury and other heavy metals are especially harmful to brain cells. Restrict your intake of large-mouth fish such as grouper, tuna, and bass to only a few servings a month. Eat swordfish and shark only very rarely, if at all. (See Chapter 5.)
- *View the simple sugars in the American diet as toxins and avoid them.* Corn syrup and table sugar (sucrose) are terrible for your metabolism. Sweetened beverages are the worst of the worst.
- *Avoid trans fats.* While common in french fries, cookies, and chips, trans fats increase your risk of heart attack, strokes, diabetes, and cancer. Read labels to ensure you aren't ingesting these nasty hydrogenated fats. (See Chapter 5.)
- *Limit holding a cell phone to your head, as there are concerns about electromagnetic radiation exposure.* It's much better (and safer, especially when driving) to use a headset.

- *Supplements can improve detoxification.* For details, visit my Web site, www.tenyearsyounger.net.

Just remember this: You can eat well, exercise daily, and manage your stress, but if you don't put a limit on toxins, you will still accelerate aging. Including these simple steps to enhance detoxification will ensure that you enjoy optimal health for decades to come.

# CHAPTER 9

# Skin Rejuvenation

n the United States alone, people spend billions of dollars annually in the pursuit of younger-looking skin. Some of the products on the market are helpful, some are pointless, and others may actually be harmful. What you need is no-nonsense information about the best ways to protect and enhance the texture of your skin. The following six easy steps to Ten Years Younger skin can, over the course of the ten-week program, make your skin appear shinier, healthier, less wrinkled, and more radiant. Now, isn't that exactly what you're after?

## Step 1: Stop Sunlight From Aging Your Skin

Tanned skin is a sign of damage, not health. Both sunburns and suntans deplete the antioxidants in your skin. They also diminish your body's total antioxidant reserve, potentially speeding the aging process. Avoiding sun damage is more than a cosmetic issue; it is important for your overall health.

That having been said, you should know that up to 80 percent of facial skin aging is attributable to sun exposure. But if you want to have skin that's younger, softer, creamier, and less wrinkled, then you must start protecting it. I recommend that you apply a sunscreen every morning. Start your day by gently washing your face and applying a moisturizing cream containing sunscreen. This is the most important thing you can do to keep your skin looking younger and staying healthier. You should also wear a hat when you're outside for extended periods of time, even if cloud cover seems to be blocking the sun. The sun can damage your skin on overcast days too. This is especially true in the tropics, in northern latitudes during summer months, and at higher elevations.

Sunlight contains two types of ultraviolet rays that impact your skin. UVB are the burning rays that cause sunburn to the epidermis—your skin's outermost layer—turning your skin hot and red. Not only do these rays accelerate skin aging, but they can also cause skin cancer by damaging your skin cells' DNA.

UVA rays don't cause sunburn, but they do age the deeper dermis layers (beneath the epidermis) of your skin. In particular, UVA rays damage collagen. Collagen is one of the strongest protein fibers in your body, and it provides the scaffolding that supports skin shape and structure. Without collagen, your skin would sag and wrinkle. Many sunscreens are rated to provide only UVB protection; without UVA protection as well, you may not burn, but you will be inflicting damage to the deeper skin layers. Therefore, you should be sure to choose a sunscreen brand that combines agents that block both UVA and UVB rays. Since the goal isn't just to avoid burning but to avoid damaging your skin (and preventing those ugly sun spots from developing in the future), an SPF of 25 is likely the minimum you'll need to receive full skin protection.

For information on specific skin product lines that follow my recommendations in this chapter, visit my Web site at www.tenyearsyounger.net.

## Step 2: Increase Your Antioxidants

It's not only what you put *on* your skin that's important; what goes into your mouth makes a big difference too. Antioxidants in the form of plant pigments not only decrease bodywide aging but also have great potential to slow the aging of the skin. As we saw in Chapter 5, the orange-red pigment called lycopene, found in tomatoes and tomato paste, actually slows burning by blocking the free radical damage to your skin that occurs with sun exposure. In contrast, people who smoke and inhale thousands of oxidants rapidly deplete their antioxidant system and thus have skin that is far more wrinkled. Following the antioxidant-rich Ten Years Younger Diet is the best way to enhance your skin. The Sweet Sixteen Vitality Foods, including 5 cups daily of colorful fruits and vegetables, deliver great results. Green tea also contains antioxidants that are potentially good for your skin.

You can apply antioxidants directly to your skin as well. Vitamins C and E, alpha lipoic acid, the supplement coenzyme $Q_{10}$, ferulic acid, and green tea are potent topical antioxidants that have the potential to slow skin aging. None of these agents has actually been shown to reverse existing deep wrinkles, but all have the potential to put the brakes on skin damage and wrinkle formation, and they are unlikely to do any harm except to your pocketbook. However, researchers are still working on enhancing penetration of these topical creams into skin cells. If they don't penetrate, they won't work!

## Step 3: Hydrate Your Skin

The outer layer of the skin should contain about 10 percent water, but as your skin dehydrates, it becomes rough, itchy, and cracked. And as you probably know, dry skin looks old and saggy. The most important step in moisturizing is making sure your skin holds on to water. You get this from using the proper moisturizers.

Moisturizers can help the outer skin layers retain fluid. They come in two forms: agents that block moisture loss from the skin into the air and agents that add moisture to the skin. The best products combine both. Some people put moisturizers only on their face, leaving the rest of their skin dry and flaky. Don't limit moisturizers to your face alone; skin all over your body benefits from and appreciates getting hydrated!

I recommend lotions with lanolin, propylene glycol, and paraffin. You'll see these listed in many moisturizing products. Lanolin comes from sheep skin secretions, and it hydrates and softens the skin nicely.

However, some people can develop allergic reactions to it. You can be
allergic to propylene glycol too, so pay attention to how your skin
responds to these agents.

The best hydrating agents are glycerin, propylene glycol, urea, and
alpha hydroxy acids. You'll find these in many moisturizing products.

In contrast, excessive use of soaps and detergents depletes the water
content of your skin. The more you bathe and the more soap you use,
the drier your skin becomes. If you follow the TV commercials trying to
sell you body soap, you'll create mountains of lather when you shower.
This is unwarranted. You only need enough soap to wash areas that
require cleaning: your hands, armpits, groin, feet, and face. Unless your
arms, legs, or torso are dirty, sweat should rinse away from these areas
in the shower without soap. Use a nonfoaming cleanser that has less
detergent and is less drying. As for the soap itself, I prefer unscented
varieties, especially for the face and hands, since they're less drying and
irritating.

Finally, your skin will also become dry with forced-air heating and
air-conditioning, as these climate-control devices decrease the humidity
in the air. When the humidity drops below 30 percent, it might be worth-
while to invest in a humidifier, especially if you suffer from dry skin. But
be careful. Humidity greater than 40 percent can promote the growth of
mildew, mold, and dust mites. Aim for a humidity level between 30 and
40 percent in your home and office to enhance your skin's moisture without increasing your exposure to allergens.

## Step 4: Add Vitamin A

Vitamin A (also known as retinol or retinoids) skin creams have been
used for years to improve skin appearance. If you apply vitamin A to
your skin over the long term, it will be shinier, less wrinkled, and pinker,
and it will show less irregular discoloration. The best news is that not
only do these products make your skin look younger, they make it
healthier and reduce your risk of skin cancer, too.

Retinol-containing products provide many benefits to your skin.

Teenagers know that they improve acne. And they boost skin cycle turnover, removing old cells and increasing the number and percentage of new skin cells in the epidermis layer for a fresher look. Finally, they improve collagen production, especially in sun-damaged skin. They also prevent collagen breakdown.

The most common side effects of retinol products are redness, irritation, and peeling. You can minimize this problem most of the time by selecting lower-strength products or using them less often. In fact, when first starting on a retinol regimen, you'll have fewer side effects if you use it only two or three nights a week and apply it to dry (not wet) skin. If your skin turns red, make sure you aren't using other products, such as hydroxy acid creams or vitamin C, that might be irritating. Over several weeks, your skin will tolerate the retinol better, and you can gradually increase the dosage. With time, you may be able to use these other skin treatment products along with the retinol.

Most people can tolerate Renova (by prescription only) fairly well, but it can cause some temporary peeling and irritation. It was the first agent approved to reverse sun damage and is clearly more effective than the over-the-counter retinol products. Newer versions of retinol creams (Tazorac or tararotene) cause less irritation. They are now available by prescription, but they're more expensive.

Milder forms of retinol creams are also on the market. Although they take longer to work, they cause less skin irritation than Renova. However, the lower the dosage, the less the effectiveness. Clearly some cosmetics advertised as containing retinol are just not strong enough to enhance skin cycling or collagen formation. Also, some that claim to have retinol really have retinyl palmitate, which is less effective. Be sure you read the labels carefully.

One big caveat: When taken orally or absorbed through your skin, retinol can cause birth defects. Whether milder topical retinol creams run this risk is debated. If you are a sexually active woman of childbearing age, check with your physician to see if retinol therapy is right for you. I recommend that pregnant women as well as those who may become pregnant avoid potent retinol products altogether.

## Step 5: Use Hydroxy Acids

Cleopatra applied sour goat's milk to her skin. Marie Antoinette used wine. Both women benefited from the ability of hydroxy acids to make their skin look younger. Because hydroxy acids speed the skin cell cycle and accelerate cell turnover, they stimulate your skin to shed older surface cells. The net result is younger skin cells, which are more uniform in reflecting light, making the skin look pinker, fresher, and smoother.

Alpha hydroxy acids are found in fruit juice, wine, and milk products. Beta hydroxy acids (salicylic acid) come from willow bark and wintergreen leaves. Weak concentrations of these agents are sold over the counter and can be used to freshen the skin, making it look younger. Many salons and department stores sell creams and lotions that contain weak concentrations of citric acid (from grape, papaya, or apple juice) or lactic acid (from sour milk products)—both forms of alpha hydroxy acids—in moisturizing preparations. You can use them long-term.

A mild treatment can smooth rough and dry skin, improve skin texture, and help control acne. But medical providers can perform skin peels with stronger solutions of hydroxy acids to smooth tiny wrinkles, fade sun spots, and repair damaged skin. These chemical peels can also remove precancerous skin lesions, making their benefits more than just cosmetic. To make a substantial difference in your skin's appearance, you would need to undergo two to four chemical peel treatments several weeks apart. Skin peels essentially remove the glue that holds dead skin cells on the skin's surface. The skin reddens and the older skin layer actually peels away. Stronger chemical peels can also improve collagen and elastin fiber formation in the dermis. Just be aware that if you select stronger and more intense peels for greater results, there is also more risk of inflammation, scarring, and *hyperpigmentation*—excessive pigment formation, especially in people of color.

Like vitamin A, alpha and beta hydroxy acids (and other agents used for skin peels) thin the skin and make it burn more quickly when exposed to the sun. Here's where your hat and sunscreen come in! In fact, if you can't use a sunscreen, then don't even try to rejuvenate your skin with alpha and beta hydroxy skin products. You'll do more harm than good. You must protect your skin from the sun if you use these products.

## Step 6: Develop a Simple Routine You Can Follow

As you are no doubt aware, hundreds of product lines are available for your skin, from over-the-counter cosmetics you can buy at a drug or department store to prescription preparations available only through a dermatologist or primary physician. After reading the first five steps in this chapter, you should be much better equipped to choose a product line with ingredients that will be effective and meet your needs. For more help deciding which skin care products are right for your unique skin needs, consult *The Skin Type Solution* by Dr. Leslie Baumann, chief of the Division of Cosmetic Dermatology at the University of Miami.

However, none of these products will help you if you don't use them on a regular basis! The most important aspect of choosing a skin care program is to keep it simple enough that you can follow it regularly. Here are my recommendations for devising a personal skin care regimen.

*First thing in the morning*
- Wash your face gently with a nondrying cleanser.
- While your skin is still moist, apply a moisturizer that contains a SPF 15–30 sunscreen (with UVB and UVA protection). Men who shave should do so before applying skin lotions. Moisturizing creams with vitamin C, alpha lipoic acid, and/or green tea (in addition to the SPF protection) are available and may provide added benefits for your skin.
- If you use specific vitamin C or other skin rejuvenation compounds, apply them after the cleanser, but before or with your moisturizer with sunscreen.
- If you venture out into direct sunlight during the day, especially if you play sports, wear a hat and apply extra sunscreen with UVA and UVB protection.

- While I always recommend sunscreen on your face and forearms to protect your long-term appearance, I'm comfortable with exposing your legs and trunk to sunshine for a limited 15-to-20 minute period to enhance vitamin D production. (More on vitamin D in Chapter 10.)

*In the evening*
- Wash your face with a nondrying, non-foaming cleanser.
- Apply retinol cream. After several weeks of adjusting to its initial effects, you can add an alpha hydroxy acid cream (in the form of glycolic acid, lactic acid, and/or citric acid). The combined action of the retinol and alpha hydroxy acid will keep your skin moist and younger-appearing, inhibit acne formation, and reduce the risk of skin cancer. If your skin becomes irritated after combining these products, try applying them on alternate evenings. Some people put on their retinol and/or alpha hydroxy acid creams after dinner, rinsing them off at bedtime. Others apply it just before retiring.
- Lastly, add a moisturizer over the other medicinal creams.

## Other Therapies That Can Rejuvenate Your Skin

While the six steps I've outlined above will help you achieve Ten Years Younger skin, there are other products and procedures you might also consider trying.

### Estriol and Estradiol

Studies have shown that for women who have reached menopause, treating the skin with estrogen in cream form improves thickness, increases collagen formation, and makes the skin look younger. Comparison photos after six months of therapy show less wrinkling and better skin texture. Estradiol 0.01 percent cream and estriol 0.3 percent cream appear to be equally effective. The estradiol preparation, however, seems to have more side effects than estriol, and both treatments are absorbed into the bloodstream.

Since estrogen therapy adds a potential risk for cancer, strokes, and other health problems, you should discuss these options with your physician before adapting them to your skin care regimen. A prescription is required.

## Depigmenting Agents

Several products are available to bleach brown age spots on the skin. Recently, these agents have also been used to decrease overall coloration. *Hydroquinone* and *kojic acid* are both effective. But they can also cause skin allergies or other safety issues, so I suggest you work with a physician experienced with these products rather than experimenting on your own. Topical soy and niacinamide may help prevent pigment formation.

Although less effective, hydroxy acid and retinol products will achieve some modest skin fading if used long-term.

## Botox

Botox injections are the most popular cosmetic procedure performed today. Botox is derived from the exotoxin of *Clostridium botulinum*

### REJUVENATE YOUR GUMS

We've been focusing on your skin, but don't forget your gums too. Believe it or not, bad gums are an aging accelerator. The surface area of your gums is much bigger than you may realize. Stretched out, it's nearly as big as your entire arm. When your gums are inflamed, such a large surface area will noticeably increase your total body inflammation and can significantly increase CRP levels. People with inflamed gums run a higher risk of heart attacks and strokes because of this inflammation. As inflammation is one of the primary causes of accelerated aging, proper tooth and gum care is an important part of the Ten Years Younger Program.

Three Steps to Healthy Gums and Teeth:
- Brush your teeth twice daily.
- Floss at bedtime.
- Rinse with a mouthwash such as Listerine to kill bacteria around your gums daily. Listerine does kill germs that cause inflammation and plaque.

bacteria—the one that causes botulism. This toxin, when highly diluted, prevents facial muscles from contracting and wrinkling the skin. Botox injections block muscle contractions for three to six months and must be repeated two to four times a year to suppress wrinkling.

The effectiveness of Botox depends on the skill of the physician injecting it, how the product was diluted and stored, and how long it has been stored—fresh Botox (used within a few days of being diluted) is better than old Botox.

Not only do Botox injections make your skin look smoother, but if used for many years, they will help prevent future wrinkles from forming, eventually yielding skin that appears younger even after you've stopped the injections. But in contrast to retinol and hydroxy acids, which make your skin younger and block skin cancer formation, Botox only provides cosmetic benefits.


Rejuvenating your skin is more than a skin-deep cosmetic issue. Younger skin makes you feel better about yourself, decreases your risk of future skin cancer, and leads to better overall health. By following the six easy steps I've outlined earlier, you'll be well on your way to a younger face— what a pleasure every time you look in the mirror!

# CHAPTER 10

# Anti-Aging Supplements

When I first started working as a physician, I was leery of supplements. I hadn't learned anything about them in medical school or residency training, and none of the literature I read at the time was devoted to them. Furthermore, I was afraid supplements would give my patients an excuse for living an unhealthy lifestyle. They might assume they were getting everything they needed from a pill or capsule and not eat as well. Over the years, however, my attitude changed dramatically. When I began doing public speaking, I was inundated with questions about supplements. If I didn't know an answer, I promised to research the question and contact the person later. Once I started investigating the subject, the possibilities seemed staggering. It was hard to understand why medical school hadn't taught us more about nutrition and the ways in which supplements could enhance our health. Since then, I have become board certified in nutrition and have developed supplement programs for health care companies, lectured to the public, and given presentations to health care providers on this topic. Everywhere I go, people are eager to learn more about supplements, and they have become an integral part of my Ten Years Younger Program.

Supplements have not been shown to make you younger, but if used properly can slow aging. Adequate vitamin D and calcium can slow bone loss and prevent osteoporosis. Ensuring adequate B vitamins slows artery damage and protects brain cells from aging. Glucosamine can slow joint degeneration. And fish oil can help reverse aging from metabolic syndrome. I believe everyone should be on a personalized supplement program to meet their unique needs. None of us eats well *all* the time, and while supplements can't make up for chronically poor habits, they can provide some nutrients otherwise lost. Not only that, but nutrient content continues to drop in our food supply. Selenium, for instance, an important mineral for your immune system and blood sugar control, is involved in hundreds of anti-aging reactions in your body. But selenium has decreased by nearly 40 percent in our food supply over the past twenty years. Unfortunately, current farming methods don't replace nutrients and minerals taken from the soil, and selenium's presence has diminished.

Supplements may also boost your health in ways that actual foods can't. Glucosamine sulfate, for example, helps mildly arthritic joints. It comes from ground-up crab and shrimp shells. The basic compound from which these shells are composed is also the building block that cartilage cells in your joints use to repair themselves. In several studies it has been shown that if people with early arthritis take glucosamine sulfate regularly, their joints break down more slowly over time and give them less pain. Surely, no one is going to enjoy a big plateful of shrimp and crab *shells* for lunch, so the best solution is to take a glucosamine supplement.

Ginger is an example of a food that needs to be taken at a supplement dosage in order to give you maximal benefit. Ginger is good for joint pain and nausea, but for it to work medicinally, you need doses well beyond what you would normally find in your favorite Asian food—at least 500 mg daily, usually in capsule form. Ginger is my favorite seasickness remedy, and I routinely carry it when traveling by boat in case any guests or family members suffer from this condition. At this dosage, ginger also has anti-inflammatory properties, and it has been shown to be helpful for treating arthritis pains.

Medications, your diet, activities, and health conditions such as diabetes, high blood pressure, and memory loss all impact which vitamins and supplements you should include, especially magnesium, calcium, and vitamin D. And you want to be careful about jumping on supplement trends or fads. All too often, you read in the paper that supplement A is terrific, so you start on it; then a friend mentions that supplement B is wonderful, so you add that too. Soon you're taking fifteen to twenty pills a day, but without any real guidance. In fact, some supplements can be dangerous if combined inappropriately with others or with certain medications. Your first step is to educate yourself.

In the Ten Years Younger Program, everyone should be taking at least a basic multivitamin to ensure adequate intake of vitamin D, B vitamins, and minerals such as selenium. I also believe that depending on diet, lifestyle, age, and medical needs, we should all ensure adequate calcium, magnesium, fiber, garlic, ginger, and omega-3 either from food or from supplements in addition to our multivitamins. But first I want to share the importance of choosing the right source for these supplements.

## Safety First

Supplements are an unregulated industry in the United States, and sources can vary tremendously. The extremes run from an outdoor lab in China or India that produces pills filled with contaminants but few real ingredients to a pristine pharmaceutical laboratory that produces pills that contain the exact dosages stated. Unfortunately, the bottles may look alike, despite the difference in content. The bottom line: Quality varies tremendously. Fortunately some companies still provide excellent products. Here's what to look for:

- *The highest standard is to choose vitamins that can be sold in Europe.* If a product is sold there, especially when produced in Germany, France, or Switzerland, it has druglike quality. All the ingredients for every batch are tested, and these vitamins are produced under strict laboratory conditions. Europeans demand pharmaceutical production standards for their supplements, a level of precision we don't have in the United States. If an American-produced supplement is sold in Europe, it also meets these higher standards. How can you tell? The product will state specifically on the label that it was approved for sale in Europe. Just be aware that these products are hard to come by.

- *USP (US Pharmocopoeia) is another quality standard set up by the government to qualify ingredients that have met tough requirements for safety and quality.* These ingredients are often used in supplements, foods, and beverages and can be independently tested right off the shelves by approved laboratories. The products I stand behind, which are found on my Web site, utilize USP quality ingredients when possible and meet or exceed this level of quality.

- *What you can also look for on product labels is a GMP stamp or logo.* This indicates quality regulation of the manufacturing behind the product. Companies with GMP logos are following Good Manufacturing Practices (GMP) as set out by the FDA. The best companies have not only quality GMP manufacturing processes but also have clinicians and scientists on board choosing the best absorbed and safest ingredients to start with. These companies are research based and adhere to the medical slogan "First do no harm."

- *Check to see if an outside source has tested the supplement you're considering.* Consumerlab.com performs independent testing on a variety of supplement products and can give you reliable information on the active agents and confirm that there are no contaminants in the product as well.

There are a few other general safety guidelines you can follow. With single vitamin supplements, the quality is generally very good. Nearly 90 percent of the world's supply of vitamins C, D, and E is produced by companies like Hoffman-LaRoche under pharmaceutical conditions. Mineral supplements (such as calcium, magnesium, zinc, and selenium) are usually dosed accurately too. One problem with mineral supplements, however, is that they can be full of contaminants. Vitamins are made from scratch, so it's easier to make them clean. But minerals must be extracted from other materials and compounds, so it's much likelier for them to be contaminated. In a study published in the *Journal of the American Medical Association* a few years ago, 30 percent of the calcium supplements tested contained excess lead. In fact, the most commonly sold form of calcium, calcium carbonate, was often contaminated. Fortunately, calcium citrate—a better choice—is fairly lead-free.

The other concern about mineral supplements is that they can be toxic when taken in excess. Selenium, for example, has narrow boundaries between inadequate, beneficial, and toxic doses. One hundred to 200 mcg taken to enhance immunity can be very helpful, but more than 400 mcg taken over the long term can be quite harmful. If you're taking two to four supplement formulations, you can easily swallow too much selenium. Optimally, you would always avoid duplicating your supplement dosages and work with a knowledgeable health professional in choosing a proper regimen.

## What About Herbs?

Quality is the biggest problem with the current uncontrolled distribution of herbs, and herbal products vary tremendously. Many lack active ingredients or are contaminated with unwelcome toxins. Unfortunately, with our current unregulated herbal product system, a simple listing of the contents isn't a guarantee, but only a start. In order to minimize the frustrations associated with these quality concerns, if you find reasons for using herbs as outlined on my Web site, then look for products that have at least GMP or USP labels.

# RDA and Optimal Doses

One thing's for sure: The RDAs (Recommended Daily Allowances) that the government has established don't meet your Ten Years Younger health needs. These were set up as estimates to prevent a disease state in 98 percent of healthy people depending on their age and gender. But these dosages are far below what you would take for the best immune function and tissue repair. Since our goal is not just preventing disease but turning back the clock and promoting a long and healthy life, you'll notice that my recommendations often exceed the RDAs. Not to worry—the doses I suggest here are safe and effective. Even so, be sure to review your supplement program with your medical provider, who knows all your health issues, before starting a supplement program.

## Choosing a Multivitamin: Key Ingredients from A to Zinc

A daily multivitamin is part of the Ten Years Younger Program, and I recommend that you take one. But there are thousands of multivitamins on the market. Which one is the right one for you? Below, I'll clarify the basics that I look for in choosing a proper multivitamin for daily use. To make your life easier, you should know that some multivitamins on the market contain all or most of the important nutrients I've listed in one or two pills a day.

The brands that most closely match my Ten Years Younger supplement list of ingredients include Solgar Multivitamins for men or women, Prothera's VitaPrime, the multivitamin by Designs for Health, and the Metagenics multivitamin.

You'll also find a useful chart in Appendix E to help you compare your current multivitamin with my recommendations and/or to help you choose a more effective regimen.

### Vitamin A

Vitamin A is essential for healthy eyes and skin, night vision, wound healing, and immunity. But in excess, vitamin A can be toxic and is associated with an increased cancer risk. Dosages above 5,000 IU may also inhibit normal bone formation and have been associated with an increased risk for hip and spinal fractures. The most common source of vitamin A overdose is supplements.

I recommend that you take 2,000 to 5,000 IU of vitamin A daily. But don't become confused. You can safely maximize your vitamin A intake simply by adding beta-carotene. Your body is smart; it won't convert so much beta-carotene into vitamin A as to cause toxicity—only taking too much straight vitamin A in supplement form can do that. A vitamin label might state, for instance, "vitamin A 8,000 IU (75 percent as beta-carotene)." This means the pill contains 2,000 IU of vitamin A and 6,000 IU of beta-carotene. This would fall within the safe range.

## Beta-Carotene and Other Carotenoids

Beta-carotene is a potent antioxidant and appears helpful in preventing cancer and cardiovascular disease. As noted in Chapter 5, carotenes, also called carotenoids, are plant pigments that give plants color and protect them from sun damage.

There are 600 carotenoids in the human diet, but taking one type of carotene in excess can block absorption of many of the other important ones, such as lycopene, lutein, and alpha-carotene. I always aim for mixed carotenoids, not just beta-carotene, in a supplement. The label should state that it contains mixed carotenoids, not just beta-carotene, to be optimal.

Smokers who take large dosages of beta-carotene may actually increase their risk for cancer. So smokers should of course quit smoking, but if they continue they should be careful to avoid taking extra beta-carotene in supplement form.

## B Vitamins

B vitamins are critical for your brain, cardiovascular health, cancer prevention, and slowing the aging process. The key B vitamins you should look for in a multivitamin are folic acid, $B_{12}$, $B_6$, and biotin.

Folic acid decreases your risk of heart attacks, strokes, Alzheimer's, and cancer. I recommend at least 400 to 600 mcg daily. Folic acid also lowers homocysteine levels (see Chapter 2), but to do so it must be taken in conjunction with $B_{12}$ and $B_6$. You should take folic acid with the $B_{12}$ and $B_6$ doses noted below.

To clarify your folic acid requirement, ask your medical provider to check your homocysteine level. If it's greater than 9 mg/dl, I recommend you increase your folic acid intake. Some people may require 2,000 to 4,000 mcg (2 to 4 mg) daily. You should also be aware that 20 percent of the population with very high homocysteine levels has difficulty converting folic acid into its most active form. They require a folic acid metabolite called 5-methyl-tetrahydrofolate in addition to folic acid, $B_{12}$, and $B_6$ to lower homocysteine levels adequately. Fortunately, 5-methyl-tetrahydrofolate is available as a supplement, and for those people who need it, adding 400 mcg of folic acid with 400 mcg of 5-methyl-tetrahydrofolate should be sufficient. But be sure to review this protocol with a health professional who knows you well.

$B_{12}$ (cobalamine) is essential for hundreds of reactions in your body, but it can be poorly absorbed, especially as you age, or if you take heartburn medications (such as Tums, Zantac, Pepcid, or any of the acid-blocking medications). Since $B_{12}$ in high doses is safe and inexpensive, and since absorption problems are common, I favor putting more $B_{12}$ in a multivitamin than average people might need. I'd prefer a multivitamin that has at least 100 mcg of $B_{12}$. If you have absorption problems or use heartburn medications, 250 to 1,000 mcg would be appropriate.

I also like to see at least 15 mg of $B_6$ (pyridoxine) and 300 mcg of biotin in a multivitamin to ensure adequate doses for these other key B vitamins.

## Vitamin C

Vitamin C is essential for collagen formation and immunity. The optimal dosage ranges from 500 mg to 1,000 mg daily. You can get 500 to 750 mg of vitamin C daily from the Ten Years Younger Diet since it's rich in fruits and vegetables. But if you eat poorly, you should take a 500 to 1,000 mg supplement daily. Healthier eaters can aim for 250 to 500 mg of vitamin C in their supplement.

## Vitamin D

Vitamin D facilitates calcium absorption to build strong bones. Sunshine helps form vitamin D, and those few individuals who get thirty minutes of direct sunshine on their arms, legs, and face at least three to four days a week *year round* without wearing sunscreen should produce on average about 400 IU vitamin D daily through their skin. Since very few people actually receive this amount of sunshine every month, and as I prefer that you cover at least your face and forearms with sunscreen, I recommend vitamin D supplements.

Low vitamin D levels are also associated with cancer risk, as low vitamin D levels seem to enhance cancer cell progression and growth, especially prostate cancer. Receiving 1,000 IU of vitamin D daily, either through sun exposure or supplements and food, appears to decrease cancer risk in men and women.

Lastly, low vitamin D levels are associated with an increased risk of autoimmune diseases caused by abnormal inflammation. In particular, multiple sclerosis (MS) has a very strong relationship to low vitamin D levels. Again, getting 500–1,000 IU of vitamin D daily is associated with a much lower risk of autoimmune disease, including MS.

Most multivitamin supplements contain 400 IU of vitamin D daily, although, as you can guess, I favor 500–1,000 IU. Either take a regular multivitamin and ensure adequate sunlight, or if you prefer to follow my advice and maximize your skin protection, add enough vitamin D in both supplements and foods to reach 1,000 IU daily.

## Vitamin E

In some individuals, vitamin E supplements (400 to 800 IU) appear to lower healthy HDL cholesterol levels. In fact, a recent study showed that taking more than 200 IU of vitamin E daily increases the chance of death among average Americans. So in a multivitamin I recommend 50 to 150 IU of mixed forms of vitamin E, including d-alpha-, delta-, and gamma-tocopherols. Avoid supplements that contain only alpha-tocopherol in their formula. Some people may need additional mixed vitamin E supplements for memory loss, immune function enhancement, clotting problems, or to relieve oxidative stress. Weigh these benefits against the risk associated with HDL reductions with your medical provider.

## Chromium

Chromium is a mineral that improves insulin activity. While widely sold as a weight loss supplement, it appears most useful to people who suffer from chromium deficiency because of poor diet and diabetes. Chromium is safe in doses up to 800 mcg daily. You should find 100 to 400 mcg in your multivitamin, but if you want extra weight loss help, you can try adding some separately. Higher doses (200 to 800 mcg) may improve body composition by enhancing insulin sensitivity, helping to shift weight from fat to muscle in people following a weight loss program. I prefer chromium polynicotinate over chromium picolinate. Chromium picolinate has benefited from incredible marketing, but I urge you to avoid this product, as picolinate has the potential to form unhealthy by-products when metabolized.

## Iron

Not everyone needs additional iron. Women who menstruate need the extra iron (about 8 to 20 mg daily) to build red blood cells, and growing children also need additional iron. But men and postmenopausal women with a decent diet generally don't need to supplement their iron intake. In fact, it not only causes constipation and gastrointestinal complaints, but it can age you more quickly. Iron in excess is a free radical stimulator. I avoid iron in my supplements, but ensure that my wife and growing boys get a 16-mg dose of iron in their vitamin formula.

## Selenium

Selenium is found in whole-grain products, but in several areas of the country (eastern Washington and Oregon and the southeastern United States) soils are selenium deficient, which results in reduced levels of this valuable mineral in food products. Selenium is important for immunity and blood sugar control and is involved in hundreds of anti-aging reactions in the human body.

The best daily dose for selenium is 200 mcg. A healthy diet rich in a variety of beans, whole grains, and nuts (Brazil nuts are an excellent source of selenium) produced in various parts of the country will provide about 100 mcg daily. If you follow such a diet, you need only supplement with 100 mcg more. With an average to poor American diet, I suggest 200 mcg daily.

Remember, selenium can cause toxicity with just 500 mcg daily. Be careful when taking several different supplement products, as many contain selenium. Check the label—you don't want to overdo it.

## Zinc

Zinc is a critical mineral for immunity, wound healing, growth, and a variety of anti-aging functions. A healthy diet should supply 12 to 15 mg of zinc daily. As the optimal total dose per day is 20 to 30 mg, aim for 15 to 20 mg daily in your multivitamin.

# Ten Years Younger Supplements

There are thousands of supplements on the market, and there are many good reasons for taking more than what you can get in a single multivitamin or packet. In addition to a high-quality multivitamin that meets my recommendations, the following five supplements are part of the Ten Years Younger Program. But read the indications carefully since, depending on your age, lifestyle, diet, and health, you may need to adjust the dosage. Indeed, if you're in good health and eat optimally, you may not have to take these supplements at all! You can receive all of their anti-aging benefits from your diet.

## Calcium and Magnesium

Before you decide whether you need a calcium and/or magnesium supplement, please refer back to Chapter 5 to determine how much calcium you should take based on your age, gender, and diet. And while we're on the subject, you may also discover some calcium and magnesium in your daily multivitamin pill. Just bear in mind that since these are large molecules, it is not practical to add them to a multivitamin in significant amounts. So you may still need additional calcium and magnesium to reach your targets. If so, supplement separately with calcium and magnesium pills.

Calcium as a true chelate is the best-absorbed of all the calcium supplements and doesn't have the problems with lead contamination that the commonly sold calcium carbonate does. With regard to magnesium, I recommend that you opt for a magnesium chelate form. Avoid magnesium oxide, the cheapest form of magnesium, since it can cause gastrointestinal problems.

## Fiber

I've been singing the praises of fiber throughout these pages, and you should know by now that your diet should have more than 30 mg of fiber daily. By following the Ten Years Younger Diet, you can achieve this goal, with at least half the fiber coming from fruits, nuts, and vegetables. Check Appendix B to ensure you are reaching this fiber intake on most days. But if for various reasons your diet contains less fiber than this, you should add a fiber supplement to reach your total fiber goals.

An excellent fiber supplement on the market is a brand called PGX, a dietary fiber source that Dr. Vladimir Vuksan and his team in Toronto have researched extensively. PGX comes in a capsule. Once it enters your intestinal tract it becomes very viscous—something akin to Jell-O—and holds a tremendous amount of water. Its viscosity permits it to lower blood sugar and cholesterol levels by slowing blood sugar from emptying from the intestinal tract into the bloodstream. It also binds to cholesterol, blocking its absorption. And since it helps you feel full and aids with blood sugar regulation, it isn't surprising that it helps with weight loss, too. Other sources of fiber include psyllium and bran.

## Garlic

Fresh garlic is truly a wonder Vitality Food. The trick is knowing how to use it, and you'll find more detailed recommendations in Chapter 4. My preference is for you to eat 1 to 2 cloves of garlic daily in your food.

I don't recommend deodorized garlic pills, largely because studies in Germany have shown that they don't work. Nondeodorized garlic should state that it contains allicin on the label. Products that list only alliin on the label may be inactive, as only allicin is fully therapeutic. If you must take garlic supplements, you will need 1 to 2 grams daily to help lower your cholesterol level. But avoid taking more than 4 grams daily in a supplement without discussing this with your medical provider, as it can increase your risk for serious bleeding problems.

## Ginger

When used regularly, ginger is effective in relieving joint pain and arthritis symptoms. In contrast to most anti-inflammatory medications, it doesn't increase the risk for stomach ulcers. In fact, people use ginger to treat ulcers. For the average person, the Ten Years Younger Diet provides all the ginger you'll need to benefit from its anti-aging properties. If you have arthritis, adding an extra 500 mg daily with your supplement regimen may relieve joint pain.

## Omega-3 Fats (EPA/DHA)

As you will recall from Chapter 5, these are essential fats that regulate inflammation and clotting, improve mental function, and prevent cancer and sudden death. As part of the Ten Years Younger Diet, I recommend that you eat 2 to 3 servings a week of seafood rich in omega-3 fats and low in mercury. If you don't or can't eat seafood, another way to get omega-3s is to take 1 gram of distilled fish oil daily. Be sure your fish oil supplement contains close to 360 mg of EPA (eicosapentaenoic acid) and 240 mg of DHA (docosahexaenoic acid).

When considering fish oil supplements, I find that many of the brands go rancid quickly and as a result taste horrible. Not only can they give you an unpleasant burp and aftertaste, but rancid fish oil may be quite harmful to your overall health. I choose fish oil brands that have been independently tested for lipid peroxide levels, an excellent measure of rancidity. Visit my Web site at www.tenyearsyounger.net for details on fish oil supplements.

Dosing with fish oil varies depending on why you're taking it. If you're seeking overall health enhancement, then 1 gram daily is enough, which is the dosage obtained from eating 2 to 3 servings weekly of seafood rich in omega-3 fats. If you're hoping to heal significant inflammation or a disc herniation or to lower triglyceride levels, then you should aim for 3 grams daily. Esteemed surgeons working with National Football League teams recommend fish oil at 3 to 4 grams daily for top athletes who suffer from nerve impingements and/or disc herniations. The fish oil supplements block the inflammatory cascade and may also help nourish nerve tissue, since that type of tissue is partly made of omega-3 fats. However, always speak to your medical provider before taking more than 2 gm of fish oil daily as it can increase the risk of bleeding.

If you don't or can't use seafood products, you can substitute 1 tablespoon of ground flaxseed daily. Sprinkle it over cereal or salad, or mix it into a smoothie. But while flaxseed is an excellent omega-3 supplement, it doesn't provide the anti-inflammatory effect of long-chain omega-3 fats. Organic eggs from flaxseed-fed chickens can also be helpful in increasing long-chain omega-3 levels. If you eat eggs, buy those that are free-range and omega-3 enriched. You get up to 300 mg of omega-3 fats from each of these eggs, which is excellent.

For additional supplement recommendations with regard to specific medical conditions such as diabetes, arthritis, and cognitive impairment, visit my Web site at www.tenyearsyounger.net.

## How and When to Take Your Supplements

So how do you make your way through what can seem like a confusing maze of choices and products? Here are my summary guidelines for designing your personal supplement regimen in three easy steps:

1. Be sure to take a quality multivitamin with enough B vitamins, selenium, zinc, and vitamin D.
2. Clarify your calcium and magnesium, fiber, fish oil, garlic, and ginger needs to guarantee that you're taking enough but not too much.
3. Review the additional recommendations for supplements at www.tenyearsyounger.net to see if other choices are warranted.

The best time to take your supplements is when you'll remember to take them. For years I swallowed my supplements at bedtime, simply because it was easy to make them part of my nighttime routine. Recently I've split the doses into two parts and started taking them in the morning and at bedtime. Splitting the dosage improves absorption and helps to maintain steadier blood levels in my system. And if I forget the morning dose, I can still take both at bedtime.

I recommend having your supplements packaged for convenience. Many companies perform this service, as do I in my clinical practice, or you can do it yourself. I have my morning pills all placed in one easy-to-open plastic packet, and I have another packet for the evening. This saves me from having to open several pill bottles. It also ensures that I drink a glass of water with each packet, giving me two of the eight glasses of water I need to drink daily. And when traveling out of town, it makes it easy to take just the supply I need for the number of days I'll be away.

Always remember, supplements were never intended to replace exercise, a healthy diet, stress reduction, or elimination of toxins—all steps in the Ten Years Younger Program. Yet when used properly, they can enhance your health and help you slow the aging process. If you're taking many supplements or supplements with medications, always check with your medical provider to prevent any adverse interactions.

# PART III

---

# THE TEN YEARS YOUNGER PROGRAM

For most of my patients, the biggest challenge in beginning a new anti-aging lifestyle is the question "Where should I start?" The problem is that everyone is biochemically and socially unique, and while one person might be a couch potato, another might already be naturally active, working out occasionally if not on a regular basis. Similarly, two active people might have very different eating habits.

So before you begin, spend a moment clarifying where you should dive into each of the various components of this program. The three that deserve the most attention are the eating, activity, and skin care plans. Too much fiber too quickly and you could end up feeling gassy, bloated, and crampy. Too much activity all at once, and you might injure yourself and wind up needing a month to recover. And if you rush to introduce a host of new skin care products, you risk irritating or burning your skin. On the other hand, if you choose a phase with too little exercise when you're already jogging and lifting weights, you'll quickly become bored with the suggestions I make. In fact, any of these outcomes can cause you to back away from your commitment to the program. The three phases of the program are designed to ease you in at the level that's right for you. The first two phases last two weeks each, and Phase Three lasts six weeks.

## Choose the Right Meal Phase

Deciding where to start the eating plan is simple. You simply use the fiber tables on pages 353–354. If you now eat less than 20 grams of fiber daily—probably like the majority of people reading this book—start with the eating plan for Phase One. If your daily fiber intake is between 20 and 30 grams, start with Phase Two. If you already eat more than 30 grams daily, congratulations! You can enjoy any of the recipes in this book.

As you move forward through the three eating plans, you don't have to give up any recipes you enjoyed in the earlier stages. Just be sure that by Phases Two and Three you substitute nonfat cheese or dairy ingredients for reduced-fat products.

## Choose the Right Exercise Phase

To identify the right exercise phase, clarify your current activity level—and remember, it's not how you *used* to work out years or months ago, but what you've been doing in the last four weeks. (See Chapter 3.) Be realistic. Your goal is to prevent injuries, and a slower start is worth the couple of extra weeks to do it right.

From my experience, most people should start with Phase One Age-Busting Fitness activities, but if you're in good shape, I don't want you to lose ground. If you already work out for up to 30 minutes with your heart rate above 70 percent of your maximum achieved heart rate zone *and* you do strength training at least twice a week, then you're ready for Phase Two. And if you engage in strength training at least twice a week and have already added intervals to your aerobic workout (see Chapter 6 about interval training), go straight to Phase Three. It only gets better from there!

## Choose the Right Skin Care Phase

If you don't already apply a skin moisturizer with sunscreen daily, then Phase One is right for you. If you do, then you can move to Phase Two and add a retinol skin product daily. If you have already been using sunscreen and retinol products, you can add a hydroxy acid skin product in Phase Three. Choose accordingly.

Your goal in beginning this program is to take the credit you deserve and modify your starting point based on a customized assessment. And now you're ready to dive in and begin the Ten Years Younger Program!

# Getting Started

I n the following pages, you'll find daily food plans that combine and incorporate Vitality Foods into lively and varied meals. As many of my study participants have found, *you will not feel hungry on this diet*. To ensure you don't, I've included an optional morning snack, a recommended afternoon snack, and what I like to call Rescue Snacks for when you just absolutely have to have something to munch on! You'll also note that I encourage a nutrient-packed dessert daily, so enjoy the treat after your evening meal. It's good for you and an essential part of my optimal nutritional plan.

In Phase One, you'll find that I've kept the level of fiber to 20 to 25 grams a day. This will increase gradually in Phases Two and Three so that eventually you'll be eating more than 30 grams a day without any discomfort.

I've included my favorite recipes here, but I want you to keep in mind that flexibility is key. You will likely need to make some adjustments on account of your and your family's various likes and dislikes, the availability of particular ingredients, and your daily schedule. In Phase One, for instance, there are many opportunities to substitute chicken or shrimp for tofu. Some recipes are quicker than others, so save the more complex (but delicious) dinners and desserts like Cioppino, Paella, and Chocolate Mousse with Grand Marnier for evenings when you have more time to enjoy cooking. This, of course, will vary from person to person, but I like to prepare these meals on the weekends.

Breakfast needs vary greatly depending on work schedules and personal preferences. Many of my patients won't take more than three or four minutes for breakfast, so cooking oatmeal won't work for them. If you find yourself in this dilemma, a high-fiber (at least 4 grams), low-saturated-fat (less than 1.5 grams) granola bar may be what you need to grab as you run out the door. Or you could whip up and freeze a batch of Mini Mushroom Cheese Frittatas or Oat Bran Muffins (you'll find the recipe for the latter in Phase Two) on the weekend and quickly heat and eat these treats as you get going on your busy day. You want to adapt the diet to *your* schedule, and not the other way around. Similarly, while I like a different breakfast three or four times a week, my wife, Nicole, enjoys eating the same thing every day. The meal plan offers lots of choices, but you can choose to have the same thing every day if that works best for you. And if the optional morning snacks suit you better than the breakfasts I offer, then go with the morning snack. All the choices are healthy.

Likewise, for lunch, choose meals that meet your likes and your schedule. If you don't have time to prepare an elaborate lunch, then cook extra for dinner and fill a lunch container before you serve the meal (so you don't eat tomorrow's lunch at the dinner table). This way, you'll have a nutritious age-busting meal for the next day. If you often eat out for lunch, almost any restaurant nowadays offers a mixed salad with grilled chicken, turkey, shrimp, or salmon. Ask for a vinaigrette dressing (olive oil and vinegar base) and you'll have made an excellent choice.

You should be able to accomplish most of your food shopping once a week, especially if you read through a week's worth of food plans and recipes in advance. (You'll find suggested weekly shopping lists in Appendix F that will help you organize your dinners and desserts for one week at a time.) A clear exception, however, is seafood. Fresh from the store is always best! In fact, I don't buy seafood more than twenty-four hours in advance, and I usually pick it up the same day I'm going to cook it. It loses something when frozen. The exception is vacuum-packed fish fillets. For example, wild-caught salmon fillets that were carefully vacuum packed, frozen, and properly shipped can be quite good, especially when prepared with recipes I've included. While fresh is almost always better, I accept that if you have a busy schedule you have to be practical, and vacuum-packed seafood can even be delivered to your door.

When selecting fresh seafood, you'll also want to choose items that look good. Clams and mussels should still be alive and responsive to stimuli—if you tap them, they should close quickly. Fish fillets should be shiny and glistening, not dry or wrinkled. When cooking with fish, be adventurous. Recipes that require fillet of sole can be made with flounder, tilapia, or cod if the sole looks off or is out of season. Vacuum-packed Alaskan salmon may be better than fresh if the only fresh salmon you can find at the fish market is "farm-raised with color added." Your best bet for salmon, though, is wild, line-caught Alaskan salmon, more expensive but better for you.

You can also change the recipes to fit the types of produce that are available and are freshest. If the broccoli in your store looks yellow, choose cauliflower or kale instead.

While a serving of alcohol daily is associated with a lower risk for memory loss, heart disease, and diabetes, I believe everyone can benefit from a short break from alcohol to prevent alcohol dependence. Additionally, dropping alcohol for a short period gives you a sense of commitment and will cut your calorie intake while your ability to burn calories is increasing. During Phase One, I recommend no alcohol for one week. During the second week, limit yourself to one serving or none a day. During Phases Two and Three, enjoy 1 to 2 servings of alcohol daily, preferably red wine, as I noted in Chapter 4. However, because drinking alcohol every day can cause chemical or emotional dependency, it would be wise to skip alcohol one or two times a week. If you have trouble following these limits, I encourage you to explore your relationship with alcohol carefully.

Along with the daily food plans, you'll also find daily Age-Busting Fitness plans. Most people do their aerobic exercise Monday through Saturday and take off Sunday, but if Sunday is a better day for you or if you're really busy some other day of the week, adjust your workout schedule accordingly. Mix up your aerobic workouts so that you engage in different activities during the week. A diverse workout routine is more fun and helps prevent injuries, because using the same joints and muscles over and over again risks wearing them out. You have many choices in strength-training options, so turn back to Chapter 6 for specific exercise instructions. I typically choose Tuesday, Thursday, and Saturday for these kinds of activities, but pick the three days that work best for you.

There are a host of relaxation, supplement, and detoxification routines to follow over the ten weeks. Refer back to Chapters 7, 8, and 10 to stimulate your thinking on which options you can adopt. Choose those that seem the most realistic for you with the time you have.

Ultimately, the Ten Years Younger Program should flex to meet your needs and your lifestyle. Just remember to keep the essential principles intact.

I wish you bon appétit, optimal health, and long life!

# DAILY MEAL AND ACTIVITY PLANS

## Day 1 (Monday)

FOOD PLAN: Vitality Foods

**Breakfast**
Oatmeal with Apples and Blueberries
Tea or coffee

**Optional Morning Snack**
Hard-boiled egg (omega-3, free-range, organic)

Lunch
Grilled chicken breast, 4–6 oz
Mixed green salad, 2–3 cups
Vinaigrette Dressing, 2 tbsp
Iced tea

**Afternoon Snack**
Baby carrots, 1 cup
Almonds, 1 oz
Pure water

**Dinner**
Salmon with Ginger-Chili Sauce
Brown rice, ¾ cup
Sautéed broccoli and shiitake mushrooms, 1 cup
Fresh spinach salad, 2 cups with ½ cucumber, sliced, and 2 tbsp Vinaigrette Dressing
Seltzer

**Dessert**
Berry-Banana Smoothie
Herbal tea

**Optional Rescue Snack**
Smoked oysters, 1½ oz
Rye crispbread, 2

## *AGE-BUSTING FITNESS PLAN*

### Aerobic Training

- 3-5 minutes of warming up
- Reach 70-80% of your max heart rate, 20-30 minutes with brisk walking, jogging, elliptical machine options
- 3-5 minutes of cooling down, heart rate less than 60% max

### Strength Training

- Rest day from strength training

### Stretching

- 4-6 body parts, 5-10 minutes of stretching time

## RELAXATION ROUTINE

- Choose a calming activity for 10-20 minutes

## SUPPLEMENT ROUTINE

- Take your customized multivitamin pack
- Skin moisturizer with SPF 15

## DETOX ROUTINE

- Choose purified water
- Go alcohol free for one week
- Clean out the junk food from your kitchen cupboards

# Day 2 (Tuesday)

FOOD PLAN: Vitality Foods

**Breakfast**
Omelet with Veggies
Whole-wheat toast, 1 slice
Tea or coffee

**Optional Morning Snack**
Nonfat, sugar-free yogurt, 4–6 oz

**Lunch**
Veggie burger with sliced tomato, lettuce, mustard, and whole-wheat pita bread
Mixed green salad, 2 cups
Vinaigrette Dressing, 2 tbsp
Iced tea

**Afternoon Snack**
Carrots and/or celery sticks, 1 cup
Pure water

**Dinner**
Sichuan Stir-Fry
Cucumber Salad with Ginger Dressing
Decaf green or black tea

**Dessert**
Nonfat, sugar-free ice cream with 3/4 cup berries and 2–3 tbsp pecans
Hot Cocoa

**Optional Rescue Snack**
Baby carrots, 1–2 cups
Nuts, 1 oz

### AGE-BUSTING FITNESS PLAN

**Aerobic Training**
- 3-5 minutes of warming up
- Reach 70-80% of your max heart rate for 20-30 minutes total activity with brisk walking, jogging, elliptical machine options
- 3 minutes of cooling down, heart rate less than 60% max

**Strength Training**
- 12 body parts, 1 set, 10-16 reps
- Mixture of ball and free weight activities

**Stretching**
- 4-6 body parts, 5-10 minutes of stretching time

## RELAXATION ROUTINE
- Choose a calming activity for 10-20 minutes

## SUPPLEMENT ROUTINE
- Take your customized multivitamin pack
- Skin moisturizer with SPF 15

## DETOX ROUTINE
- Choose purified water
- Go alcohol free for one week
- Clean out the junk food from your kitchen cupboards

# Day 3 (Wednesday)

FOOD PLAN: Vitality Foods

## Breakfast
Grits, $3/4$–1 cup cooked
Soy sausage, 1–2
Tea or coffee

## Optional Morning Snack
Nonfat, sugar-free yogurt, 4–6 oz

## Lunch
Turkey wrap
Carrot and/or celery sticks, 1 cup
Apple
Seltzer

## Afternoon Snack
Nonfat cottage cheese, 4 oz ($1/2$ cup)
Pure water

## Dinner
Sole with Almond Crust
Wild Rice with Red Onions and Shiitake Mushrooms
Mixed green salad, 2–3 cups
Vinaigrette Dressing, 2 tbsp
Seltzer

## Dessert
Melon
Hot Cocoa

## Optional Rescue Snack
Veggie chicken nuggets, 4 pieces

## *AGE-BUSTING FITNESS PLAN*

### Aerobic Training
- 3–5 minutes of warming up
- Reach 70–80% of your max heart rate for 20–30 minutes total activity with brisk walking, jogging, elliptical machine options
- 3 minutes of cooling down, heart rate less than 60% max

### Strength Training
- Rest day from strength training

### Stretching
- 4–6 body parts, 5–10 minutes of stretching time

## RELAXATION ROUTINE
- Enjoy a massage

## SUPPLEMENT ROUTINE
- Take your customized multivitamin pack
- Skin moisturizer with SPF 15

## DETOX ROUTINE
- Choose purified water
- Go alcohol free for one week
- Clean out the junk food from your kitchen cupboards

# Day 4 (Thursday)

FOOD PLAN: Vitality Foods

## Breakfast
Oatmeal with Apples and Blueberries
Tea or coffee

## Optional Morning Snack
Hard-boiled egg (omega-3, free-range, organic)

## Lunch
Crab with Mixed Salad
Seltzer

## Afternoon Snack
Pear
Walnuts, 1 oz
Pure water

## Dinner
Thai Stuffed Cabbage Rolls
Decaf tea

## Dessert
Cubed apple dipped in 1–2 oz melted chocolate
Herbal tea

## Optional Rescue Snack
Sardines, 1½–3 oz
Rye crispbread, 2–3 pieces

## *AGE-BUSTING FITNESS PLAN*

### Aerobic Training
- 3–5 minutes of warming up
- Reach 70–80% of your max heart rate for 20–30 minutes total activity with brisk walking, jogging, elliptical machine options
- 3 minutes of cooling down, heart rate less than 60% max

### Strength Training
- 12 body parts, 1 set, 10–16 reps
- Mixture of ball and free weight activities

### Stretching
- 4–6 body parts, 5–10 minutes of stretching time

### RELAXATION ROUTINE
- Choose a calming activity for 10–20 minutes

### SUPPLEMENT ROUTINE
- Take your customized multivitamin pack
- Skin moisturizer with SPF 15

### DETOX ROUTINE
- Choose purified water
- Go alcohol free for one week
- Clean out the junk food from your kitchen cupboards

# Day 5 (Friday)

FOOD PLAN: Vitality Foods

**Breakfast**
Bran cereal with blueberries and nonfat milk
Tea or coffee

**Optional Morning Snack**
Nonfat, sugar-free yogurt, 4-6 oz

**Lunch**
Salmon Spread with Pita
Orange
Iced tea

**Afternoon Snack**
Baby carrots, 1 cup
Almonds, 1 oz
Pure water

**Dinner**
Chicken Breasts with Ginger, Garlic, and Chili
Brown rice, ¾ cup
Sautéed carrots and cauliflower, 1-2 cups
Mixed green salad, 2-3 cups
Vinaigrette Dressing, 2 tbsp

**Dessert**
Chocolate Mousse with Grand Marnier
Hot Cocoa

**Optional Rescue Snack**
Veggie chicken nuggets, 4 pieces

## *AGE-BUSTING FITNESS PLAN*

### Aerobic Training
- 3-5 minutes of warming up
- Reach 70-80% of your max heart rate for 20-30 minutes total activity with brisk walking, jogging, elliptical machine options
- 3 minutes of cooling down, heart rate less than 60% max

### Strength Training
- Rest day from strength training

### Stretching
- 4-6 body parts, 5-10 minutes of stretching time

## RELAXATION ROUTINE
- Choose a calming activity for 10-20 minutes

## SUPPLEMENT ROUTINE
- Take your customized multivitamin pack
- Skin moisturizer with SPF 15

## DETOX ROUTINE
- Choose purified water
- Go alcohol free for one week
- Clean out the junk food from your kitchen cupboards

# Day 6 (Saturday)

FOOD PLAN: Vitality Foods

**Breakfast**
Mushroom Cheese Frittata
Berry-Banana Smoothie
Tea or coffee

**Optional Morning Snack**
Hard-boiled egg (omega-3, free-range, organic)

**Lunch**
Turkey breast, 5–6 oz
Mixed green salad, 2–3 cups
Vinaigrette Dressing, 2 tbsp
Apple
Seltzer

**Afternoon Snack**
Veggie chicken nuggets, 4 pieces
Pure water

**Dinner**
Cioppino
Mixed green salad, 2–3 cups
Vinaigrette Dressing, 2 tbsp
Seltzer

**Dessert**
Strawberries, ½ pint, dipped in 1 oz melted dark chocolate, with ¼ cup vanilla
    nonfat yogurt
Herbal tea

**Optional Rescue Snack**
Nuts, 1 oz
1 apple

## *AGE-BUSTING FITNESS PLAN*

### Aerobic Training
- 3-5 minutes of warming up
- Reach 70-80% of your max heart rate for 20-30 minutes total activity with brisk walking, jogging, elliptical machine options
- 3 minutes of cooling down, heart rate less than 60% max

### Strength Training
- Rest day from strength training

### Stretching
- Yoga class or a 20-30 minute stretch with 10-12 body parts

### RELAXATION ROUTINE
- Choose a calming activity for 10-20 minutes

### SUPPLEMENT ROUTINE
- Take your customized multivitamin pack
- Skin moisturizer with SPF 15

### DETOX ROUTINE
- Choose purified water
- Go alcohol free for one week
- Clean out the junk food from your kitchen cupboards

# Day 7 (Sunday)

FOOD PLAN: Vitality Foods

**Breakfast**
Omelet with Veggies
Soy sausage, 1
Tea or coffee

**Optional Morning Snack**
None

**Lunch**
Gazpacho
Iced tea

**Afternoon Snack**
Air-popped popcorn, 2 cups, sprinkled with 1 tbsp brewer's yeast
Pure water

**Dinner**
Grilled Salmon with Lemon and Dill
Steamed broccoli, 1 cup
Sweet Potato Fries with Cinnamon
Iced mint tea

**Dessert**
Nonfat, sugar-free ice cream, $\frac{1}{2}$–$\frac{3}{4}$ cup
Pecans, 2–3 tbsp
Hot Cocoa

**Optional Rescue Snack**
Almonds, 1 oz

## *AGE-BUSTING FITNESS PLAN*

### Aerobic Training
- Aerobic rest day

### Strength Training
- Rest day from strength training

### Stretching
- 4-6 body parts, 5-10 minutes of stretching time

## RELAXATION ROUTINE
- Choose a calming activity for 10-20 minutes

## SUPPLEMENT ROUTINE
- Take your customized multivitamin pack
- Skin moisturizer with SPF 15

## DETOX ROUTINE
- Choose purified water
- Go alcohol free for one week
- Clean out the junk food from your kitchen cupboards

# Day 8 (Monday)

FOOD PLAN: Vitality Foods

### Breakfast
Mini Mushroom Cheese Frittatas
Whole-wheat toast, 1 slice, or 1 soy sausage
Tea or coffee

### Optional Morning Snack
Nonfat yogurt, 4–6 oz

### Lunch
Veggie burger with pita bread, sliced tomato, mustard, and lettuce
Mixed green salad, 2 cups, with 1 cup extra veggies
Vinaigrette Dressing, 2 tbsp
Iced tea

### Afternoon Snack
Pear
Pure water

### Dinner
Garlic Shrimp Burritos
Roasted Bell Peppers, 1–2 pieces
Seltzer
Red wine

### Dessert
Mango Frozen Yogurt

### Optional Rescue Snack
Almonds, 1 oz

## *AGE-BUSTING FITNESS PLAN*

### Aerobic Training
- 3-5 minutes of warming up
- Reach 70-80% of your max heart rate for 20-30 minutes total activity with brisk walking, jogging, elliptical machine options
- 3 minutes of cooling down, heart rate less than 60% max

### Strength Training
- Rest day from strength training

### Stretching
- 4-6 body parts, 5-10 minutes of stretching time

## RELAXATION ROUTINE
- Choose a calming activity for 10-20 minutes

## SUPPLEMENT ROUTINE
- Take your customized multivitamin pack
- Skin moisturizer with SPF 15

## DETOX ROUTINE
- One alcohol serving per day or none
- Add plants to your work and home
- Shun hydrogenated fats, corn syrup, and other added sweeteners in your diet
- Avoid processed sandwich meats that have nitrites or other chemicals

# Day 9 (Tuesday)

FOOD PLAN: Vitality Foods

**Breakfast**
Bran cereal, 1 cup, with ½ cup berries and ½ cup nonfat milk
Tea or coffee

**Optional Morning Snack**
Hard-boiled egg (omega-3, free-range, organic)

**Lunch**
Shrimp Bisque
Apple
Iced Tea

**Afternoon Snack**
Pecans, 1 oz
Pure water

**Dinner**
Whole-wheat spaghetti, 1–1½ cups cooked, with 1 cup Tomato Sauce, 2 tbsp
    reduced fat or nonfat grated cheese
Mixed green salad, 2–3 cups
Vinaigrette Dressing, 2 tbsp

**Dessert**
Coffee Flan

**Optional Rescue Snack**
Almonds, 1 oz

## *AGE-BUSTING FITNESS PLAN*

### Aerobic Training
- 3-5 minutes of warming up
- Reach 70-80% of your max heart rate for 20-30 minutes total activity with brisk walking, jogging, elliptical machine options
- 3 minutes of cooling down, heart rate less than 60% max

### Strength Training
- 12 body parts, 1 set, 10-16 reps
- Mixture of ball and free weight activities

### Stretching
- 4-6 body parts, 5-10 minutes of stretching time

## RELAXATION ROUTINE
- Choose a calming activity for 10-20 minutes

## SUPPLEMENT ROUTINE
- Take your customized multivitamin pack
- Skin moisturizer with SPF 15

## DETOX ROUTINE
- One alcohol serving per day or none
- Add plants to your work and home environment
- Shun hydrogenated fats, corn syrup, and other added sweeteners in your diet
- Avoid processed sandwich meats that have nitrites or other chemicals

# Day 10 (Wednesday)

FOOD PLAN: Vitality Foods

## Breakfast
Mini Mushroom Cheese Frittatas
Soy sausage, 1
Tea or coffee

## Optional Morning Snack
Nonfat yogurt, 4–6 oz

## Lunch
Chicken wrap
Carrot and/or celery sticks, 1 cup
Orange
Iced tea

## Afternoon Snack
Pecans, 1 oz
Pure water

## Dinner
Spinach Soufflé
Wild Rice with Red Onions and Shiitake Mushrooms
Seltzer
Red wine

## Dessert
Blueberry and Port Frozen Yogurt

## Optional Rescue Snack
Sardines, 1½–3 oz can, with rye crispbread, 2

## *AGE-BUSTING FITNESS PLAN*

### Aerobic Training
- 3-5 minutes of warming up
- Reach 70-80% of your max heart rate for 20-30 minutes total activity with brisk walking, jogging, elliptical machine options
- 3 minutes of cooling down, heart rate less than 60% max

### Strength Training
- Rest day from strength training

### Stretching
- 4-6 body parts, 5-10 minutes of stretching time

## RELAXATION ROUTINE
- Enjoy a massage

## SUPPLEMENT ROUTINE
- Take your customized multivitamin pack
- Skin moisturizer with SPF 15

## DETOX ROUTINE
- One alcohol serving per day or none
- Add plants to your work and home environment
- Shun hydrogenated fats, corn syrup, and other added sweeteners in your diet
- Avoid processed sandwich meats that have nitrites or other chemical agents

# Day 11 (Thursday)

FOOD PLAN: Vitality Foods

**Breakfast**
Oatmeal with Apples and Blueberries
Tea or coffee

**Optional Morning Snack**
Hard-boiled egg (omega-3, free-range, organic)

**Lunch**
Mixed green salad with grilled fish or chicken or turkey
Vinaigrette Dressing, 2 tbsp
Iced tea

**Afternoon Snack**
Almonds, 1 oz
Pure water

**Dinner**
Chicken with Hazelnut Crust
Barley with Celery, Parsley, and Mushrooms
Sautéed mixed vegetables, 1–2 cups
Seltzer
Red wine

**Dessert**
Mixed fresh fruit, 1 cup
Nonfat vanilla yogurt, ½ cup

**Optional Rescue Snack**
Veggie chicken nuggets, 4 pieces

## *AGE-BUSTING FITNESS PLAN*

### Aerobic Training
- 3-5 minutes of warming up
- Reach 70-80% of your max heart rate for 20-30 minutes total activity with brisk walking, jogging, elliptical machine options
- 3 minutes of cooling down, heart rate less than 60% max

### Strength Training
- 12 body parts, 1 set, 10-16 reps
- Mixture of ball and free weight activities

### Stretching
- 4-6 body parts, 5-10 minutes of stretching time

## RELAXATION ROUTINE
- Choose a calming activity for 10-20 minutes

## SUPPLEMENT ROUTINE
- Take your customized multivitamin pack
- Skin moisturizer with SPF 15

## DETOX ROUTINE
- One alcohol serving per day or none
- Add plants to your work and home environment
- Shun hydrogenated fats, corn syrup, and other added sweeteners in your diet
- Avoid processed sandwich meats that have nitrites or other chemical agents

# Day 12 (Friday)

FOOD PLAN: Vitality Foods

**Breakfast**
Omelet with Veggies
Soy sausages, 1–2
Tea or coffee

**Optional Morning Snack**
Nonfat yogurt, 4–6 oz

**Lunch**
Veggie burger with pita bread, tomato slice, mustard, and lettuce
Sweet Potato Fries with Cinnamon, 1–2 cups
Apple
Iced tea

**Afternoon Snack**
Mixed nuts, 1 oz
Pure water

**Dinner**
Paella
Mixed green salad, 2 cups
Vinaigrette Dressing, 2 tbsp
Seltzer
Red wine

**Dessert**
Nonfat, sugar-free ice cream, 1/2–3/4 cup
Pecans, 2–3 tbsp
Hot Cocoa

**Optional Rescue Snack**
Almonds, 1 oz

## *AGE-BUSTING FITNESS PLAN*

### Aerobic Training

- 3–5 minutes of warming up
- Reach 70–80% of your max heart rate for 20–30 minutes total activity with brisk walking, jogging, elliptical machine options
- 3 minutes of cooling down, heart rate less than 60% max

### Strength Training

- Rest day from strength training

### Stretching

- 4–6 body parts, 5–10 minutes of stretching time

## RELAXATION ROUTINE

- Choose a calming activity for 10–20 minutes

## SUPPLEMENT ROUTINE

- Take your customized multivitamin pack
- Skin moisturizer with SPF 15

## DETOX ROUTINE

- One alcohol serving per day or none
- Add plants to your work and home environment
- Shun hydrogenated fats, corn syrup, and other added sweeteners in your diet
- Avoid processed sandwich meats that have nitrites or other chemical agents

# Day 13 (Saturday)

FOOD PLAN: Vitality Foods

**Breakfast**
Oatmeal Waffles with Fruit
Tea or coffee

**Optional Morning Snack**
Nonfat yogurt (4–6 oz)

**Lunch**
Mixed green salad with grilled sliced chicken or turkey breast
Vinaigrette Dressing, 2 tbsp
Iced tea

**Afternoon Snack**
Almonds, 1 oz
Pure water

**Dinner**
Tilapia with Pistachio Crust
Broccoli, 1 cup
Mixed green salad, 2 cups
Vinaigrette Dressing, 2 tbsp
Seltzer
Red wine

**Dessert**
Strawberries, ½ pint, dipped in 1 oz dark melted semi-sweet chocolate, with ¼ cup
vanilla nonfat yogurt

**Optional Rescue Snack**
Smoked oysters, 1½–3 oz can

### AGE-BUSTING FITNESS PLAN

**Aerobic Training**
- 3-5 minutes of warming up
- Reach 70-80% of your max heart rate for 20-30 minutes total activity with brisk walking, jogging, elliptical machine options
- 3 minutes of cooling down, heart rate less than 60% max

**Strength Training**
- 12 body parts, 1 set, 10-16 reps
- Mixture of ball and free weight activities

**Stretching**
- Yoga class or a 20-30 minute stretch with 10-12 body parts

## RELAXATION ROUTINE
- Choose a calming activity for 10-20 minutes

## SUPPLEMENT ROUTINE
- Take your customized multivitamin pack
- Skin moisturizer with SPF 15

## DETOX ROUTINE
- One alcohol serving per day or none
- Add plants to your work and home environment
- Shun hydrogenated fats, corn syrup, and other added sweeteners in your diet
- Avoid processed sandwich meats that have nitrites or other chemical agents

# Day 14 (Sunday)

FOOD PLAN: Vitality Foods

## Breakfast
Huevos Rancheros
Guacamole, 2 tbsp
Nonfat sour cream, 1 tbsp
Whole-wheat toast, 1 slice

## Optional Morning Snack
None

## Lunch
Gazpacho
Mixed green salad, 2 cups
Vinaigrette Dressing, 2 tbsp

## Afternoon Snack
Pecans, 1 oz
Pure water

## Dinner
Broccoli, Shiitaké, and Tofu Stir-Fry
Brown rice, ¾ cup
Seltzer
Red wine

## Dessert
Air-popped popcorn, 2 cups with 1–2 tbsp brewer's yeast
Berry-Banana Smoothie

## Optional Rescue Snack
Almonds, 1 oz

## *AGE-BUSTING FITNESS PLAN*

### Aerobic Training
- Aerobic rest day

### Strength Training
- Rest day from strength training

### Stretching
- 4-6 body parts, 5-10 minutes of stretching time

## RELAXATION ROUTINE
- Choose a calming activity for 10-20 minutes

## SUPPLEMENT ROUTINE
- Take your customized multivitamin pack
- Skin moisturizer with SPF 15

## DETOX ROUTINE
- One alcohol serving per day or none
- Add plants to your work and home environment
- Shun hydrogenated fats, corn syrup, and other added sweeteners in your diet
- Avoid processed sandwich meats that have nitrites or other chemical agents

## Breakfast Recipes

### HUEVOS RANCHEROS

*A traditional breakfast I enjoyed often in northern Mexico, featuring fried eggs, black beans, salsa, and corn tortillas.*

Serves: 2

2 teaspoons extra-virgin olive oil
4 large eggs (omega-3, free-range, organic)
⅛ teaspoon sea salt
Dash black pepper
1 cup canned black beans, rinsed and
    drained

4 medium corn tortillas
2 tablespoons grated nonfat cheese
    (or soy cheese)
½ cup Salsa (page 236)
Cilantro sprigs

Heat a skillet or sauté pan. Add oil and fry eggs, sunny side up or over easy. Season with salt and pepper.

While eggs are cooking, heat black beans in a saucepan. Heat tortillas in a skillet and keep warm.

To serve, place a tortilla on a plate and top with beans and egg. Garnish with cheese, Salsa, and cilantro sprigs.

*Per Serving*
Calories: 369 · Fiber: 10g · Saturated fat: 2.3g · Sodium: 680mg ·
Protein: 22g · Total fat: 11.5g · Carbs: 48g · Calories from fat: 27%

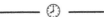

### MINI MUSHROOM CHEESE FRITTATAS

*A dozen frittatas can be made in advance in a muffin pan, refrigerated for later use. Eat them cold, or pop them in the microwave or toaster oven for a quick, easy, and tasty breakfast.*

Makes: 6 servings (2 mini frittatas per serving)

12 large eggs (omega-3, free-range, organic)
½ cup nonfat milk (or calcium-fortified
    soy milk)
1 cup grated reduced-fat or nonfat cheese
1 teaspoon extra-virgin olive oil
1 small sweet onion, diced

1½ cups sliced mushrooms
1 teaspoon Italian seasoning
¼ teaspoon sea salt
¼ teaspoon black pepper
1 large red bell pepper, finely diced
Olive oil spray

Preheat oven to 400° F.

Whisk eggs with nonfat milk in a large bowl. Add grated cheese and set aside.

Heat a sauté or omelet pan over medium-high heat. Add oil. Sauté onions and mushrooms with Italian seasoning, salt, and pepper. When onions are nearly translucent and mushrooms soft, add peppers and cook 1 more minute, stirring occasionally. Remove from heat.

Insert 12 cupcake liners into a muffin pan and spray liners with olive oil, or spray muffin pan liberally with olive oil. Divide sautéed vegetables among muffin cups and ladle egg-cheese mixture on top of the vegetables.

Slip onto the middle rack of the oven and bake until the eggs are set and browned, 15 to 20 minutes.

*Serving suggestion:* Serve with a slice of whole-grain toast or soy sausage.

*Per Serving*
Calories: 167 · Fiber: 2g · Saturated fat: 1.8g · Sodium: 404mg ·
Protein: 18g · Total fat: 7.5g · Carbs: 7.5g · Calories from fat: 40%

# MUSHROOM CHEESE FRITTATA

*An easy, hearty breakfast for a leisurely morning or a quick dinner.*

Serves: 2

| | |
|---|---|
| 4 large eggs (omega-3, free-range, organic) | 1 cup sliced mushrooms |
| ¼ cup nonfat milk | ¼ teaspoon sea salt |
| ½ cup grated reduced fat or nonfat cheese | ⅛ teaspoon black pepper |
| | ½ teaspoon Italian seasoning |
| ½ teaspoon extra-virgin olive oil | ½ medium red bell pepper, diced |
| ½ medium sweet onion, diced | Parsley sprigs |

Preheat oven to 400° F.

Whisk eggs with milk. Add cheese and set aside.

Heat an ovenproof sauté or omelet pan over medium-high heat. Add oil. Sauté onions and mushrooms with salt, pepper, and Italian seasoning. After 2 to 3 minutes, add peppers and sauté another 1 to 2 minutes. When onions are translucent and mushrooms soft, add bell pepper, cook another 1 to 2 minutes, then pour in egg mixture. As frittata cooks, gently lift edges and tilt pan, allowing the uncooked mixture to run under the edges. Slip onto the middle rack of the oven and bake until the eggs are set and browned, 15 to 20 minutes.

*Serving suggestion:* Serve with whole-grain toast and garnish with sprigs of parsley. As a dinner entrée, serve with Salsa, Guacamole, and Sweet Potato Fries.

*Per Serving*
Calories: 205 · Fiber: 2g · Saturated fat: 1.9g · Sodium: 631mg ·
Protein: 22g · Total fat: 9g · Carbs: 11g · Calories from fat: 38%

🕐

# OATMEAL WAFFLES WITH FRUIT

*Easy to prepare, and a breakfast my family looks forward to on weekends.
Topped with fresh fruit and sugar-free syrup, it's packed with fiber and
nutrients—and makes a real treat. Wrap and freeze any extras
to toast another morning.*

Serves: 4

2 cups quick-cooking oats
1 cup whole-wheat pastry flour
2 teaspoons baking powder
¼ teaspoon sea salt
2 tablespoons freshly ground flaxseed
¼ cup chopped pecans
3 large eggs (omega-3, free-range,
    organic)
1½ cups nonfat milk

1 tablespoon canola oil (organic, expeller-
    pressed)
Canola oil spray
2 cups berries (or other fruit such as
    sliced bananas, chopped apples, or
    chopped pears)
¼ cup sugar-free maple-flavored syrup
    (or sugar-free jam or unsweetened
    applesauce)

Preheat a waffle iron.

Combine oats, flour, baking powder, salt, flaxseed, and pecans in a bowl.
Separate eggs and whisk yolks, milk, and oil together. Gently mix into dry
ingredients.

Beat egg whites until stiff and fold into batter. Spray canola oil on waffle
iron and pour in batter (the amount will vary with size of your waffle iron),
aiming to cover ⅔ to ¾ of the iron's surface before closing. Cook until golden
brown.

Top waffles with berries and syrup and serve.

*Variation:* Add ½ cup of berries to the batter; top cooked waffles with
remaining berries.

*Per Serving*
Calories: 481 · Fiber: 11.6g · Saturated fat: 2g · Sodium: 418mg ·
Protein: 20g · Total fat: 16.5g · Carbs: 69g · Calories from fat: 29%

# OATMEAL WITH APPLES AND BLUEBERRIES

*Simple, hearty, and heart-healthy. The oatmeal lowers your cholesterol level while the blueberries block your cholesterol from being converted into plaque.*

Serves: 2

1 cup quick-cooking (5-minute) oats
⅛ teaspoon sea salt
¼ teaspoon cinnamon
1 medium apple, cored and cut into
    ½-inch cubes

½ cup blueberries
½ cup nonfat milk (or calcium-fortified
    soy milk)

Combine oats, 2 cups water, salt, cinnamon, and apple. Cook for five minutes on stovetop or in microwave. Top with blueberries and milk and serve.

*Per Serving*
Calories: 362 · Fiber: 9.3g · Saturated fat: 0.8g · Sodium: 71mg ·
Protein: 19g · Total fat: 7.6g · Carbs: 81g · Calories from fat: 12%

# OMELET WITH VEGGIES

*An easy-to-prepare and hearty start to the day. Adding veggies to an omelet increases your fiber and nutrient intake, and leaves you feeling more satisfied.*

Serves: 2

4 large eggs (omega-3, free-range, organic)
1 teaspoon extra-virgin olive oil
½ cup diced red onion
1 cup sliced mushrooms
½ cup diced bell peppers, any color, to
    taste

¼ teaspoon sea salt
⅛ teaspoon black pepper
¼ cup chopped parsley
Olive oil spray

Beat eggs in a bowl. Heat a sauté pan over medium-high heat, then add oil and sauté onion, mushrooms, and peppers. Add salt and pepper. When vegetables are 80 percent cooked, remove from heat and mix with eggs. Add parsley. Quickly wipe sauté pan with a paper towel, spray with olive oil for 2 seconds, and pour egg and vegetable mixture back into the hot pan. Lift edges of omelet as it cooks so uncooked mixture can flow underneath. When done, fold in half and serve.

*Serving suggestion:* Serve with a slice of whole-grain toast or soy sausage.

*Per Serving*
Calories: 145 · Fiber: 2g · Saturated fat: 1.9g · Sodium: 403mg ·
Protein: 8g · Total fat: 7.6g · Carbs: 8g · Calories from fat: 45%

PHASE ONE

## Lunch Recipes

## CRAB WITH MIXED SALAD

### Serves: 2

½ pound crabmeat, picked over for shells and cartilage
2 cups mixed organic greens
1 cup grated or finely chopped red cabbage
2 medium carrots, grated or finely diced
1 cup cherry tomatoes

One 15-ounce can corn, rinsed
4 tablespoons Vinaigrette Dressing (page 233)
Juice of 1 lemon
2 tablespoons chopped cilantro (or parsley)

Rinse crab with water in a colander and drain.

Toss greens, cabbage, carrots, tomatoes, and corn with Vinaigrette Dressing. Divide among two plates and top with crab. Drizzle lemon juice over and garnish with cilantro.

*Per Serving*
Calories: 323 · Fiber: 6.6g · Saturated fat: 1.9g · Sodium: 445mg ·
Protein: 27g · Total fat: 12g · Carbs: 27g · Calories from fat: 34%

## GAZPACHO

*This is a wonderful chilled soup, especially delightful on a hot summer day, and it is packed with anti-aging ingredients. This dish originates in southern Spain, and while in restaurants it is usually served in bowls, traditionally it is drunk from a glass.*

### Serves: 4

1 tablespoon extra-virgin olive oil
1 tablespoon balsamic vinegar
1 medium cucumber, chopped, divided
2 garlic cloves
2 pounds tomatoes (about 6 medium)
½ cup whole-wheat bread crumbs
Juice of 1 lemon
½ teaspoon sea salt

½ teaspoon paprika
¼ cup mint
¼ cup flat-leaf parsley
¼ cup basil
½ medium red onion, diced
1 medium green bell pepper, diced
1 medium tomato, diced

Place olive oil, vinegar, half the cucumber, garlic, 2 pounds tomatoes, bread crumbs, lemon juice, salt, paprika, mint, parsley, and basil in a food processor and pulse until smooth. Add up to 1 cup water to thin if needed.

To serve, pour gazpacho into bowls or glasses, and top with onion, remaining cucumber, pepper, and diced tomato.

*Per Serving*
Calories: 90 · Fiber: 3.6g · Saturated fat: 0.3g · Sodium: 220mg ·
Protein: 3g · Total fat: 2.3g · Carbs: 17.5g · Calories from fat: 20%

## SALMON SPREAD WITH PITA

*This healthy spread is great in pita bread. Try various substitutes for the usual mayo.*

Serves: 4

7 ounces canned salmon, preferably
    wild Alaskan
2 medium scallions, chopped
1 teaspoon Dijon mustard
3 tablespoons Tomato Sauce (page 237)
    (or nonfat cottage cheese or soy
    mayonnaise)

2 teaspoons capers
¼ cup diced celery
4 pita breads
Lettuce or spinach leaves

Flake salmon and mix with scallions, mustard, tomato sauce, capers, and celery. Stuff a pita bread with lettuce or spinach leaves and a scoop of the spread.

*Per Serving*
Calories: 251 · Fiber: 6g · Saturated fat: 1g · Sodium: 643mg ·
Protein: 17g · Total fat: 5g · Carbs: 31g · Calories from fat: 20%

## SHRIMP BISQUE

*Simple, smooth, flavorful. For added color and heartiness, try adding corn, spinach, and/or chopped tomatoes.*

Serves: 4

1 tablespoon canola oil (organic, expeller-
    pressed)
1 medium onion, minced
2 tablespoons whole-wheat pastry flour
¼ cup sherry (or white wine)
2 cups (low-sodium) vegetable stock (or
    chicken stock)

¼ cup tomato paste
1 pound shrimp, shelled, deveined, and cut
    into bite-sized pieces
2 cups nonfat milk, warmed (or calcium-
    fortified soy milk)
Chopped chives (or parsley)

Heat a saucepan over medium-high heat, add canola oil, and sauté onion about 2 minutes, until soft. Add flour and cook 2 minutes, stirring occasionally. Add

*(continued)*

sherry a tablespoon at a time, stirring continuously until flour mixture thickens and becomes smooth. Add stock and tomato paste and mix well. Bring to a boil, reduce heat, and simmer 10 minutes. Add shrimp and simmer 10 minutes more, until shrimp are pink. Add milk; do not boil soup after this point or it may curdle. Garnish with chives and serve.

*Per Serving*
Calories: 257 • Fiber: 2g • Saturated fat: 0.8g • Sodium: 494mg •
Protein: 30g • Total fat: 6g • Carbs: 17g • Calories from fat: 21%

## Dinner Recipes

### BROCCOLI, SHIITAKE, AND TOFU STIR-FRY

*I like the color in this meal. Shiitakes are incredible mushrooms, vastly more nutritious than regular mushrooms and with cancer-fighting and blood-sugar-lowering properties. Substitute shrimp or chicken for tofu if you prefer.*

Serves: 4

| | |
|---|---|
| 1 teaspoon low-sodium soy sauce | 1 tablespoon canola oil (organic, expeller-pressed) |
| 2 tablespoons sake (or white wine) | |
| 2 tablespoons rice vinegar | 1 tablespoon grated ginger |
| 1 tablespoon kuzu root powder (or cornstarch) | 2 cups shiitake mushrooms, stemmed and sliced |
| 14 ounces extra-firm tofu, cut into 1-inch cubes | 3 medium carrots, sliced |
| | 2 cups sliced broccoli |
| 1 tablespoon miso | 4 garlic cloves, minced |
| 2 tablespoons tomato paste | 4 cups cooked soba noodles (about 8 ounces dry) |
| ½ teaspoon Asian chili paste or to taste | ¼ cup cashews, toasted |

Mix soy sauce, sake, vinegar, and kuzu in a bowl. Add tofu and toss to coat. Dissolve miso, tomato paste, and Asian chili paste in ¼ cup hot water and add to tofu.

Heat a sauté pan, add canola oil, and sauté ginger and mushrooms for 3 minutes, stirring occasionally. If it seems dry, add 2 tablespoons sake or water. Add carrots and broccoli and sauté 3 minutes. Add garlic, tofu, and marinade, cover, and steam for 3 minutes, stirring occasionally.

Arrange soba noodles on a serving platter, top with tofu-vegetable mixture, and garnish with cashews.

*Per Serving*
Calories: 441 • Fiber: 7.5g • Saturated fat: 3g • Sodium: 441mg •
Protein: 17.5g • Total fat: 16g • Carbs: 62g • Calories from fat: 31%

# CHICKEN BREASTS WITH GINGER, GARLIC, AND CHILI

### Serves: 2

2 teaspoons grated ginger
2 garlic cloves, minced
⅛ teaspoon cayenne or to taste
1 teaspoon low-sodium soy sauce
Juice of 1 lime

1 teaspoon sesame oil
2 skinless, boneless chicken breasts
(about 5 ounces each)
Olive oil spray

Combine ginger, garlic, cayenne, soy sauce, lime juice, and sesame oil in a large bowl. Add chicken and marinate in the refrigerator 30 to 60 minutes.

Heat sauté pan over medium-high heat and spray with olive oil. Cook chicken 4 to 5 minutes. Turn chicken and drizzle a spoonful of marinade over each breast. Cook 4 to 5 minutes more or until done.

*Serving suggestion:* Serve with brown rice, sautéed vegetables, and a mixed salad with Ginger-Sesame Dressing (page 233).

*Per Serving*
Calories: 229 · Fiber: 1g · Saturated fat: 0.3g · Sodium: 191mg ·
Protein: 42g · Total fat: 5g · Carbs: 4g · Calories from fat: 20%

# CHICKEN WITH HAZELNUT CRUST

### Serves: 2

1 large egg (omega-3, free-range, organic)
⅓ cup ground hazelnuts
¼ teaspoon sea salt
⅛ teaspoon black pepper

½ teaspoon dried rosemary, chopped
2 skinless, boneless chicken breasts
(about 5 ounces each)
Olive oil spray

Preheat oven to 400° F.

Beat egg in a shallow bowl. In another shallow bowl mix hazelnuts with salt, pepper, and rosemary. Dip chicken breasts first in egg and then into nut mixture. Spray baking pan with olive oil and place chicken on pan. Spray top of chicken with oil. Bake 20 minutes, until golden.

*Serving suggestion:* Pair with Roasted Beets, Carrots, and Parsnips (page 291).

*Per Serving*
Calories: 317 · Fiber: 2g · Saturated fat: 2g · Sodium: 409mg ·
Protein: 39g · Total fat: 16g · Carbs: 4g · Calories from fat: 45%

# CIOPPINO

*This is a San Francisco version of an Italian seafood stew, a favorite in our home. Make sure you use the freshest fish and shellfish. Feel free to vary the ingredients according to availability.*

Serves: 4

1 tablespoon extra-virgin olive oil
1 medium onion, chopped
¼ teaspoon sea salt
1 cup sliced mushrooms
¼ teaspoon dried rosemary
¼ teaspoon dried thyme
¼ teaspoon dried oregano
¼ teaspoon dried basil
¼ teaspoon black pepper
3 large carrots, chopped
3 celery stalks, chopped

1 cup dry red wine
2 medium potatoes, cut into 1-inch cubes
1 cup tomato sauce
2 cups low-sodium vegetable broth
1 pound mussels in the shell
¾ pound salmon, cut into 1-inch pieces
⅔ pound shrimp, peeled and deveined
8 large scallops (or ¼ pound bay scallops)
½ cup chopped parsley

Heat a large pot over medium-high heat. Add oil, onion, salt, mushrooms, rosemary, thyme, oregano, basil, and pepper and stir. Cook 2 minutes. Add carrots and celery and cook another 2 minutes. Add wine and simmer for 30 seconds, stirring. Add potatoes, tomato sauce, and broth, reduce heat, and let simmer for 15 to 20 minutes, until carrots and potatoes are nearly cooked.

Meanwhile, bring water to a boil in a pan with a steamer insert. Add mussels and steam until they open. Drain and set aside.

Increase heat under stew to medium-high and add salmon, shrimp, and scallops. Cook 3 minutes or until shrimp turn pink. Add drained mussels and simmer 1 minute more. Garnish with parsley and serve.

*Per Serving*
Calories: 444 • Fiber: 8g • Saturated fat: 1.7g • Sodium: 736mg •
Protein: 51g • Total fat: 8.5g • Carbs: 30g • Calories from fat: 17%

---

# GARLIC SHRIMP BURRITOS

*When looking for a quick meal, burritos come to the rescue! Extras can easily be refrigerated and saved for lunch the next day.*

Serves: 4

8 whole-wheat tortillas (or corn tortillas)
1 tablespoon extra-virgin olive oil
1 pound shrimp, shelled and deveined
8 garlic cloves, minced
⅛ teaspoon sea salt

⅛ teaspoon cayenne or to taste
1 cup Roasted Pepper Salsa (page 236)
2 cups shredded cabbage
Guacamole (page 234)
¼ cup chopped cilantro (or parsley)

Heat tortillas in a skillet and keep warm. Meanwhile, heat a sauté pan over medium-high heat, add oil, and sauté shrimp and garlic until shrimp is pink. Add salt and cayenne.

Lay one tortilla flat. Place one-eighth each of shrimp mixture, Roasted Pepper Salsa, cabbage, Guacamole, and cilantro at bottom of tortilla. Roll up, tucking sides in. Repeat with other tortillas.

*Per Serving*
Calories: 376 · Fiber: 18g · Saturated fat: 2.4g · Sodium: 768mg ·
Protein: 30g · Total fat: 15g · Carbs: 32g · Calories from fat: 35%

# GRILLED SALMON WITH LEMON, GARLIC, AND DILL

*Fresh dill is great with salmon, but dried dill works too.*

Serves: 4

1½ pounds salmon (preferably wild
  Alaskan coho)
Juice of 1 lemon
¼ teaspoon sea salt

4 garlic cloves, minced
¼ cup chopped fresh dill
Lemon wedges
Dill sprigs

Rinse salmon and pat dry. Mix lemon juice, salt, garlic, and dill and add fish; refrigerate for 30 minutes, turning salmon once. Grill salmon 5 minutes on one side; turn and top with garlic and dill from marinade. Grill for 5 more minutes or until done. Garnish with lemon wedges and dill sprigs.

*Per Serving*
Calories: 245 · Fiber: 0.5g · Saturated fat: 1.8g · Sodium: 381mg ·
Protein: 41.5g · Total fat: 7.5g · Carbs: 2.5g · Calories from fat: 28%

# PAELLA

*This dish from southern Spain originally was called "para ella" (for her) and was essentially the leftovers after the men ate. The ladies would add bits of seafood, chicken, and/or sausage to rice, onions, and peppers, and spice up their dish with a wonderful but now expensive spice, saffron.*

Serves: 4

2 tablespoons extra-virgin olive oil
1 medium sweet onion, chopped
2 teaspoons paprika
½ teaspoon dried thyme
2 tablespoons tomato paste
½ teaspoon saffron (or turmeric)
1½ cups brown rice
1 medium red bell pepper, diced

1 medium green bell pepper, diced
1 pound red snapper fillets (or cod or
  other white fish), cut into 1-inch pieces
¾ pound large shrimp
1 pound mussels and/or clams, shells
  scrubbed clean
1 cup peas (fresh or frozen)

*(continued)*

Heat a large sauté pan over medium-high heat, add oil, and sauté onion for 2 minutes. Add paprika, thyme, tomato paste, saffron, and rice; cook, stirring, 1 to 2 minutes. Add 1½ cups water and peppers, stir, and bring to a boil. Reduce heat and simmer, covered, for 20 to 25 minutes over low heat, until most of the liquid is absorbed.

Stir in fish, shrimp, and mussels and/or clams and cover. Simmer over low heat another 20 minutes, or until rice is cooked and clams and mussels have opened. Add peas and simmer 3 to 5 minutes more. If the paella appears dry, add 2 tablespoons of water; if too wet, simmer uncovered until most of the liquid is absorbed.

*Per Serving*
Calories: 559 · Fiber: 7.3g · Saturated fat: 1.8g · Sodium: 500mg ·
Protein: 49g · Total fat: 12g · Carbs: 64g · Calories from fat: 19%

## SALMON WITH GINGER-CHILI SAUCE

*Wild Alaskan salmon is one of the healthiest protein sources. If you can't get fresh Alaskan salmon, then look for vacuum-packed frozen salmon. This sauce is also terrific with white-fleshed fish, scallops, and shrimp dishes. You can grill or broil this meal.*

Serves: 4

½ teaspoon lime zest
Juice of 1 lime
2 tablespoons rice vinegar
1 tablespoon low-sodium soy sauce
2 tablespoons brown sugar (or 5 packets of Splenda)

2 tablespoons tomato paste
1 tablespoon grated ginger
4 garlic cloves, minced
¼ teaspoon cayenne or to taste
1 teaspoon sesame oil
1½ pounds salmon

Rinse salmon and pat dry. Combine zest, juice, vinegar, soy sauce, sugar, tomato paste, ginger, garlic, cayenne, and sesame oil in a bowl. Add salmon and marinate for at least 30 minutes, turning salmon once.

Grill or broil salmon for 5 to 7 minutes on each side until fish is cooked through but not dry.

*Per Serving*
Calories: 298 · Fiber: 0.5g · Saturated fat: 2.3g · Sodium: 354mg ·
Protein: 38g · Total fat: 11g · Carbs: 9g · Calories from fat: 35%

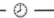

## SICHUAN STIR-FRY

*The Sichuan region of China relies on garlic, red pepper, leeks, ginger, and vinegar to flavor its cuisine. This dish is also excellent with shrimp or chicken in place of tofu.*

Serves: 4

1 tablespoon miso dissolved in ⅓ cup
   hot water
1 teaspoon Asian chili sauce or to taste
1 teaspoon low-sodium soy sauce
1 lime, juiced
1 tablespoon tomato paste
4 garlic cloves, minced
1 tablespoon grated ginger
2 teaspoons kuzu root powder (or
   cornstarch)
2 tablespoons rice vinegar
14 ounces firm tofu, cut into ½-inch cubes
3 medium Japanese eggplants (or 1
   regular eggplant)

1 teaspoon canola oil (organic, expeller-
   pressed)
2 medium leeks, diced
1 cup stemmed and sliced shiitake
   mushrooms
2 cups chopped broccoli
2 medium red bell peppers, sliced in thin
   strips
1 teaspoon sesame oil
4 cups cooked soba noodles (about
   8 ounces dry)
⅔ cup cashews, toasted
¼ cup chopped cilantro (or parsley)

Combine miso mixture, chili sauce, soy sauce, lime juice, tomato paste, garlic, and ginger. Dissolve kuzu in rice vinegar and add to marinade. Add tofu and marinate at least 30 minutes at room temperature or all day in the refrigerator.

Slice eggplant lengthwise into finger-sized pieces. Microwave or steam for 5–6 minutes to precook.

Heat a sauté pan or wok over medium-high heat, add oil, then sauté leeks and mushrooms for 2 to 3 minutes, until softened. Add broccoli, bell peppers, eggplant, and tofu with marinade and sauté 4 to 5 minutes covered, stirring occasionally. Stir in sesame oil. Serve over soba and garnish with cashews and cilantro.

*Per Serving*
Calories: 485 · Fiber: 9.5g · Saturated fat: 2.9g · Sodium: 658mg ·
Protein: 19.5g · Total fat: 18.3g · Carbs: 60.5g · Calories from fat: 34%

## SOLE WITH ALMOND CRUST

*Fish with a nut crust is very tasty. Try almonds, pistachios, or hazelnuts. Choose the freshest fish you can find—flounder, tilapia, or cod also works well here.*

Serves: 4

1½ pounds sole (in 4 fillets)
1 large egg (omega-3, free-range, organic)
1 cup almonds, coarsely ground
½ teaspoon sea salt

⅛ teaspoon black pepper
Canola oil spray
4 lemon wedges

Preheat oven to 425° F.

Rinse sole fillets and pat dry. Beat the egg in a bowl. In a separate shallow bowl, combine ground almonds with salt and pepper. Dip the fish first in the

*(continued)*

PHASE ONE

egg, then in the almond mixture. Spray a baking dish with oil and place fish on it. Lightly spray the top of each fillet.

Bake about 20 minutes, until tender and flaky. Garnish with a wedge of lemon.

*Per Serving*
Calories: 355 · Fiber: 5g · Saturated fat: 1.6g · Sodium: 561mg ·
Protein: 36.5g · Total fat: 20g · Carbs: 8g · Calories from fat: 50%

# SPINACH SOUFFLÉ

*This easy-to-make dish is colorful and flavorful, though it rises less than other soufflés. You can even make a double batch, allow one soufflé to collapse, and serve it chilled for a brunch or breakfast entrée.*

Serves: 4

1 tablespoon extra-virgin olive oil
1 medium onion, diced
¼ teaspoon sea salt
1 teaspoon Italian seasoning
2 tablespoons whole-wheat pastry flour
½ cup nonfat milk
4 garlic cloves, minced
¼ cup chopped basil
1¼ cups spinach, cooked and drained, chopped

½ cup grated reduced-fat mozzarella or Swiss cheese
4 egg yolks (omega-3, free-range, organic)
8 egg whites
1 slice whole-wheat bread, toasted and processed into crumbs (½ cup)
Olive oil spray
2 tablespoons Parmesan cheese
Basil sprigs

Preheat oven to 400° F. Heat sauté pan over medium-high heat, add oil, then sauté onion with salt and Italian seasoning for 3 to 4 minutes, until onion softens. Stir in flour and cook for 2 minutes, stirring occasionally. Pour in half the milk, stir to mix, and let thicken. Add remaining milk and garlic and cook until the sauce is the consistency of heavy cream. Remove from heat and mix in chopped basil, spinach, grated cheese, and egg yolks.

Whip egg whites until stiff. Fold bread crumbs into egg whites, then gently fold the sauce and spinach mixture into the egg whites, adding one-quarter of the sauce at a time. Be careful not to overmix or the soufflé will not rise.

Spray a soufflé dish with olive oil and pour mixture in. Sprinkle Parmesan on top and bake on the middle rack in the oven 30 minutes, until top is golden and a toothpick inserted in the center comes out clean. Garnish with basil sprigs and serve immediately.

*Per Serving*
Calories: 188 · Fiber: 3.3g · Saturated fat: 2.5g · Sodium: 667mg ·
Protein: 9g · Total fat: 9g · Carbs: 11g · Calories from fat: 42%

# SWEET AND TANGY TOFU

*This is my favorite way to serve tofu.*

Serves: 4

14 ounces extra-firm tofu
2 garlic cloves, minced
1½ tablespoons grated ginger
1 tablespoon sesame oil

¼ cup rice vinegar
2 tablespoons low-sodium soy sauce
1 tablespoon sugar (or 2 packets Splenda)

Preheat oven to 425° F. Rinse tofu, pat dry, and cut into strips the size of french fries.

Mix remaining ingredients and pour over tofu. Marinate for 30 minutes. Drain tofu, spread on a nonstick baking pan, and bake for 20 minutes, until brown and firm.

*Per Serving*
Calories: 112 · Fiber: 1g · Saturated fat: 0g · Sodium: 602mg ·
Protein: 8g · Total fat: 4.7g · Carbs: 9g · Calories from fat: 39%

# THAI STUFFED CABBAGE ROLLS

*This dish is a bit messy but lots of fun to eat—especially nice on a warm sunny day.*
*You can substitute cooked cold shrimp or chicken strips for the tofu.*

Serves: 4

12 large cabbage leaves, red or green
2 cups shredded cabbage, red or green
Sweet and Tangy Tofu (above)
2 medium carrots, grated
1 large green bell pepper, julienned
1 large yellow or orange bell pepper,
    julienned

1 cup fresh mint, chopped
½ cup Thai basil (or regular basil),
    chopped
1 cup Spicy Peanut Sauce (page 237)
¼ cup Thai sweetened chili sauce
½ cup Oyster and Lime Sauce
    (page 235)

Steam cabbage leaves and shredded cabbage for 4 minutes, until somewhat softened. Place tofu, cabbage, carrots, peppers, mint, basil, Spicy Peanut Sauce, sweetened chili sauce, and Oyster and Lime Sauce in separate bowls. Guests assemble their own rolls by using a cabbage leaf as a wrapper for the other ingredients. The sauces can be spooned onto the other ingredients before rolling or used as dipping sauces.

*Per Serving*
Calories: 275 · Fiber: 11g · Saturated fat: 1.7g · Sodium: 293mg ·
Protein: 17g · Total fat: 12g · Carbs: 32g · Calories from fat: 35%

# TILAPIA WITH PISTACHIO CRUST

*I really enjoy the tilapia-pistachio combo. Always choose the freshest fish you can find (you can substitute sole, flounder, or cod), and try a variety of nut crusts—almonds, hazelnuts, or pecans—to find your favorite combination.*

Serves: 2

1 pound tilapia (in 2 fillets)
1 large egg (omega-3, free-range, organic)
½ cup coarsely ground pistachios
¼ teaspoon sea salt

⅛ teaspoon black pepper
Canola oil spray
2 lemon wedges
½ recipe Mango Salsa (page 235)

Preheat oven to 400° F.

Rinse fish and pat dry. Beat the egg in a bowl. In a separate shallow bowl, combine pistachios with salt and pepper. Dip the fish first in the egg, then in the pistachio mixture. Spray a baking dish with oil and place fish on it. Lightly spray the top of each fillet.

Bake about 20 minutes, until tender and flaky. Garnish with a wedge of lemon and serve with Mango Salsa.

*Per Serving*
Calories: 466 · Fiber: 3.3g · Saturated fat: 2g · Sodium: 304mg ·
Protein: 55g · Total fat: 26g · Carbs: 19g · Calories from fat: 48%

## Side Dish Recipes

# BARLEY WITH CELERY, PARSLEY, AND MUSHROOMS

*Barley is packed with anti-aging compounds and fiber and has the lowest glycemic load of the common grains. It has a delightful nutty and chewy texture.*

Serves: 4

1 cup hulled barley
1 tablespoon extra-virgin olive oil
½ medium red onion, chopped
2 cups sliced mushrooms
¼ teaspoon sea salt
⅛ teaspoon black pepper

1 teaspoon dried oregano
2 celery stalks with tops, chopped
1 medium carrot, grated
2 scallions, diced
2 garlic cloves, minced
½ cup chopped flat-leaf parsley

Bring barley and 3 cups water to a boil. Simmer 40 minutes, until barley is tender but still al dente (chewy and firm to the bite).

When barley is 10 minutes from being done, heat a sauté pan over medium-high heat, add oil, and sauté onion and mushrooms with salt, black pepper, and oregano. After 2 minutes, add celery and cook 1 minute. Add carrot, scallions, garlic, and parsley and cook 1 to 2 minutes.

When barley is cooked, drain any remaining liquid. Mix vegetables into barley and serve hot.

*Variations:* Use pearl barley, reduce water to 2 cups, and simmer for 15 to 20 minutes.

To serve chilled, rinse barley with cold water, drain, mix with sautéed vegetables, and refrigerate for at least 30 minutes.

You can add chicken, shrimp, beans, baked or marinated tofu and serve as an entrée.

*Per Serving*
Calories: 270 · Fiber: 11g · Saturated fat: 0.7g · Sodium: 170mg ·
Protein: 7g · Total fat: 4.5g · Carbs: 55g · Calories from fat: 14%

# SWEET POTATO FRIES
# WITH CINNAMON

*Simple, wonderful.*

Serves: 4

2 large sweet potatoes
Canola oil spray
¼ teaspoon sea salt

¼ teaspoon black pepper
½ teaspoon cinnamon

Preheat oven to 425° F.

Peel sweet potatoes and cut into strips. Spray with oil. Season with salt, pepper, and cinnamon. Spread on a baking sheet and bake 15 minutes. Serve warm or cold.

*Per Serving*
Calories: 69 · Fiber: 2g · Saturated fat: 0g · Sodium: 149mg ·
Protein: 1g · Total fat: 0.2g · Carbs: 16g · Calories from fat: 3%

## WILD RICE WITH RED ONIONS AND SHIITAKE MUSHROOMS

*Wild rice is one of my favorite grains, very nutritious and also fragrant.*
*I like to make a double batch of this recipe and save the extra in the refrigerator for*
*another meal. You can mix wild rice with quinoa, brown rice, or other grains—*
*adding different textures, colors, and nutrients. Add white beans and chopped*
*tomatoes to the leftovers, and it makes a nice cold salad lunch.*

Serves: 4

| | |
|---|---|
| 1½ cups wild rice | ½ teaspoon sea salt |
| 2 teaspoons extra-virgin olive oil | ¼ teaspoon black pepper |
| 1 medium red onion, cut into thin slices or diced | 1 teaspoon Italian seasoning |
| 1 cup stemmed and sliced shiitake mushrooms | 4 scallions, chopped |
| | ½ cup chopped flat-leaf parsley |
| | 2 tablespoons slivered almonds |

Bring wild rice and 4 cups water to a boil. Simmer 40 to 50 minutes until tender but still al dente (chewy and firm to the bite). Drain remaining liquid.

When rice is 10 minutes from being done, heat a sauté pan over medium-high heat, add oil, and sauté onion and mushrooms with salt, black pepper, and Italian seasoning until onion is translucent and mushrooms are soft. Add three-quarters of the scallions and cook 1 to 2 minutes.

Mix vegetables into cooked wild rice. Garnish with remaining scallion, parsley, and almonds.

*Per Serving*
Calories: 258 · Fiber: 6g · Saturated fat: 0.5g · Sodium: 302mg ·
Protein: 9g · Total fat: 5.5g · Carbs: 46g · Calories from fat: 18%

## Salad Recipes

## CUCUMBER SALAD WITH GINGER-SESAME DRESSING

Serves: 4

| | |
|---|---|
| 2 medium cucumbers, thinly sliced | 4 cups spinach |
| Ginger-Sesame Dressing (page 233) | 8 cherry tomatoes |

PHASE ONE

Mix cucumbers and dressing and marinate for 10 to 30 minutes. Rinse and dry spinach leaves and tear into bite-sized pieces. Divide spinach among individual salad plates. Arrange cucumber over spinach, drizzling remaining dressing over the cucumber and spinach. Garnish with cherry tomatoes. Serve chilled.

*Per Serving*
Calories: 30 · Fiber: 2g · Saturated fat: 0g · Sodium: 28mg ·
Protein: 2g · Total fat: 0.3g · Carbs: 5.8g · Calories from fat: 9%

## GINGER-SESAME DRESSING

*A great dressing with Asian cuisine.*

Serves: 4

1 tablespoon sherry (or white wine or apple juice)
2 tablespoons canola oil (organic, expeller-pressed)
3 tablespoons rice vinegar

1 tablespoon sesame oil
1 tablespoon grated ginger
½ teaspoon low-sodium soy sauce
1 or 2 garlic cloves, minced

Mix all ingredients and blend until smooth. Chill. Shake before serving.

*Per Serving*
Calories: 104 · Fiber: 0g · Saturated fat: 0.5g · Sodium: 24mg ·
Protein: 0.2g · Total fat: 10.5g · Carbs: 1.3g · Calories from fat: 91%

## VINAIGRETTE DRESSING

*This is my basic salad dressing. Make a double or triple batch and store up to one week refrigerated.*

Serves: 4

3 tablespoons extra-virgin olive oil
2 tablespoons balsamic vinegar
1 tablespoon dry white wine
1 tablespoon lime juice

1 teaspoon Dijon mustard
½ teaspoon low-sodium soy sauce
1 garlic clove, finely minced, or to taste
½ teaspoon Italian seasoning

Mix all ingredients.

*Variation:* Add blueberries or raspberries for variety.

*Per Serving*
Calories: 102 · Fiber: 0g · Saturated fat: 1g · Sodium: 27mg ·
Protein: 0.1g · Total fat: 10g · Carbs: 11g · Calories from fat: 91%

PHASE ONE

## CREAMY VINAIGRETTE SALAD DRESSING

*This produces a thicker, smoother vinaigrette dressing.*
*Make a double or triple batch and store up to one week refrigerated.*

Serves: 4

3 tablespoons extra-virgin olive oil

2 tablespoons red wine vinegar (or rice vinegar)

1 tablespoon wine

2 tablespoons nonfat sour cream

1 teaspoon Dijon mustard or to taste

1 garlic clove, finely minced, or to taste

Mix all ingredients. Serve chilled.

*Per Serving*
Calories: 100 · Fiber: 0g · Saturated fat: 1g · Sodium: 11mg ·
Protein: 0.5g · Total fat: 10.8g · Carbs: 2.5g · Calories from fat: 90%

## Condiment Recipes

## GUACAMOLE

*This is a frequent side dish in our home, best prepared just before serving.*
*To store for a few hours, drizzle extra lime juice over the top,*
*cover, and refrigerate.*

Serves: 4

1 large avocado

Juice of 1 lime

1/4 medium red onion, minced

1 garlic clove, minced

1/4 cup chopped cilantro

1/2 teaspoon paprika

1/4 teaspoon cayenne or to taste

Cilantro sprigs

Peel, pit, and mash avocado. Add lime juice, onion, garlic, chopped cilantro, paprika, and cayenne and mix well. Garnish with cilantro sprigs.

*Per Serving*
Calories: 93 · Fiber: 4.6g · Saturated fat: 1.3g · Sodium: 146mg ·
Protein: 1.4g · Total fat: 6.8g · Carbs: 9.2g · Calories from fat: 59%

# MANGO SALSA

*Terrific on fish.*

Serves: 4

2 cups diced mango
½ cup finely diced red onion
Juice of 1 lime
¼ teaspoon sea salt
¼ teaspoon paprika

1 garlic clove, minced, or to taste
¼ cup chopped cilantro
1 medium apple, peeled, cored, and cut
into ½-inch cubes

Combine ingredients and refrigerate at least 30 minutes.

*Per Serving*
Calories: 87 · Fiber: 3.3g · Saturated fat: 0g · Sodium: 145mg ·
Protein: 1g · Total fat: 0.5g · Carbs: 23g · Calories from fat: 5%

# OYSTER AND LIME SAUCE

*Oyster and lime sauce adds tanginess to Asian cuisine.*
*This sauce is terrific for dipping Thai Stuffed Cabbage Rolls,*
*or for marinating either tofu, shrimp, or fish.*

Makes: ½ cup

2 tablespoons oyster sauce
3 tablespoons lime juice
1 tablespoon sherry (or white wine or
sake)

1 teaspoon low-sodium soy sauce
1 garlic clove, minced
¼ cup chopped cilantro
¼ teaspoon lime zest (optional)

Combine all ingredients. Refrigerate and serve chilled.

*Per Serving*
Calories: 9 · Fiber: 0.1g · Saturated fat: 0g · Sodium: 100mg ·
Protein: 0.2g · Total fat: 0.1g · Carbs: 1.4g · Calories from fat: 2%

# ROASTED BELL PEPPERS

*Roasted peppers freeze well. They are much sweeter than cooked peppers*
*and are lovely in many Mexican and Latin American dishes.*

12 or more bell peppers (any color)          Olive oil spray

*(continued)*

Preheat broiler. Cut off pepper crown and scoop out seeds. Spray peppers and a rimmed baking pan with olive oil spray. Broil on the top rack until peppers are evenly charred, turning occasionally, a total of about 12 minutes.

Allow to cool a few minutes and remove skin. Serve immediately, or cool completely and freeze.

*Serving suggestion:* You can chop peppers for a stir-fry, bake them in cornbread, fill them with rice and beans, or purée them for a dip.

## ROASTED PEPPER SALSA

*A terrific flavor, different from ordinary salsa. The roasted peppers and lime create a sweet-tart taste that is great with seafood.*

Serves: 4 (makes 2 cups)

2 medium plum tomatoes
Juice of 1 lime
½ medium onion, chopped
1 garlic clove
1 teaspoon extra-virgin olive oil

¼ teaspoon sea salt
¼ cup chopped cilantro (or diced scallions)
3 medium red bell peppers, roasted and diced (page 234)

Mix tomatoes, lime juice, onion, garlic, olive oil, and salt. Purée in a blender or food processor. Stir in cilantro and peppers and chill.

*Per Serving*
Calories: 44 · Fiber: 2g · Saturated fat: 0.2g · Sodium: 284mg ·
Protein: 1g · Total fat: 1.4g · Carbs: 8g · Calories from fat: 25%

## SALSA

Serves: 4 (makes 2 cups)

4 medium plum tomatoes
Juice of 1 lime
½ medium onion, chopped
1 garlic clove
1 teaspoon extra-virgin olive oil
½ teaspoon sea salt

¼ teaspoon black pepper
⅛ teaspoon cayenne or to taste (or 1 jalapeño pepper, seeded)
¼ cup chopped cilantro (or diced scallions)

Mix tomatoes, lime juice, onion, garlic, olive oil, salt, pepper, and cayenne and purée in a blender or food processor. Stir in cilantro and chill.

*Per Serving*
Calories: 23 · Fiber: 1.3g · Saturated fat: 0g · Sodium: 288mg ·
Protein: 0.8g · Total fat: 0.3g · Carbs: 5.5g · Calories from fat: 8%

# SPICY PEANUT SAUCE

*This can be used with Southeast Asian cuisine, or as a dip for veggies.*

Makes: 1 cup

⅓ cup natural peanut butter
⅔ cup calcium-fortified soy milk (or nonfat milk)

½ teaspoon Asian chili sauce or to taste

Combine ingredients in a saucepan and warm over low heat, stirring until blended. Serve warm or at room temperature.

*Per Serving*
Calories: 109 · Fiber: 2.2g · Saturated fat: 1.5g · Sodium: 183mg ·
Protein: 5.4g · Total fat: 8.5g · Carbs: 4.5g · Calories from fat: 66%

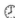

# TOMATO SAUCE

*The soy-based veggie crumbles provide a nice meaty texture, are filling, and help to lower rather than raise your cholesterol. You can substitute tofu or ground sirloin.*

Makes: 8 cups (16 servings)

1 tablespoon extra-virgin olive oil
1 medium onion, diced
2 celery stalks, finely diced
2 teaspoons Italian seasoning
2 bay leaves

6 garlic cloves, chopped
4 cups puréed tomatoes
¾ cup tomato paste (6 ounces)
½ cup dry red wine
1 pound veggie crumbles

In a pot, heat oil over medium-high heat. Add onion, celery, and Italian seasoning and sauté until onion is translucent. Add bay leaves and garlic and sauté 1 minute. Add tomato sauce, tomato paste, wine, and veggie crumbles. Simmer at least 30 minutes. (This sauce tastes even better if simmered several hours and refrigerated overnight.) Remove bay leaves before serving.

*Per Serving*
Calories: 93 · Fiber: 3g · Saturated fat: 0.2g · Sodium: 413mg ·
Protein: 7.5g · Total fat: 1.8g · Carbs: 10.5g · Calories from fat: 17%

PHASE ONE

PHASE ONE

## Dessert Recipes

### BERRY-BANANA SMOOTHIE

*Great with breakfast, for a snack, or as dessert.*

Serves: 2

2 cups nonfat milk (or calcium-fortified
   soy milk)
1 cup frozen berries (blueberries,
   raspberries, cherries, etc.)

1 medium banana, frozen
1 to 2 packets Splenda (optional)

Combine ingredients in a blender and process until smooth.

*Per Serving*
Calories: 177 · Fiber: 2.5g · Saturated fat: 0.3g · Sodium: 133mg ·
Protein: 9.4g · Total fat: 1g · Carbs: 35g · Calories from fat: 6%

### BLUEBERRY AND PORT FROZEN YOGURT

*This is one of my favorite desserts, and for less than 100 calories.
It's quick, easy, and delicious.*

Serves: 4

2 cups nonfat plain yogurt (16 ounces)
1 cup frozen blueberries (or other berries)
3-4 tablespoons sugar (to taste)
3 tablespoons port

⅛ teaspoon sea salt
Juice of 1 lime
Grated lime zest for garnish

Combine yogurt, berries, sugar, port, salt, and juice in a food processor or
blender and process until smooth. Freeze in an ice cream maker according to
manufacturer's directions. Or freeze in a bowl for 3 to 5 hours until solid, then
process until smooth and refreeze. Sprinkle with lime zest and serve in chilled
bowls.

*Per Serving*
Calories: 96 · Fiber: 1g · Saturated fat: 0.1g · Sodium: 78mg ·
Protein: 6g · Total fat: 0.3g · Carbs: 17g · Calories from fat: 2%

# CHOCOLATE MOUSSE WITH GRAND MARNIER

*This is one of my favorite desserts, created by my wife, Nicole, and so healthy you should eat it often. Half the saturated fat in chocolate is not bad for you, so enjoy with a clear conscience. It stores well in the refrigerator, covered, for several days.*

### Serves: 6

12 ounces silken tofu
4 ounces semisweet dark chocolate chips
²/₃ cup maple syrup
1 shot espresso or ¹/₄ cup strong coffee
¹/₈ teaspoon sea salt

¹/₂ cup cocoa, unsweetened
3 tablespoons Grand Marnier
2 tablespoons grated orange zest, divided
6 thin slices orange

Rinse and drain the tofu. Set aside.

In a food processor, process chocolate until finely chopped.

In a saucepan, heat maple syrup until gently bubbling. Remove from heat and stir in coffee and salt. With the food processor running, slowly pour in the hot syrup and process for 1 to 2 minutes, until the chocolate has melted.

Add tofu, cocoa, Grand Marnier, and 1 tablespoon orange zest and process until smooth. Pour into a serving bowl or 6 individual dessert bowls and garnish with orange zest. Chill until ready; serve with orange slices.

*Per Serving*
Calories: 261 · Fiber: 3.6g · Saturated fat: 3.7g · Sodium: 56mg ·
Protein: 5.3g · Total fat: 7.7g · Carbs: 42.3g · Calories from fat: 25%

# COFFEE FLAN

*My wife grew up making flan in Mexico. This healthy version of traditional flan is easy to make and delicious.*

### Serves: 6

4 large eggs (omega-3, free-range, organic)
One 15-ounce can evaporated nonfat milk
¹/₂ cup sugar (or 8 packets Splenda) plus ¹/₃ cup sugar

¹/₄ cup strong coffee or 1 shot espresso
1 teaspoon vanilla

Preheat oven to 375° F. Fill an ovenproof casserole half full with very hot water and place in the oven.

*(continued)*

Combine eggs, milk, 1 can water, ½ cup sugar, coffee, and vanilla in a blender or food processor and blend until smooth. Set aside.

Dissolve ⅓ cup sugar in ¼ cup water and heat in a saucepan over medium-high heat until sugar caramelizes and turns slightly brown. Pour hot caramel into a large ovenproof serving bowl (or six smaller ovenproof bowls). Pour egg mixture on top of caramel. Place bowl in the water bath and bake for 1 hour. Cool until warm to the touch. Run a knife or spatula around the sides of the bowl. Place a plate over the top of the bowl and invert. Gently tap the top and sides of the bowl, allowing flan to drop onto the plate with the caramel on top. Refrigerate at least 1 hour.

*Serving suggestion:* Accompany with fresh berries.

*Per Serving*
Calories: 208 · Fiber: 0g · Saturated fat: 0.8g · Sodium: 124mg ·
Protein: 9g · Total fat: 2g · Carbs: 37g · Calories from fat: 10%

# HOT COCOA

*Cocoa is a fabulous treat to end a day—satisfying and calming.*
*Cocoa powder is also great for your health, as long as you don't*
*add too much sugar to it.*

Serves: 1

1 cup nonfat milk (or calcium-enriched soy milk)
1½ tablespoons cocoa (preferably Dutch-process)

1 to 2 tablespoons soy creamer (optional)
1 to 2 packets Splenda (or 1 teaspoon sugar) (optional)
Dash cinnamon (optional)

Heat milk for 80 seconds in the microwave or over medium heat on the stovetop for 6 minutes. Do not allow to boil. Vigorously stir in cocoa powder. Add soy creamer, Splenda (or other sweetener), and cinnamon if using.

*Per Serving*
Calories: 104 · Fiber: 2.5g · Saturated fat: 0.5g · Sodium: 129mg ·
Protein: 9.8g · Total fat: 1.5g · Carbs: 16.3g · Calories from fat: 11%

# MANGO FROZEN YOGURT

*This is a light, delicate dessert, especially nice with Asian cuisine.*
*You can substitute any orange-flavored liqueur or orange extract*
*for the Grand Marnier.*

Serves: 4

1 cup nonfat plain yogurt
3 tablespoons sugar
2 tablespoons Grand Marnier
⅛ teaspoon sea salt

½ teaspoon vanilla
1 medium mango, peeled, seeded, and
    chopped
Grated orange zest

Combine yogurt, sugar, Grand Marnier, salt, vanilla, and half the mango in a
food processor or blender and process until smooth. Add the remaining mango
and blend briefly, so some chunks of mango remain. Pour into an ice cream
maker and freeze according to manufacturer's directions, or freeze in a bowl for
3 to 5 hours until solid, then process until smooth and refreeze. Garnish with
orange zest and serve in chilled bowls.

*Per Serving*
Calories: 81 · Fiber: 1g · Saturated fat: 0g · Sodium: 109mg ·
Protein: 109g · Total fat: 0.1g · Carbs: 14g · Calories from fat: 1%

# Revving It Up

Now that you're in Phase Two, you'll find that the fiber content in your diet increases and the reduced-fat cheeses (which are still very high in saturated fat) disappear. During the next two weeks, you'll also enjoy more foods that help whisk away toxins, including cruciferous vegetables (cabbage, bok choy, broccoli, kale, cauliflower, and Brussels sprouts), turmeric (often found in curry powder), garlic, rosemary, and soy products. These are all part of the Ten Years Younger Diet.

You can now enjoy wine or other alcoholic beverages with dinner, but don't drink more than one to two restaurant-sized servings a day. I'll have you skip alcohol two days a week—I've listed those days between Monday and Thursday, but you can pick any two days you wish.

Your Age-Busting Fitness plan will help you increase the level of weights you've been using for strength training. Once you reach the point where you can smoothly lift a weight for 16 reps, it's time to up the ante. Your exercise and calorie-burning ability will continue to rise, and during the second week, you'll raise your heart rate to 70 to 85% of your maximum rate during your aerobic activities. Plus, you'll also start interval training during the second week with your aerobic workouts once or twice a week. (See Chapter 6.) Remember, interval training is great for improving aerobic fitness and rejuvenating you biochemically.

For mental peace and calm, you should schedule yourself for 20 minutes daily of a relaxing activity that you enjoy. Also, be sure to arrange for a massage during Phase Two; with all the hard work you've been doing, you deserve it!

# DAILY MEAL AND ACTIVITY PLANS

## Day 1 (Monday)

FOOD PLAN: Vitality Foods

### Breakfast
Oatmeal with Apples and Blueberries
Tea or coffee

### Optional Morning Snack
Edamame, ½ cup

### Lunch
Spinach Salad with Sautéed Shrimp and Orange Vinaigrette Dressing
Iced tea

### Afternoon Snack
Baby carrots, 1 cup
Almonds, 1 oz
Pure water

### Dinner
Grilled Mahi Mahi Soft Tacos
Roasted peppers
Black beans, ½ cup
Mexican Rice, ¾ cup
Seltzer
Beer or red wine

### Dessert
Blueberry–Soy Milk Smoothie
Herbal tea

### Optional Rescue Snack
Smoked oysters, 1½ oz
Rye crispbread, 2

## AGE-BUSTING FITNESS PLAN

### Aerobic Training

- 3–5 minutes of warming up
- Reach 70–80% of your max heart rate for 30–40 minutes total activity with brisk walking, jogging, elliptical machine options
- 3–5 minutes of cooling down, heart rate less than 60% max

### Strength Training

- Rest day from strength training

### Stretching

- 4–6 body parts, 5–10 minutes of stretching time

## RELAXATION ROUTINE

- Choose a calming activity for 20 minutes

## SUPPLEMENT ROUTINE

- Take your customized multivitamin pack
- Skin moisturizer with SPF 15
- Apply retinol skin product every other day

## DETOX ROUTINE

- Look for organic food products
- Soak all produce in water with a couple of drops of dish soap, then rinse
- Don't cook or heat with plastic
- Limit largemouth fish intake to less than 2–3 servings per month

---

# Day 2 (Tuesday)

FOOD PLAN: Vitality Foods

**Breakfast**
Oatmeal Waffles with Fruit
Tea or coffee

**Optional Morning Snack**
Nonfat, sugar-free yogurt, 4–6 oz

**Lunch**
Gazpacho
Mixed green salad, 2 cups
Vinaigrette Dressing, 2 tbsp
Iced tea

**Afternoon Snack**
Carrot and/or celery sticks, 1 cup
Hummus, 3–4 tbsp
Pure water

**Dinner**
Black Beans and Rice
Mixed green salad, 2 cups
Vinaigrette Dressing, 2 tbsp
Decaf green or black tea

**Dessert**
Nonfat, sugar-free ice cream with ¼ cup berries and 2–3 tbsp pecans
Hot Cocoa

**Optional Rescue Snack**
Nuts, 1 oz

## AGE-BUSTING FITNESS PLAN

### Aerobic Training
- 3-5 minutes of warming up
- Reach 70-80% of your max heart rate for 30-40 minutes total activity with brisk walking, jogging, elliptical machine options
- 3 minutes of cooling down, heart rate less than 60% max

### Strength Training
- Retest your push-up and sit-up ability
- 12 body parts, 2 sets, 10-16 reps
- Use a mixture of ball and free weight activities

### Stretching
- 4-6 body parts, 5-10 minutes of stretching time

## RELAXATION ROUTINE
- Choose a calming activity for 20 minutes

## SUPPLEMENT ROUTINE
- Take your customized multivitamin pack
- Skin moisturizer with SPF 15

## DETOX ROUTINE
- Look for organic food products
- Soak all produce in water with a couple of drops of dish soap, then rinse
- Don't cook or heat with plastic
- Limit largemouth fish intake to less than 2-3 servings per month

---

# Day 3 (Wednesday)

FOOD PLAN: Vitality Foods

## Breakfast
Grits, 1 cup cooked
Soy sausage, 1–2 pieces
Tea or coffee

## Optional Morning Snack
Nonfat cottage cheese, ½ cup with celery sticks, 1 cup

## Lunch
Turkey wrap
Carrot and celery sticks, 1 cup
Apple
Seltzer

## Afternoon Snack
Almonds, 1 oz
Pure water

## Dinner
Pepperonata
Mixed green salad, 2–3 cups
Vinaigrette Dressing, 2 tbsp
Seltzer
Red wine

## Dessert
Fruit salad, 1 cup with nonfat vanilla yogurt, ½ cup
Hot Cocoa

## Optional Rescue Snack
Veggie chicken nuggets, 4 pieces

## *AGE-BUSTING FITNESS PLAN*

### Aerobic Training
- 3-5 minutes of warming up
- Reach 70-80% of your max heart rate for 30-40 minutes total activity with brisk walking, jogging, elliptical machine options
- 3 minutes of cooling down, heart rate less than 60% max

### Strength Training
- Rest day from strength training

### Stretching
- 4-6 body parts, 5-10 minutes of stretching time

## RELAXATION ROUTINE
- Schedule a massage

## SUPPLEMENT ROUTINE
- Take your customized multivitamin pack
- Skin moisturizer with SPF 15
- Apply retinol skin product every other day

## DETOX ROUTINE
- Look for organic food products
- Soak all produce in water with a couple of drops of dish soap, then rinse
- Don't cook or heat with plastic
- Limit largemouth fish intake to less than 2-3 servings per month

PHASE TWO

# Day 4 (Thursday)

FOOD PLAN: Vitality Foods

**Breakfast**
Oatmeal with Apples and Blueberries
Tea or coffee

**Optional Morning Snack**
Hard-boiled egg (omega-3, free-range, organic)

**Lunch**
Veggie burger with sliced tomato, lettuce, mustard, and whole-wheat pita bread
Mixed green salad, 2 cups
Vinaigrette Dressing, 2 tbsp
Iced tea

**Afternoon Snack**
Pear
Walnuts, 1 oz
Pure water

**Dinner**
Chicken with Hazelnut Crust
Roasted Beets, Carrots, and Parsnips
Seltzer
Red wine

**Dessert**
Cherry and Orange Juice Smoothie
Herbal tea

**Optional Rescue Snack**
Sardines, 1½–3 oz
Rye crispbread, 2–3 pieces

## *AGE-BUSTING FITNESS PLAN*

### Aerobic Training

- 3-5 minutes of warming up
- Reach 70-80% of your max heart rate for 30-40 minutes total activity with brisk walking, jogging, elliptical machine options
- 3 minutes of cooling down, heart rate less than 60% max

### Strength Training

- 12 body parts, 1 set, 10-16 reps
- Use a mixture of ball and free weight activities

### Stretching

- 4-6 body parts, 5-10 minutes of stretching time

## RELAXATION ROUTINE

- Choose a calming activity for 20 minutes

## SUPPLEMENT ROUTINE

- Take your customized multivitamin pack
- Skin moisturizer with SPF 15

## DETOX ROUTINE

- Look for organic food products
- Soak all produce in water with a couple of drops of dish soap, then rinse
- Don't cook or heat with plastic
- Limit largemouth fish intake to less than 2-3 servings per month

---

# Day 5 (Friday)

FOOD PLAN: Vitality Foods

## Breakfast
Bran cereal, 1 cup, with ½ to 1 cup nonfat milk and ½ cup blueberries
Tea or coffee

## Optional Morning Snack
Edamame, ½ cup

## Lunch
Canned Salmon Spread with Pita
Orange
Iced tea

## Afternoon Snack
Pecans, 1 oz
Pure water

## Dinner
Scallops with Soy-Chili Sauce
Snow Peas with Bok Choy
Wild Rice with Red Onions and Shiitake Mushrooms
Seltzer
Red wine

## Dessert
Chocolate Mousse with Grand Marnier
Hot Cocoa

## Optional Rescue Snack
Veggie chicken nuggets, 4 pieces

## *AGE-BUSTING FITNESS PLAN*

### Aerobic Training
- 3-5 minutes of warming up
- Reach 70-80% of your max heart rate for 30-40 minutes total activity with brisk walking, jogging, elliptical machine options
- 3 minutes of cooling down, heart rate less than 60% max

### Strength Training
- Rest day from strength training

### Stretching
- 4-6 body parts, 5-10 minutes of stretching time

## RELAXATION ROUTINE
- Choose a calming activity for 20 minutes

## SUPPLEMENT ROUTINE
- Take your customized multivitamin pack
- Skin moisturizer with SPF 15
- Apply retinol skin product every other day

## DETOX ROUTINE
- Look for organic food products
- Soak all produce in water with a couple of drops of dish soap, then rinse
- Don't cook or heat with plastic
- Limit largemouth fish intake to less than 2-3 servings per month

# Day 6 (Saturday)

FOOD PLAN: Vitality Foods

## Breakfast
Oat Bran Muffin with 2 tsp sugar-free apricot jam
Blueberry–Soy Milk Smoothie
Tea or coffee

## Optional Morning Snack
Hot Cocoa

## Lunch
Tabbouleh
Iced mint tea

## Afternoon Snack
Spicy Baked Garbanzo Beans
Pure water

## Dinner
Crab Cakes
Sweet Potato Fries
Brussels Sprouts with Vinaigrette Dressing
Seltzer
Red wine

## Dessert
Strawberries, 1 cup, dipped in 1 oz melted semi-sweet dark chocolate, with 1/4 cup
    vanilla nonfat yogurt
Herbal tea

## Optional Rescue Snack
Apple
Nuts, 1 oz

### *AGE-BUSTING FITNESS PLAN*

## Aerobic Training
- 3–5 minutes of warming up
- Reach 70–80% of your max heart rate for 30–40 minutes total activity with brisk walking, jogging, elliptical machine options
- 3 minutes of cooling down, heart rate less than 60% max

## Strength Training
- 12 body parts, 2 sets, 10–16 reps
- Use a mixture of ball and free weight activities

## Stretching
- 4–6 body parts, 5–10 minutes of stretching time

## RELAXATION ROUTINE
- Choose a calming activity for 20 minutes

## SUPPLEMENT ROUTINE
- Take your customized multivitamin pack
- Skin moisturizer with SPF 15

## DETOX ROUTINE
- Look for organic food products
- Soak all produce in water with a couple of drops of dish soap, then rinse
- Don't cook or heat with plastic
- Limit largemouth fish intake to less than 2–3 servings per month

# Day 7 (Sunday)

FOOD PLAN: Vitality Foods

## Breakfast
Mini Fennel and Tomato Frittatas
Soy sausage, 1 piece
Tea or coffee

## Optional Morning Snack
None

## Lunch
Almond Soup
Turkey wrap
Iced tea

## Afternoon Snack
Air-popped popcorn, 2 cups, sprinkled with 1 tbsp brewer's yeast
Pure water

## Dinner
Grilled Shrimp Kabobs
Barley with Celery, Parsley, and Mushrooms
Steamed broccoli with 2 tbsp Vinaigrette Dressing
Seltzer
Red wine

## Dessert
Peach and Raspberry Crumble
Mint tea

## Optional Rescue Snack
Almonds, 1 oz

## *AGE-BUSTING FITNESS PLAN*

### Aerobic Training
- Aerobic rest day
- Go for a 20-30 minute casual walk with family or friends

### Strength Training
- Rest day from strength training

### Stretching
- 4-6 body parts, 5-10 minutes of stretching time

## RELAXATION ROUTINE
- Choose a calming activity for 20 minutes

## SUPPLEMENT ROUTINE
- Take your customized multivitamin pack
- Skin moisturizer with SPF 15
- Apply retinol skin product every other day

## DETOX ROUTINE
- Look for organic food products
- Soak all produce in water with a couple of drops of dish soap, then rinse
- Don't cook or heat with plastic
- Limit largemouth fish intake to less than 2-3 servings per month

# Day 8 (Monday)

FOOD PLAN: Vitality Foods

**Breakfast**
Mini Fennel and Tomato Frittatas
Whole-wheat toast, 1 slice, or soy sausage, 1–2
Tea or coffee

**Optional Morning Snack**
Nonfat yogurt, 4–6 oz

**Lunch**
Tabbouleh
Iced mint tea

**Afternoon Snack**
Pear
Walnuts, 1 oz
Pure water

**Dinner**
Garbanzo, Cauliflower, and Red Pepper Curry
Indian Rice
Raita
Decaf tea

**Dessert**
Mango Frozen Yogurt

**Optional Rescue Snack**
Almonds, 1 oz

## AGE-BUSTING FITNESS PLAN

### Aerobic Training
- 3–5 minutes of warming up
- Reach 70–85% of your max heart rate for 30–40 minutes total activity with brisk walking, jogging, elliptical machine options
- Include 10 minutes of interval training
- 3 minutes of cooling down, heart rate less than 60% max

### Strength Training
- Rest day from strength training

### Stretching
- 4–6 body parts, 5–10 minutes of stretching time

PHASE TWO

## RELAXATION ROUTINE
- Choose a calming activity for 20 minutes

## SUPPLEMENT ROUTINE
- Take your customized multivitamin pack
- Skin moisturizer with SPF 15
- Apply retinol skin product every other day

## DETOX ROUTINE
- In restaurants, confirm no use of hydrogenated fats; ask, "How is it prepared?"
- Double-check that you've removed all products with hydrogenated fat, corn syrup, and white flour from your pantry

# Day 9 (Tuesday)

FOOD PLAN: Vitality Foods

**Breakfast**
Bran cereal, 1 cup, with ½ cup berries and ½ cup nonfat milk
Tea or coffee

**Optional Morning Snack**
Edamame

**Lunch**
Almond Soup
Canned Salmon Spread with Pita
Iced tea

**Afternoon Snack**
Hummus, 3–4 tbsp, with 1 cup baby carrots
Pure water

**Dinner**
Couscous with Chicken
Raita
Seltzer
Red wine

**Dessert**
Fruit Salad, 1 cup with nonfat yogurt, ½ cup

**Optional Rescue Snack**
Almonds, 1 oz

## AGE-BUSTING FITNESS PLAN

### Aerobic Training
- 3–5 minutes of warming up
- Reach 70–85% of your max heart rate for 30–40 minutes total activity with brisk walking, jogging, elliptical machine options
- 3 minutes of cooling down, heart rate less than 60% max

### Strength Training
- 12 body parts, 2 sets, 10–16 reps
- Use a mixture of ball and free weight activities

### Stretching
- 4–6 body parts, 5–10 minutes of stretching time

## RELAXATION ROUTINE
- Choose a calming activity for 20 minutes

## SUPPLEMENT ROUTINE
- Take your customized multivitamin pack
- Skin moisturizer with SPF 15

## DETOX ROUTINE
- In restaurants, confirm no use of hydrogenated fats; ask, "How is it prepared?"
- Double-check that you've removed all products with hydrogenated fat, corn syrup, and white flour from your pantry

# Day 10 (Wednesday)

FOOD PLAN: Vitality Foods

## Breakfast
Oatmeal Muffin with sugar-free apricot jam, 2 tsp
Blueberry-Soy Milk Smoothie
Tea or coffee

## Optional Morning Snack
Nonfat yogurt, 4-6 oz

## Lunch
Chicken wrap
Carrot and/or celery sticks, 1 cup
Orange
Iced tea

## Afternoon Snack
Pecans, 1 oz
Pure water

## Dinner
Sole with Oyster and Lime Sauce
Brown rice, $^{3}/_{4}$-1 cup
Snow Peas with Bok Choy, 2 cups
Seltzer
Red wine or beer

## Dessert
Blueberry and Port Frozen Yogurt

## Optional Rescue Snack
Sardines, $1^{1}/_{2}$-3 oz can, with rye crispbread, 2

## AGE-BUSTING FITNESS PLAN

### Aerobic Training
- 3-5 minutes of warming up
- Reach 70-85% of your max heart rate for 30-40 minutes total activity with brisk walking, jogging, elliptical machine options
- Include 10 minutes of interval training
- 3 minutes of cooling down, heart rate less than 60% max

### Strength Training
- Rest day from strength training

### Stretching
- 4-6 body parts, 5-10 minutes of stretching time

## RELAXATION ROUTINE
- Choose a calming activity for 20 minutes

## SUPPLEMENT ROUTINE
- Take your customized multivitamin pack
- Skin moisturizer with SPF 15
- Apply retinol skin product every other day

## DETOX ROUTINE
- In restaurants, confirm no use of hydrogenated fat; ask, "How is it prepared?"
- Double-check that you've removed all products with hydrogenated fat, corn syrup, and white flour from your pantry

---

# Day 11 (Thursday)

FOOD PLAN: Vitality Foods

**Breakfast**
Mini Mushroom Cheese Frittatas
Soy sausage, 1 piece
Tea or coffee

**Optional Morning Snack**
Nonfat cottage cheese, ½ cup with celery sticks, 1 cup

**Lunch**
Mixed Green Salad with Salmon, Apple, and Corn
Iced tea

**Afternoon Snack**
Almonds, 1 oz
Pure water

**Dinner**
Falafel
Tabbouleh
Sliced tomatoes, ½ cup
Mint tea

**Dessert**
Mixed fresh fruit, 1 cup
Nonfat vanilla yogurt, ½ cup

**Optional Rescue Snack**
Veggie chicken nuggets, 4 pieces

## AGE-BUSTING FITNESS PLAN

### Aerobic Training
- 3-5 minutes of warming up
- Reach 70-85% of your max heart rate for 30-40 minutes total activity with brisk walking, jogging, elliptical machine options
- 3 minutes of cooling down, heart rate less than 60% max

### Strength Training
- 12 body parts, 1 set, 10-16 reps
- Use a mixture of ball and free weight activities

### Stretching
- 4-6 body parts, 5-10 minutes of stretching time

PHASE TWO

## RELAXATION ROUTINE
- Choose a calming activity for 20 minutes

## SUPPLEMENT ROUTINE
- Take your customized multivitamin pack
- Skin moisturizer with SPF 15

## DETOX ROUTINE
- In restaurants, confirm no use of hydrogenated fat; ask, "How is it prepared?"
- Double-check that you've removed all products with hydrogenated fat, corn syrup, and white flour from your pantry

---

# Day 12 (Friday)

FOOD PLAN: Vitality Foods

## Breakfast
Oatmeal with Apples and Blueberries
Tea or coffee

## Optional Morning Snack
Nonfat yogurt, 4–6 oz

## Lunch
Veggie burger with pita bread, sliced tomato, mustard, and lettuce
Sweet Potato Fries with Cinnamon
Iced tea

## Afternoon Snack
Miso Soup
Green tea

## Dinner
Garlic Shrimp Burritos
Roasted Bell Peppers, 1–2 pieces
Seltzer
Red wine

## Dessert
Nonfat, sugar-free ice cream, 1/2–3/4 cup
Pecans, 2–3 tbsp
Hot Cocoa

## Optional Rescue Snack
Almonds, 1 oz

## AGE-BUSTING FITNESS PLAN

### Aerobic Training
- 3-5 minutes of warming up
- Reach 70-85% of your max heart rate for 30-40 minutes total activity with brisk walking, jogging, elliptical machine options
- 3 minutes of cooling down, heart rate less than 60% max

### Strength Training
- Rest day from strength training

### Stretching
- 4-6 body parts, 5-10 minutes of stretching time

## RELAXATION ROUTINE
- Choose a calming activity for 20 minutes

## SUPPLEMENT ROUTINE
- Take your customized multivitamin pack
- Skin moisturizer with SPF 15
- Apply retinol skin product every other day

## DETOX ROUTINE
- In restaurants, confirm no use of hydrogenated fat; ask, "How is it prepared?"
- Double-check that you've removed all products with hydrogenated fat, corn syrup, and white flour from your pantry

---

# Day 13 (Saturday)

FOOD PLAN: Vitality Foods

## Breakfast
Buckwheat and Pecan Pancakes
Apricot, Ginger, and Pear Sauce
Tea or coffee

## Optional Morning Snack
Nonfat yogurt, 4–6 oz

## Lunch
Pasta Salad with Veggies, White Beans, and Pine Nuts
Iced tea

## Afternoon Snack
Almonds, 1 oz
Pure water

## Dinner
Minestrone, $3/4$ cup
Marinated Salmon with Pecan Crust
Brown rice, $3/4$ cup
Broccoli, 1 cup
Mixed green salad, 2 cups
Vinaigrette Dressing, 2 tbsp
Seltzer
Red wine

## Dessert
Strawberries, $1/2$ pint, dipped in 1 oz melted semi-sweet dark chocolate, with $1/4$ cup
    vanilla nonfat yogurt
Herbal tea

## Optional Rescue Snack
Smoked oysters, $1 1/2$–3 oz
Rye crispbread, 2

## AGE-BUSTING FITNESS PLAN

### Aerobic Training

- 3-5 minutes of warming up
- Reach 70-85% of your max heart rate for 30-40 minutes total activity with brisk walking, jogging, elliptical machine options
- 3 minutes of cooling down, heart rate less than 60% max

### Strength Training

- 12 body parts, 2 sets, 10-16 reps
- Use a mixture of ball and free weight activities

### Stretching

- 4-6 body parts, 5-10 minutes of stretching time

## RELAXATION ROUTINE

- Choose a calming activity for 20 minutes

## SUPPLEMENT ROUTINE

- Take your customized multivitamin pack
- Skin moisturizer with SPF 15

## DETOX ROUTINE

- In restaurants, confirm no use of hydrogenated fat; ask, "How is it prepared?"
- Double-check that you've removed all products with hydrogenated fat, corn syrup, and white flour from your pantry

# Day 14 (Sunday)

FOOD PLAN: Vitality Foods

**Breakfast**
Crêpes with Blueberries and Nonfat Yogurt
Tea or coffee

**Optional Morning Snack**
None

**Lunch**
Shrimp Bisque
Mixed green salad, 2 cups
Vinaigrette Dressing, 2 tbsp

**Afternoon Snack**
Minestrone
Pure water

**Dinner**
Chiles Rellenos
Mixed salad, 2 cups
Vinaigrette, 2 tbsp
Seltzer
Red wine or beer

**Dessert**
Air-popped popcorn, 2 cups, sprinkled with 1 tbsp brewer's yeast
Blueberry–Soy Milk Smoothie

**Optional Rescue Snack**
Almonds, 1 oz

## *AGE-BUSTING FITNESS PLAN*

### Aerobic Training
- Aerobic rest day
- Take a walk with a friend or loved one

### Strength Training
- Rest day from strength training

### Stretching
- 4–6 body parts, 5–10 minutes of stretching time

## RELAXATION ROUTINE
- Choose a calming activity for 20 minutes

## SUPPLEMENT ROUTINE
- Take your customized multivitamin pack
- Skin moisturizer with SPF 15
- Apply retinol skin product daily

## DETOX ROUTINE
- In restaurants, confirm no use of hydrogenated fat; ask, "How is it prepared?"
- Double-check that you've removed all products with hydrogenated fat, corn syrup, and white flour from your pantry

## Breakfast Recipes

### BUCKWHEAT AND PECAN PANCAKES

*Buckwheat is a wholesome, nutrient-rich flour and makes terrific pancakes.
While all flour products cause a jump in blood sugar, the nuts and
cinnamon in this recipe help to minimize this rise.*

Makes: 4 servings

2 cups buckwheat flour
1 tablespoon baking powder
½ teaspoon cinnamon
⅛ teaspoon sea salt
⅓ cup chopped pecans
2 large eggs (omega-3, free-range, organic)

2 cups calcium-fortified soy milk
¼ cup unsweetened applesauce
2 tablespoons canola oil (organic, expeller-pressed)
Canola oil spray

Mix flour, baking powder, cinnamon, salt, and pecans in a large bowl. In a separate bowl, whisk eggs, soy milk, applesauce, and oil. Gently fold wet ingredients into dry ingredients. Spray griddle or pan with oil. Pour batter into pan and cook until bottom is golden; flip and cook other side.

*Serving suggestion:* Serve with fresh fruit; Apricot, Ginger, and Pear Sauce (page 292); raspberry sauce; or maple syrup.

*Per Serving*
Calories: 414 · Fiber: 8.5g · Saturated fat: 2g · Sodium: 397mg ·
Protein: 15g · Total fat: 19g · Carbs: 50g · Calories from fat: 40%

### CRÊPES WITH BLUEBERRIES AND NONFAT YOGURT

*Crêpes are fun to make—my boys get in line to flip them. Filled with fruit
and nonfat yogurt, these make for a great breakfast or even dessert.
Crêpes store easily—just wrap and freeze for later use.*

Serves: 4 (makes 12 six-inch crêpes)

1 cup whole-wheat pastry flour
⅛ teaspoon sea salt
1⅓ cups nonfat milk (or calcium-fortified soy milk)
2 large eggs (omega-3, free-range, organic)
1 tablespoon canola oil (organic, expeller-pressed)

Canola oil spray
1 cup blueberries
2 tablespoons port (or grape juice)
2 tablespoons blueberry jam, regular or sugar-free
1 cup nonfat yogurt, plain or vanilla

Mix flour and salt in large bowl. In a separate bowl, whisk milk, eggs, and oil. Gently fold wet into dry ingredients.

Spray crêpe or sauté pan with canola oil and pour in ¼ cup batter. Cook until bottom is golden; flip and cook other side. Keep finished crêpes warm.

Heat blueberries in a saucepan with port and jam until liquid is thickened. Mix with yogurt.

To fill, place about 3 tablespoons of blueberry-yogurt filling at the bottom of each crêpe and roll.

*Per Serving*
Calories: 255 · Fiber: 4.1g · Saturated fat: 2.3g · Sodium: 63mg ·
Protein: 12g · Total fat: 5g · Carbs: 41g · Calories from fat: 19%

---

# MINI FENNEL AND TOMATO FRITTATAS

*Fennel is loaded with anti-aging nutrients.*
*Bake a batch and enjoy them during the week.*

Serves: 6 (makes 18 mini frittatas)

12 large eggs (omega-3, free-range, organic)
½ cup nonfat milk (or calcium-fortified soy milk)
½ cup grated nonfat cheese (or soy cheese)
2 teaspoons extra-virgin olive oil

1 small sweet onion, diced
1 medium fennel bulb, finely chopped
1 teaspoon Italian seasoning
¼ teaspoon sea salt
¼ teaspoon black pepper
2 medium tomatoes, chopped
Olive oil spray

Preheat oven to 400° F.

Whisk eggs with milk in a bowl. Add grated cheese and set aside.

Heat a sauté or omelet pan over medium-high heat and add oil. Sauté onion and fennel with Italian seasoning, salt, and pepper until onion is translucent. Add tomatoes and cook 1 minute more, stirring occasionally. Remove from heat.

Insert 18 cupcake liners into a muffin pan and spray liners with olive oil or spray pan liberally with olive oil. Divide sautéed vegetables among the muffin cups and ladle egg-cheese mixture on top of the vegetables.

Bake on the middle rack of the oven until the eggs are set and browned, 15 to 20 minutes.

*Serving suggestion:* Serve with a slice of whole-grain toast or soy sausage.

*Per Serving*
Calories: 154 · Fiber: 2g · Saturated fat: 1.8g · Sodium: 242mg ·
Protein: 8g · Total fat: 6.7g · Carbs: 8g · Calories from fat: 40%

## OAT BRAN MUFFINS

*These muffins are equally good as breakfast or as a snack and are great
served with a smoothie. They also freeze well.*

Makes: 12 muffins (1 muffin per serving)

Preheat oven to 400° F.

3 cups rolled oats
1 cup oat bran
1 tablespoon baking powder
1 teaspoon cinnamon
½ teaspoon sea salt
½ cup raisins (or other dried fruit)
¾ cup calcium-fortified soy milk

3 large eggs (omega-3, free-range, organic)
¼ cup canola oil (organic, expeller-
   pressed)
¾ cup unsweetened applesauce
⅓ cup molasses (or ¼ cup Splenda plus
   additional ¼ cup applesauce)
Canola oil spray

Mix oats, bran, baking powder, cinnamon, salt, and raisins in a large bowl.
In a separate bowl, mix soy milk, eggs, oil, applesauce, and molasses. Gently
fold wet ingredients into the dry ingredients. Spray muffin pan with canola oil
and pour batter into pan. Bake for 25 to 30 minutes, until a toothpick inserted
into the center of a muffin comes out clean.

*Serving suggestion:* Serve with fresh fruit and vanilla yogurt, or sugar-free
jam.

*Per Serving*
Calories: 175 · Fiber: 3g · Saturated fat: 1g · Sodium: 196mg ·
Protein: 5g · Total fat: 7.4g · Carbs: 26g · Calories from fat: 35%

## Lunch Recipes

## ALMOND SOUP

*This is a delicious soup popular in southern Spain.
Almonds are very rich in vitamin E, calcium, and other nutrients.*

Serves: 4

1 teaspoon canola oil (organic, expeller-
   pressed)
1 medium onion, chopped
4 garlic cloves, minced
1 cup sherry (or white wine)

2 cups low-sodium vegetable stock
1 cup very finely ground almonds
½ cup toasted whole-wheat bread
   crumbs (optional)
2 teaspoons finely chopped parsley

Heat a saucepan over medium-high heat, add oil, and sauté onion 3 to 5 minutes, until soft. Add garlic and cook 30 seconds, stirring gently. Add sherry and stir for 15 seconds to deglaze. Pour into a blender or food processor and purée until smooth. Return mixture to the saucepan and add stock. Bring to a boil, then reduce heat to low. Stir in almond flour and simmer at least 20 minutes. Stir in bread crumbs, if using, just before serving. Garnish with parsley.

*Variation:* To prepare with milk rather than sherry, sauté onions and garlic and add vegetable stock and almonds. Bring to a boil, then reduce heat. Add 1 cup nonfat milk (or soy milk) and heat through. Stir in bread crumbs and parsley and serve.

*Per Serving*
Calories: 321 · Fiber: 5g · Saturated fat: 1.5g · Sodium: 540mg ·
Protein: 10g · Total fat: 20g · Carbs: 16g · Calories from fat: 54%

# MINESTRONE

*This hearty, flavorful soup is great for lunch, afternoon snacks, or dinner.
Make extra and store in the refrigerator for several days.*

Makes: 8 one-cup servings

1 tablespoon extra-virgin olive oil
1 medium onion, chopped
2 medium carrots, diced
2 celery stalks, diced
4 white or cremini mushrooms, sliced
¼ teaspoon sea salt
¼ teaspoon black pepper
1 medium zucchini, diced
½ head cauliflower, cut into 1-inch florets
½ cup chopped flat-leaf parsley
10 fresh basil leaves, sliced into thin strips
3 garlic cloves, minced
4 medium plum tomatoes, coarsely
  chopped

3 cups low-sodium vegetable stock
2 tablespoons tomato paste
1 medium russet potato (or 2 small red
  potatoes), cut into ½-inch cubes
One 15-ounce can cannellini (or other
  white beans), rinsed and drained
½ 15-ounce can garbanzo beans, rinsed
  and drained
⅛ teaspoon red pepper flakes (optional)
4 ounces whole-wheat pasta (elbows,
  shells, or similar shape)
4 tablespoons nonfat sour cream
  (optional)

Heat a large soup pot over medium-high heat and add oil. Sauté onion until translucent, 3 to 5 minutes. Add carrots, celery, mushrooms, salt, and pepper and cook 3 minutes, stirring often. Reduce heat to medium and add zucchini, cauliflower, parsley, basil, garlic, and tomatoes. Continue cooking, stirring

*(continued)*

PHASE TWO

occasionally, until the tomatoes break down and start forming a sauce, about 5 minutes.

Add the stock, 2 cups water, tomato paste, potato, cannellini, garbanzo beans, and red pepper flakes. Bring to a boil, then reduce heat to low and simmer for 20 to 25 minutes, partially covered, until potatoes are tender. Add the pasta and cook 10 minutes more. Garnish with sour cream if desired.

*Per Serving*
Calories: 191 • Fiber: 6g • Saturated fat: 0.3g • Sodium: 564mg •
Protein: 9g • Total fat: 3.3g • Carbs: 34g • Calories from fat: 15%

# MISO SOUP

*This is an easy starter for any meal. To turn leftovers into a dinner entrée, add buckwheat or udon noodles (or whole-wheat or other fiber-rich pasta) and a green leafy vegetable and you're set. Miso is packed with vitamins and nutrients; don't boil the soup, as that will destroy many of the nutrients.*

Serves: 4

2 tablespoons wakame (seaweed)
4 tablespoons miso
1 teaspoon canola oil (organic, expeller-
  pressed)
½ medium onion, diced
1 cup sliced mushrooms,
  preferably shiitakes

1 teaspoon grated ginger
4 garlic cloves, minced
½ 14-ounce package firm tofu, cut into
  ½-inch cubes
2 scallions, diced

Soak wakame in a bowl of cool water for a few minutes and cut into ½-inch pieces. Dissolve miso in 2 cups hot water.

Heat a saucepan over medium-high heat, add canola oil, and sauté onion, mushrooms, and ginger for 3 to 4 minutes, until mushrooms soften and onions become translucent.

Add garlic to saucepan and cook 30 seconds, stirring. Add 2 cups water, bring to a boil, and reduce heat to low. Add tofu and dissolved miso and simmer for 3 to 4 minutes.

Add wakame and scallions to soup. Serve immediately.

*Per Serving*
Calories: 88 • Fiber: 2.3g • Saturated fat: 0g • Sodium: 805mg •
Protein: 7g • Total fat: 3.8g • Carbs: 9g • Calories from fat: 35%

## Dinner Recipes

### BLACK BEANS AND RICE

*This meal has converted many brown rice haters into enthusiasts. The tomato-lime garnish adds just the right touch. You can also add diced chicken or turkey.*

Serves: 2

One 15-ounce can black beans, rinsed and
   drained
½ cup brown rice
2 tablespoons extra-virgin olive oil
½ medium onion, chopped
½ teaspoon dried oregano
¼ teaspoon sea salt
¼ teaspoon black pepper

1 medium bell pepper, any color, chopped
2 garlic cloves, minced
4 medium tomatoes, chopped
Juice of 1 lime
¼ cup finely chopped cilantro
¼ cup nonfat sour cream
Tabasco sauce

Bring rice and 1 cup water to a boil, then reduce heat and simmer for about 40 minutes, until nearly done.

Heat a sauté pan over medium-high heat and add 1 tablespoon oil. Sauté onion with oregano, salt, and black pepper until onion is soft. Add bell pepper and garlic and cook 2 minutes. Stir in half the tomatoes, then remove from heat and mix into the rice. Cook rice mixture another 10 minutes or until rice is tender.

In a separate bowl, mix remaining tomatoes, lime juice, remaining oil, and cilantro. To serve, spoon beans and rice onto plates and garnish with tomato-lime mixture, a dollop of sour cream, and Tabasco to taste.

*Variation:* If desired, sauté diced chicken or turkey separately and add to the vegetables before mixing with the rice.

*Per Serving*
Calories: 581 · Fiber: 18g · Saturated fat: 2.3g · Sodium: 360mg ·
Protein: 22g · Total fat: 16g · Carbs: 90g · Calories from fat: 24%

PHASE TWO

# CHILES RELLENOS

*You can choose many types of peppers to stuff. I prefer poblano chiles, which vary unpredictably from mild and sweet to quite spicy. For tender palates, consider Anaheim or bell peppers. While this recipe requires several steps, the results are rewarding. Leftover chiles store well in the refrigerator for several days.*

Serves: 6

6 medium poblano chiles
4 medium tomatoes, chopped, divided
2 small red bell peppers, roasted
   (page 235) and chopped
1 teaspoon cumin
1 teaspoon chili powder or to taste
2 garlic cloves, minced
2 teaspoons extra-virgin olive oil
1 small onion, chopped
3/4 teaspoon sea salt
1/2 teaspoon dried oregano
1 1/2 cups corn kernels, fresh or frozen
1/2 cup chopped cilantro

One 15-ounce can black beans, rinsed
   and drained
1 large egg (omega-3, free-range,
   organic), whisked
1/2 cup nonfat milk (or calcium-fortified
   soy milk)
1 tablespoon canola oil (organic,
   expeller-pressed)
2 teaspoons baking powder
1 cup cornmeal
Olive oil spray
2 tablespoons nonfat sour cream
Cilantro sprigs

Roast poblano chiles (follow directions for Roasted Bell Peppers on page 235), leaving stems on if possible, and remove skin. Slit chiles lengthwise and remove seeds. Set chiles aside. Preheat oven to 350° F.

To prepare sauce, place 2 chopped tomatoes, roasted bell pepper, 1/2 teaspoon cumin, chili powder, and garlic in a food processor or blender and purée until smooth. Pour into a saucepan and simmer 10 minutes. Set aside.

Heat a sauté pan over medium-high heat, add olive oil, and sauté onion with 1/2 teaspoon salt, oregano, and the remaining 1/2 teaspoon cumin about 2 minutes. Add 1 cup corn and remaining chopped tomatoes, cook 2 minutes, then add cilantro and beans and remove from heat.

In a food processor or blender purée egg, milk, oil, remaining 1/2 cup corn, remaining 1/4 teaspoon salt, and baking powder. Stir in the cornmeal.

Place chiles in an ovenproof pan sprayed with olive oil. Spoon cornmeal mixture into each poblano pepper and top with sauce. Bake 20 minutes. Reheat sauce and pour around baked chiles. Garnish with sour cream and cilantro sprigs.

*Per Serving*
Calories: 368 · Fiber: 10g · Saturated fat: 1g · Sodium: 348mg ·
Protein: 12g · Total fat: 7g · Carbs: 67g · Calories from fat: 17%

PHASE TWO

# COUSCOUS WITH CHICKEN

*This is a fragrant meal, good for company, and easy to prepare.*
*Shrimp or garbanzo beans can be substituted for chicken.*

Serves: 4

2 tablespoons extra-virgin olive oil
4 chicken breasts, cut into strips
½ medium sweet onion, diced
1 medium fennel bulb, chopped
2 carrots, chopped
¼ teaspoon cumin
½ teaspoon cinnamon
½ teaspoon paprika
½ teaspoon saffron (optional)

1 medium red bell pepper, chopped
¼ cup chopped dried fruit (figs, dates, and/or raisins)
2 cups low-sodium vegetable stock
1½ cups whole-grain couscous
Tabasco to taste
3 scallions, chopped
2 tablespoons slivered almonds

Heat a sauté pan over medium-high heat. Add oil and sauté chicken strips for 3 minutes or until no longer pink. Set chicken aside. In the same pan, sauté onion, fennel, carrots, cumin, cinnamon, paprika, and saffron over medium-high heat for 2 to 3 minutes, stirring occasionally, until onion softens. Add bell pepper and dried fruit and sauté for 2 to 3 minutes, stirring occasionally. Mix in chicken, cover, and set aside.

In a large pot, heat stock to boiling and add couscous. Reduce heat and simmer for 5 minutes. Add chicken mixture and cook another 5 to 10 minutes, until couscous is done. Add Tabasco and garnish with scallions and almonds.

*Variation:* Substitute 1 pound shrimp, shelled and deveined, for the chicken or one 15-ounce can rinsed and drained garbanzo beans. Add at the same time as the bell pepper and dried fruit and cook until shrimp is pink, then continue with recipe.

*Per Serving*
Calories: 603 · Fiber: 10g · Saturated fat: 2g · Sodium: 638mg ·
Protein: 47g · Total fat: 144g · Carbs: 74g · Calories from fat: 21%

# CRAB CAKES

*This meal is easy and tasty. You can sauté these cakes in a skillet with olive oil,
but they hold together better when baked in the oven. Fresh crab is best,
but this recipe works with canned crab too.*

Serves: 4

2 tablespoons freshly squeezed lemon
   juice
1 tablespoon Dijon mustard
½ cup nonfat sour cream
¼ teaspoon black pepper
2 large eggs (omega-3, free-range,
   organic), beaten
1 pound crabmeat, picked over for shells
2 teaspoons extra-virgin olive oil
½ cup sweet onion, minced

½ cup diced celery
1 cup sliced mushrooms
½ teaspoon dried thyme
2 slices whole-wheat bread, toasted and
   ground into crumbs in food processor
½ cup chopped flat-leaf parsley
¼ cup slivered almonds
Olive oil spray
1 lemon, sliced

Preheat oven to 350° F. Combine lemon juice, mustard, sour cream, pepper, and eggs in a bowl. Add crab, mix, and set aside.

Heat a sauté pan over medium-high heat, add oil, and sauté onion, celery, mushrooms, and thyme until onion is translucent. Remove from heat and add bread crumbs, parsley, and almonds. Add onion mixture to crab mixture and form into eight patties.

Place on a cookie sheet sprayed with oil. Spray the top of each patty for 1 to 2 seconds with olive oil. Let sit for 5 to 10 minutes.

Bake for 20 minutes, until cakes are golden. Serve with sliced lemon.

*Per Serving*
Calories: 290 · Fiber: 3g · Saturated fat: 1.3g · Sodium: 540mg ·
Protein: 29.5g · Total fat: 8.5g · Carbs: 24g · Calories from fat: 26%

# FALAFEL

*Falafel, tomatoes, cucumbers, lettuce, and yogurt make a great stuffing for pita bread. For an extra treat, replace tomatoes with Salsa (page 236), yogurt with Raita (page 294), and add Guacamole (page 234) in place of lettuce.*

Serves: 4

1 tablespoon extra-virgin olive oil
⅔ cup chopped onion
¼ teaspoon sea salt
½ teaspoon cumin
¼ teaspoon black pepper
2 cups chopped carrots
1 cup chopped celery
¼ cup chopped mint
¼ cup lemon juice
One 15-ounce can garbanzo beans, rinsed and drained

1 slice whole-wheat bread, toasted and processed into crumbs (½ cup)
2 large eggs (omega-3, free-range, organic)
Olive oil spray
4 medium pita breads
1 medium cucumber, diced
1 cup chopped tomatoes
2 cups Bibb lettuce, chopped
1 cup nonfat yogurt

Preheat oven to 375° F.

Heat a sauté pan over medium-high heat, add oil, then sauté onion with salt, cumin, and pepper for 2 minutes. Add carrots and celery and cook 2 to 3 minutes, until carrots and celery soften slightly but are still firm.

Put vegetables in a blender or food processor and add mint, lemon juice, garbanzo beans, bread crumbs, and eggs. Process to form a chunky paste. Form into eight patties.

Place patties on a cookie sheet sprayed with olive oil and spray tops of patties. Bake for about 25 minutes, until lightly browned.

Serve falafel patties in warmed pita halves with cucumber, tomatoes, lettuce, and yogurt.

*Per Serving*
Calories: 383 · Fiber: 9.5g · Saturated fat: 1.5g · Sodium: 563mg ·
Protein: 18g · Total fat: 8.6g · Carbs: 61g · Calories from fat: 20%

PHASE TWO

# GARBANZO, CAULIFLOWER, AND RED PEPPER CURRY

*This is a colorful, flavorful, and easy curry. Substitute chicken or shrimp for garbanzo beans as desired. Serve with Indian Rice (page 290) and Raita (page 294) for a complete meal.*

Serves: 4

1 tablespoon canola oil (organic, expeller-pressed)
½ medium onion, chopped
¼ teaspoon sea salt
2 medium carrots, sliced
1½ tablespoons curry powder
1 tablespoon grated ginger
⅛ teaspoon cayenne or to taste
1 medium potato, cut into ½-inch cubes
3 tablespoons tomato paste

1 medium head cauliflower, cut into 1-inch cubes
1 medium red bell pepper, sliced into ½-inch strips
One 15-ounce can garbanzo beans, rinsed and drained
4 garlic cloves, minced
1 cup frozen peas, thawed
1 cup nonfat yogurt
¼ cup chopped cilantro

Heat a large skillet over medium-high heat. Add canola oil, onion, salt, and carrots and cook for 2 minutes, stirring occasionally. Add curry powder, ginger, cayenne, and potato and cook for 1 to 2 minutes, stirring often. Combine tomato paste with ½ cup hot water and add to curry. Cover, reduce heat to medium, and simmer for 5 to 10 minutes, until potato is nearly tender. Add cauliflower, bell pepper, garbanzo beans, garlic, and peas and cook 2 to 4 minutes more, until potato and cauliflower are tender.

Remove from heat and set aside for 2 minutes. Stir in yogurt. Garnish with cilantro and serve.

*Variation:* Make your own curry powder with 1 teaspoon cumin, 1 teaspoon cardamom, 1 teaspoon turmeric, 1 teaspoon ground ginger, ¼ teaspoon sea salt, and ¼ teaspoon black pepper.

*Per Serving*
Calories: 271 · Fiber: 11.5g · Saturated fat: 0.3g · Sodium: 283mg ·
Protein: 15g · Total fat: 5.6g · Carbs: 42g · Calories from fat: 18%

# GRILLED MAHI MAHI SOFT TACOS

*You could substitute cod, snapper, or tilapia depending upon what's freshest at the market.*

Serves: 4

1½ pounds mahi mahi fillets
Juice of 1 lime
½ teaspoon paprika
¼ teaspoon dried oregano
¼ teaspoon sea salt
⅛ teaspoon black pepper

Olive oil spray
8 corn tortillas
4 cups shredded lettuce (or cabbage)
Mango Salsa (page 235)
4 tablespoons nonfat sour cream

Rinse and dry fish fillets. Marinate in a dish with lime juice, paprika, oregano, salt, and pepper for 10 minutes. Spray both sides of fish with olive oil and grill about 10 to 12 minutes for a 1-inch thick fillet, turning halfway through, or broil for 12 to 15 minutes, turning halfway through. Cut fish into 8 pieces.

Heat corn tortillas in a skillet and keep warm.

To serve, place one piece of fish in center of tortilla. Fold in half. Top with lettuce, Mango Salsa, and sour cream.

*Serving suggestion:* Great side dishes include Roasted Bell Peppers (page 235), black beans, and Mexican Rice (page 291).

*Per Serving*
Calories: 386 · Fiber: 5g · Saturated fat: 0.3g · Sodium: 455mg ·
Protein: 47g · Total fat: 4g · Carbs: 40g · Calories from fat: 9%

PHASE TWO

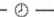

# GRILLED SHRIMP KABOBS

*Easy to make, fun to eat. You can use fish or chicken in place of shrimp*

Serves: 4 (makes 10–12 kabobs)

1 pound large shrimp, shelled and
   deveined
½ medium red onion, cut into quarters,
   each quarter separated into 4 pieces
1 large green bell pepper, cut into 1-to-2-
   inch pieces
8 ounces fresh or canned pineapple
   chunks
16 large cherry tomatoes

16 small button mushrooms
1½ tablespoons extra-virgin olive oil
1½ tablespoons balsamic vinegar
½ teaspoon sea salt
¼ teaspoon black pepper
½ teaspoon paprika
½ teaspoon cayenne or to taste
1 teaspoon Dijon mustard
Olive oil spray

*(continued)*

In a deep bowl, combine all ingredients except olive oil spray and mix well. Marinate, refrigerated, 15 to 20 minutes. Preheat grill or broiler.

Thread shrimp, onion, pepper, pineapple, cherry tomato, and mushrooms on metal skewers. (If you use bamboo skewers, soak them in water for at least 15 minutes to prevent them from burning.) Spray well with olive oil. Grill until shrimp are cooked through.

*Serving suggestion:* Serve over brown rice, wild rice, couscous, or barley, or with a tossed salad.

*Per Serving*
Calories: 258 · Fiber: 3.7g · Saturated fat: 1g · Sodium: 558mg ·
Protein: 26g · Total fat: 8g · Carbs: 22g · Calories from fat: 27%

# MARINATED SALMON WITH PECAN NUT CRUST

*Fish with nut crusts are very tasty, and this is one of my favorite fish-nut combos. Try almonds, pecans, or hazelnuts. Choose the freshest fish you can find—sole, flounder, tilapia, and cod are also delicious.*

Serves: 4

1½ pounds salmon (in 4 fillets)
2 tablespoons sherry
2 tablespoons rice vinegar
1 tablespoon low-sodium soy sauce
1 teaspoon sesame oil
1 cup pecans, toasted, finely ground in blender or food processor

2 slices whole-wheat bread, toasted and processed into crumbs (1 cup)
½ teaspoon sea salt
⅛ teaspoon black pepper
Canola oil spray
4 lemon wedges

Preheat oven to 400° F.

Rinse salmon and pat dry. Mix sherry, vinegar, soy sauce, and sesame oil in a bowl, add fish, and marinate, refrigerated, for 30 to 60 minutes, turning once or twice.

Combine pecans, bread crumbs, salt, and pepper in a shallow dish. Remove fish from marinade and dip in nut mixture. Spray a baking pan with oil and place breaded fish on it. Spray the top of each fillet.

Bake 20 to 25 minutes, until tender and flaky. Serve with a wedge of lemon.

*Per Serving*
Calories: 493 · Fiber: 3.3g · Saturated fat: 4g · Sodium: 536mg ·
Protein: 41g · Total fat: 31g · Carbs: 10.5g · Calories from fat: 57%

PHASE TWO

# PEPPERONATA

*This is a popular Italian pepper stew we enjoy serving on a bed of pasta,*
*but you can eat it with any grain dish. It's also a great topping for polenta.*

Serves: 4

1 tablespoon extra-virgin olive oil
1 medium onion, chopped
¼ teaspoon sea salt
¼ teaspoon black pepper
1 teaspoon Italian seasoning
1 medium zucchini, sliced
¼ cup dry white wine
4 medium bell peppers, various colors, julienned

4 garlic cloves, minced
2 medium tomatoes, chopped
One 15-ounce can cannellini beans, rinsed and drained
8 ounces whole-wheat, or other fiber-enriched pasta
½ cup pine nuts (or sliced almonds), toasted
½ cup chopped parsley

Heat a large sauté pan or saucepan over medium-high heat. Add oil, then sauté onion with salt, pepper, and Italian seasoning for about 3 minutes, until onion is translucent. Add zucchini and cook 2 minutes, stirring occasionally. Add wine, then mix in peppers, garlic, and tomatoes, cover, and simmer 4 to 5 minutes, until tomatoes and peppers are cooked but not overly soft. Add cannellini beans.

Spoon hot cooked pasta onto a platter and top with pepper stew. Garnish with pine nuts and parsley.

*Per Serving*
Calories: 495 · Fiber: 15.5g · Saturated fat: 2.8g · Sodium: 439mg ·
Protein: 23g · Total fat: 14g · Carbs: 71g · Calories from fat: 24%

# SCALLOPS WITH SOY-CHILI SAUCE

*In our home, this is a favorite seafood dish. The sauce is grand over scallops,*
*but if the scallops in the store don't smell absolutely fresh,*
*then try the same sauce with shrimp or salmon.*

Serves: 4

1½ pounds scallops
2 tablespoons rice vinegar
2 tablespoons brown sugar (or 6 packets of Splenda)
3 garlic cloves, minced
1 tablespoon grated ginger

1 teaspoon sesame oil
¼ teaspoon cayenne or to taste
1 teaspoon kuzu root (or cornstarch)
2 tablespoons low-sodium soy sauce
Juice of 1 lime

(continued)

PHASE TWO

Rinse scallops and pat dry. Mix vinegar, sugar, garlic, ginger, sesame oil, and cayenne in a saucepan over medium heat. Dissolve kuzu in soy sauce and lime juice and add to vinegar mixture. Cook until mixture starts to bubble and resembles thin syrup. Set aside.

Heat a sauté pan over high heat. Spray pan with oil and sear scallops 1 to 2 minutes on each side, until tender; be careful not to overcook. Serve scallops with warm sauce.

*Serving suggestion:* Serve over brown rice and/or a bed of sautéed spinach with a side dish of sautéed vegetables.

*Per Serving*
Calories: 201 · Fiber: 0.5g · Saturated fat: 0.3g · Sodium: 583mg ·
Protein: 30g · Total fat: 2.6g · Carbs: 13g · Calories from fat: 12%

# SOLE WITH OYSTER AND LIME SAUCE

*This oyster and lime marinade is great with fish, shrimp, and tofu.*

Serves: 4

1½ pounds sole (in 4 fillets)
2 tablespoons oyster sauce
Juice of 1 lime
1 tablespoon sherry (or white wine or sake)

1 teaspoon low-sodium soy sauce
1 garlic clove, minced
¼ teaspoon lime zest (optional)
¼ cup chopped cilantro

Preheat oven to 425° F. Rinse sole and pat dry, and place in an ovenproof dish. Mix oyster sauce, lime juice, sherry, soy sauce, garlic, and lime zest and pour over fish. Refrigerate for 30 to 60 minutes.

Bake sole in marinade for 20 to 25 minutes, until tender and flaky. Garnish with cilantro.

*Per Serving*
Calories: 145 · Fiber: 0g · Saturated fat: 0g · Sodium: 370mg ·
Protein: 29g · Total fat: 1.5g · Carbs: 1.5g · Calories from fat: 13%

## Salad Recipes

### MIXED GREEN SALAD WITH SALMON, APPLE, AND CORN

*For an easy lunch out on the patio, my wife and I will put these ingredients together. This meal is packed with a symphony of colors—clearly health-promoting.*

Serves: 2

3 cups mixed greens
1 cup grated or finely shredded red cabbage
2 celery stalks, chopped
One 4-ounce can corn, rinsed and drained
1 medium apple, cut into ½-inch cubes
1 medium tomato, sliced

Vinaigrette Dressing (page 233)
  (or Raspberry Vinaigrette Salad
  Dressing, page 341)
7 ounces canned Alaskan salmon, drained
  and flaked
¼ cup mixed fresh berries (or edible flowers)

Toss greens, cabbage, celery, corn, apple, and tomato in a large salad bowl with Vinaigrette Dressing. Divide salad between two plates, top with salmon, and garnish with berries.

*Per Serving*
Calories: 214 · Fiber: 5.5g · Saturated fat: 2g · Sodium: 486mg ·
Protein: 23g · Total fat: 6.7g · Carbs: 17g · Calories from fat: 27%

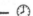

### PASTA SALAD WITH VEGGIES, WHITE BEANS, AND PINE NUTS

*Pasta salad is great for picnics and potlucks, and leftovers create easy lunches. Add turkey, chicken, or seafood to transform this into a hearty and vibrantly colored dinner.*

Serves: 4

¾ teaspoon sea salt
5 tablespoons extra-virgin olive oil
8 ounces whole-wheat or fiber-enriched
  spirals or bow ties
½ medium onion, diced
1 teaspoon Italian seasoning
¼ teaspoon black pepper
¼ cup white wine (or stock)
2 medium carrots, diced
4 cups chopped broccoli

1 medium yellow squash, chopped
3 tablespoons balsamic vinegar
1 tablespoon low-sodium soy sauce
2 garlic cloves, minced
1 teaspoon Dijon mustard
¼ cup pine nuts, toasted
20 medium cherry tomatoes
One 15-ounce can cannellini, rinsed and
  drained
½ cup chopped parsley

(continued)

PHASE TWO

Bring water to a boil in a large pot and add ½ teaspoon salt and 1 tablespoon olive oil. Add pasta, stir, and boil for 8 to 10 minutes, until al dente (do not overcook). Drain and rinse in cold water to stop the cooking. Set aside.

Heat a sauté pan to medium high, add 2 tablespoons oil, and sauté onion with Italian seasoning, ¼ teaspoon salt, and pepper for 2 to 3 minutes, until translucent. Add wine to deglaze and stir. Add carrots, broccoli, and squash and sauté 2 to 4 minutes. Mix vegetables with pasta in a serving bowl and set aside.

Whisk together vinegar, remaining 2 tablespoons oil, soy sauce, garlic, and mustard. Add to serving bowl and toss. Top with pine nuts, tomatoes, cannellini, and parsley.

*Per Serving*
Calories: 609 · Fiber: 12.5g · Saturated fat: 3g · Sodium: 349mg ·
Protein: 26g · Total fat: 20.5g · Carbs: 88g · Calories from fat: 28%

# SPINACH SALAD WITH SAUTÉED SHRIMP AND ORANGE VINAIGRETTE DRESSING

*Shrimp, ginger, mint, and oranges bring tantalizing flavors to this salad.*
*You could also try chicken or a white fish in place of the shrimp.*

Serves: 2

| | |
|---|---|
| 5½ teaspoons extra-virgin olive oil | 2 medium carrots, grated |
| 1 tablespoon grated ginger | 4 tablespoons chopped mint |
| 10 ounces large shrimp, peeled and deveined, rinsed and patted dry | 1 tablespoon balsamic vinegar |
| | 2 tablespoons orange juice |
| 2 cups mixed organic greens | ½ teaspoon Dijon mustard |
| 4 cups baby spinach leaves | ½ teaspoon grated orange zest |

Heat a sauté pan over medium-high heat, add 1 teaspoon oil and ginger, and cook for 1 minute. Add shrimp and cook, stirring, 3 to 4 minutes, until shrimp are pink and curled.

Mix greens, spinach, carrots, and mint in a large bowl. Whisk remaining oil, vinegar, juice, mustard, and orange zest and toss with salad. Top with shrimp and serve.

*Per Serving*
Calories: 339 · Fiber: 5.3g · Saturated fat: 2.2g · Sodium: 552mg ·
Protein: 31g · Total fat: 14.5g · Carbs: 22g · Calories from fat: 38%

# TABBOULEH

*This is a wholesome Middle Eastern salad with wonderful texture.*
*It makes a great side dish with chicken, fish, or falafel,*
*or can be served by itself for lunch.*

Serves: 4

1½ cups bulgur
2 tablespoons extra-virgin olive oil
½ medium onion, diced
¼ teaspoon sea salt
1 teaspoon Italian seasoning
3 garlic cloves, minced
¼ cup chopped walnuts
2 medium tomatoes, chopped

1 cup chopped parsley
½ cup chopped mint
Juice of 2 lemons (or limes)
1 tablespoon balsamic vinegar
½ 15-ounce can garbanzo beans, rinsed
   and drained (or white beans)
Lettuce for serving, optional
Parsley and mint sprigs for garnish

Combine bulgur with 1¾ cups boiling water (or vegetable broth) in a large bowl, cover, and let sit for 20 minutes, stirring occasionally.

Heat a sauté pan over medium-high heat. Add 1 tablespoon oil and sauté onion with salt and Italian seasoning for 2 to 3 minutes, until onion softens. Add garlic and walnuts and cook 1 minute, stirring frequently. Stir vegetable-nut mixture into bulgur and let sit for 20 minutes to blend flavors.

Meanwhile, in a separate bowl, combine tomatoes, parsley, mint, lemon juice, remaining olive oil, vinegar, and beans. Add tomato-bean mixture to bulgur and chill.

*Serving suggestion:* Serve either in a large salad bowl or over a bed of lettuce on a platter. Garnish with sprigs of parsley and mint.

*Per Serving*
Calories: 525 · Fiber: 17.5g · Saturated fat: 1.6g · Sodium: 165mg ·
Protein: 16g · Total fat: 16g · Carbs: 82g · Calories from fat: 27%

## Side Dish Recipes

# BRUSSELS SPROUTS WITH VINAIGRETTE DRESSING

*I had no idea I liked Brussels sprouts until I tried them steamed and
with a vinaigrette. Brussels sprouts are packed with calcium, nutrients,
and anti-aging compounds.*

Serves: 4

4 cups Brussels sprouts                     Vinaigrette Dressing (page 233)

Prepare Brussels sprouts by cutting off the base of the stems and slicing vegetables in half. Steam about 5 minutes, until tender. Toss with Vinaigrette Dressing and serve.

*Per Serving*
Calories: 138 · Fiber: 3.4g · Saturated fat: 1.5g · Sodium: 50mg ·
Protein: 3g · Total fat: 10.8g · Carbs: 9g · Calories from fat: 66%

# INDIAN RICE

*This makes an excellent side dish. Combined with beans, fish, or chicken
and a vegetable side dish, it makes a complete meal.*

Serves: 4

1 teaspoon canola oil (organic,          ¼ cup chopped dried fruit (figs, dates,
   expeller-pressed)                         and/or raisins) (optional)
¼ medium onion, chopped               ½ cup frozen peas, thawed
¼ teaspoon sea salt                     ¼ cup sliced almonds, toasted
½ teaspoon cumin                        ¼ cup chopped cilantro (optional)
1½ cups brown basmati rice

Heat a large saucepan over medium-high heat. Add oil and sauté onion, salt, and
cumin for 2 to 3 minutes, until onion softens. Add rice and sauté another 2 minutes, stirring often. Add 3 cups water and bring to a boil. Reduce heat to low and
simmer, covered, for another 35 to 40 minutes, until rice is tender. Add dried fruit,
peas, nuts and heat 2 to 3 minutes, until peas are cooked. Garnish with cilantro.

*Variation:* If you have leftovers, add ½ cup garbanzo beans or cooked cubed
chicken breast, ½ cup more peas, and refrigerate for a future lunch.

*Per Serving*
Calories: 369 · Fiber: 7.8g · Saturated fat: 1g · Sodium: 180mg ·
Protein: 9.6g · Total fat: 10.7g · Carbs: 59g · Calories from fat: 26%

# MEXICAN RICE

*This is a rice dish we like to serve with Mexican or Latin American food.*
*It's very colorful and packed with nutrients. Use it as a side dish,*
*or add beans and serve as a main course.*

Serves: 6

1 teaspoon extra-virgin olive oil
1 medium onion, chopped
½ teaspoon sea salt
1 teaspoon paprika, ground
1½ cups brown rice

1 cup corn
1 medium red bell pepper, sliced
2 medium tomatoes, chopped
¼ cup chopped fresh cilantro (optional)

Heat a large saucepan to medium high. Add oil, then onion, salt, and paprika
and sauté for 2 to 3 minutes, until onion softens. Add rice and sauté another 2
minutes, stirring often. Add 3 cups water and bring to a boil. Cover, reduce
heat to low, and simmer for 30 minutes. Stir in corn, bell pepper, and tomatoes
and simmer covered for another 5-10 minutes, until rice is al dente.

Serve and garnish with chopped cilantro.

*Per Serving*
Calories: 310 · Fiber: 2.7g · Saturated fat: 0.8g · Sodium: 204mg ·
Protein: 7g · Total fat: 5g · Carbs: 60g · Calories from fat: 15%

PHASE TWO

# ROASTED BEETS, CARROTS, AND PARSNIPS

*Roasted vegetables are much sweeter than when they are baked or sautéed.*
*You can also roast rutabagas, zucchini, asparagus, and other vegetables.*

Serves: 6

4 large beets, peeled and sliced into
    ¾-inch wedges
4 medium carrots, scrubbed, unpeeled,
    cut into 1-inch pieces
4 medium parsnips, scrubbed, unpeeled,
    cut into 1-inch pieces
1 medium red onion, cut into eighths

½ teaspoon sea salt
¼ teaspoon black pepper
1 teaspoon Italian seasoning
2 tablespoons extra-virgin olive oil
1 cup green beans (or scallions)
Olive oil spray

Preheat oven to 425° F.

Toss beets, carrots, parsnips, and onions with salt, pepper, Italian seasoning,
and 2 tablespoons olive oil. Place on a baking sheet and bake 20 to 25 minutes,

*(continued)*

until nearly tender. Spray green beans with olive oil and add to the baking sheet. Bake 10 to 15 minutes longer, until all vegetables are tender.

*Per Serving*
Calories: 181 · Fiber: 8.4g · Saturated fat: 1g · Sodium: 378mg · Protein: 3g · Total fat: 7.5g · Carbs: 28g · Calories from fat: 35%

---

## SNOW PEAS WITH BOK CHOY

*Bok choy is used often in Asian cuisine and is a lovely side dish with many meals. It is rich in calcium and has some of the same anti-aging compounds found in broccoli. Don't overcook this vegetable—it's best when it remains tender yet crunchy.*

Serves: 4

1 teaspoon canola oil (organic, expeller-pressed)
1 tablespoon grated ginger
2 cups snow peas, trimmed
1 bunch bok choy, chopped

2 garlic cloves, minced
¼ cup low-sodium vegetable stock or water
1 teaspoon low-sodium soy sauce
1 teaspoon sesame oil

Heat a sauté pan over medium-high heat, add oil and ginger, and cook 1 minute. Add snow peas, bok choy, garlic, and stock and cook, stirring occasionally, 2 to 3 minutes, until vegetables are tender but still crisp. Stir in soy sauce and sesame oil and serve.

*Per Serving*
Calories: 59 · Fiber: 2g · Saturated fat: 0.2g · Sodium: 181mg · Protein: 12g · Total fat: 1.2g · Carbs: 12g · Calories from fat: 32%

## Condiment Recipes

---

## APRICOT, GINGER, AND PEAR SAUCE

*Serving maple syrup might be quicker, but this is a lovely sauce with pancakes, French toast, waffles, or crêpes, and it's packed with nutrients and flavor.*

Serves: 4

3 tablespoons sugar (or 9 packets of Splenda)
1 teaspoon kuzu powder (or cornstarch)
⅔ cup apricot nectar (or orange juice)
½ teaspoon vanilla

1 cup chopped apricots, fresh or canned
1 medium Bosc pear, diced
2 tablespoons candied ginger, diced
1 to 2 tablespoons Grand Marnier (optional)
Chopped fresh mint

Dissolve sugar and kuzu in apricot nectar in a small saucepan. Add vanilla and bring to a boil. Add apricots, pear, and ginger and bring back to a boil. Reduce heat to low, add Grand Marnier, and simmer 10 minutes. Serve hot or chilled, garnished with mint.

*Per Serving*
Calories: 140 · Fiber: 2g · Saturated fat: 0g · Sodium: 2mg ·
Protein: 0.8g · Total fat: 0.3g · Carbs: 26.3g · Calories from fat: 2%

# EDAMAME

*Green soybeans are a fantastic snack, and they're loaded with nutrients. Frozen soybeans need just a short steaming or microwaving and they're ready to serve.*

Serves: 2

4 cups frozen soybeans in the pod
  (or 2 cups shelled)
1 tablespoon rice vinegar

1 teaspoon low-sodium soy sauce
Tabasco sauce

Heat soybeans in the microwave about 5 minutes or add to boiling water and cook 5 to 6 minutes until warm and al dente. Drain. If cooking the beans in their pods, discard pods after heating. In a bowl, mix heated soybeans with vinegar, soy sauce, and Tabasco to taste.

*Per Serving*
Calories: 185 · Fiber: 6g · Saturated fat: 0.75g · Sodium: 95mg ·
Protein: 15g · Total fat: 7.5g · Carbs: 15g · Calories from fat: 50%

# HUMMUS

*Hummus makes a lovely dip for veggies and pita bread triangles.*

Serves: 4

One 15-ounce can garbanzo beans, rinsed
  and drained
2 to 4 garlic cloves
¼ cup lemon juice
2 tablespoons sesame tahini

⅛ teaspoon cayenne or to taste
¼ teaspoon ground ginger
¼ teaspoon sea salt
3 tablespoons extra-virgin olive oil
1 medium tomato, chopped

Combine garbanzo beans, garlic, lemon juice, tahini, cayenne, ginger, salt, olive oil, and tomato in a blender or food processor. Pulse until smooth.

*Per Serving*
Calories: 284 · Fiber: 5.4g · Saturated fat: 2.5g · Sodium: 300mg ·
Protein: 9g · Total fat: 19g · Carbs: 21.6g · Calories from fat: 60%

# RAITA

*Raita is wonderful with curry and as a side dish.*
*If your mouth explodes from a hot chile, dive for the raita to recover.*

Serves: 4

1 cup plain nonfat yogurt
¼ medium onion, diced
½ medium cucumber, diced

¼ cup chopped cilantro
¼ teaspoon whole cumin seed
Dash paprika

Combine yogurt, onion, cucumber, cilantro, and cumin and refrigerate at least 20 minutes. Garnish with paprika and serve.

*Per Serving*
Calories: 143 · Fiber: 1.3g · Saturated fat: 0g · Sodium: 155mg ·
Protein: 12g · Total fat: 0.2g · Carbs: 24g · Calories from fat: 1%

# SPICY BAKED GARBANZO BEANS

*Baked garbanzo beans can make a very nice snack or can be served with*
*veggies and rice to make a complete dinner.*

Serves: 4

One 15-ounce can garbanzo beans, rinsed
    and drained
¼ teaspoon sea salt
⅛ teaspoon black pepper

¼ teaspoon cayenne or to taste
¼ teaspoon cumin, ground
2 teaspoons extra-virgin olive oil

Preheat oven to 425° F.

Mix all ingredients and spread on a baking sheet. Bake 20 to 25 minutes until garbanzo beans are crisp and chewy but not hard.

*Per Serving*
Calories: 118 · Fiber: 4g · Saturated fat: 0.3g · Sodium: 150mg ·
Protein: 6g · Total fat: 4g · Carbs: 16g · Calories from fat: 27%

## Dessert Recipes

# BLUEBERRY-SOY MILK SMOOTHIE

*A popular dessert or snack in our home.*

Serves: 2

PHASE TWO

2 cups calcium-fortified soy milk                    Juice of ½ lime
2 cups frozen blueberries

Combine all ingredients in a blender or food processor and pulse until smooth.

*Per Serving*
Calories: 172 · Fiber: 5g · Saturated fat: 0.5g · Sodium: 145mg ·
Protein: 7g · Total fat: 4g · Carbs: 30g · Calories from fat: 20%

---

# CHERRY AND ORANGE JUICE SMOOTHIE

*Simply delicious!*

Serves: 2

2 cups orange juice                                  2 tablespoons port (optional)
2 cups frozen Bing cherries, thawed                  Juice of ½ lime
    (about 12 ounces)

Combine all ingredients in a blender or food processor and pulse until smooth.

*Per Serving*
Calories: 119 · Fiber: 1.7g · Saturated fat: 0g · Sodium: 1mg ·
Protein: 2g · Total fat: 0.7g · Carbs: 26g · Calories from fat: 5%

PHASE TWO

---

# PEACH AND RASPBERRY CRUMBLE

*A simple dish that tastes great. Berries high in pectin, such as raspberries
and blackberries, are ideal for this recipe.*

Serves: 4

¼ cup maple syrup (or ¼ cup apple juice            2 tablespoons quick-cooking tapioca
    with 2 tablespoons Splenda)                     Juice of 1 lime
2 cups sliced peaches (thawed and                  1 medium green apple, peeled, cored,
    drained if frozen)                                 and cut into ½-inch cubes
½ cup unsweetened applesauce                        1 cup low-fat granola
2 cups raspberries (thawed and drained             ¼ cup sliced almonds
    if frozen)                                      ½ cup nonfat yogurt, plain (or vanilla)

Preheat oven to 375° F.

In a saucepan over medium heat, cook syrup, peaches, applesauce, raspberries, tapioca, and lime juice until bubbling, about 5 minutes. Add apple and
reduce heat to low. Simmer 5 minutes. Pour into a pie plate. Cover with granola
and almonds and bake 15 minutes. Serve in bowls topped with yogurt.

*Per Serving*
Calories: 373 · Fiber: 9g · Saturated fat: 1g · Sodium: 123mg ·
Protein: 8g · Total fat: 10g · Carbs: 67g · Calories from fat: 23%

# Taking Off the Years

Now that you're in Phase Three, you'll find your energy and concentration have improved, you sleep more soundly, your clothes fit better (you may have had to buy some new outfits!), and even your sex life has gotten noticeably zippier.

For the next six weeks, your Age-Busting Fitness plan will help you increase the weights you're using for strength training. Remember, if you're at the point where you can smoothly lift a weight 16 times, it's time to take it up a notch. Your exercise and calorie-burning ability will continue to rise, and you should maintain your interval training at least twice a week to increase your aerobic capacity. Many people find that by this phase, their exercise routine has become fairly easy—if so, it's time to retest yourself and find your new maximum heart rate. (See Chapter 3.) Pick up the pace to keep your heart rate in your new aerobic zone, as I explained in Chapter 6.

You're now in Phase Three of the Ten Years Younger Diet as well. The hydrogenated fat and corn syrup toxins should have completely disappeared from your diet by now, and you'll be enjoying an abundance of anti-aging foods daily. With the Phase Three recipes, I'll help you eat at least 30 grams of fiber a day. Cruciferous vegetables, allicin-rich foods (garlic, onions, leeks, and scallions), beans, flaxseed, and soy products are part of your eating routine too. If you're a man or woman with hor-monal symptoms (perimenopause, menopause, andropause), then I'll bet you've discovered that these annoyances have diminished, because all of these foods enhance detoxification and the metabolism of your hor-mones. Adding the Phase Three Berry, Soy Milk, and Flax Smoothie reg-ularly to your diet will help alleviate these symptoms even further.

While you may not have loved every single recipe in Phases One and Two, by now you should have found at least ten or twelve that you can enjoy regularly. That's all you really need for normal dining. In Phase Three, you'll see a few popular recipes repeated, plus many new ones to spark your interest. You can still enjoy wine or other alcoholic beverages with dinner, but don't drink more than one to two restaurant-sized serv-ings a day, and I'll still have you skip alcohol two days a week. But if you're aiming to lose weight, limit your alcohol intake to no more than 4 to 5 servings a week.

As you move through the next six weeks, your skin will be growing younger and its fine lines disappearing as you apply retinol and hydroxy acid products. Just don't forget the hat and the sunscreen! Your detox plan will continue to remove chemicals from your system. If you eat more than two to three servings a month of largemouth fish, consider checking your mercury level with your regular physician, or simply switch to a healthier form of seafood—sole, shrimp, salmon. You should also review your supplement plan to ensure you're getting enough of what you need.

For mental peace and calm, keep scheduling 20 minutes daily of a relaxing activity that you enjoy. Also, I recommend that you arrange for a massage every two to four weeks. Not only will it feel good and encourage relaxation, but it also helps you to identify stiff areas that you need to stretch more during your workouts, which will prevent exercise-limiting injuries.

While I've provided meal and activity plans for the first two weeks of Phase Three, by now the Ten Years Younger Program should feel like a habit—a new lifestyle that you've acquired. Once you've finished the ten weeks I've outlined, you will be ten years younger! Stay true to the prin-ciples I've stressed throughout this book, and a whole new, healthier world will open up for you for years to come.

# DAILY MEAL AND ACTIVITY PLANS

## Day 1 (Monday)

FOOD PLAN: Vitality Foods

**Breakfast**
Oatmeal with Apples and Blueberries plus 1 tbsp ground flaxseed
Tea or coffee

**Optional Morning Snack**
Edamame, ½ cup

**Lunch**
Spinach Salad with Sautéed Shrimp and Orange Vinaigrette Dressing
Iced tea

**Afternoon Snack**
Baby carrots, 1 cup
Almonds, 1 oz
Water

**Dinner**
Tomatoes and Artichoke Hearts with Salmon and Soba Noodles
Seltzer, wine, or beer

**Dessert**
Mixed fruit and soy milk smoothie
Herbal tea

**Optional Rescue Snack**
1½ oz smoked oysters
Rye crispbread, 2

## *AGE-BUSTING FITNESS PLAN*

### Aerobic Training
- 3-5 minutes of warming up
- Reach 70-85% of your max heart rate, 40 minutes with brisk walking, jogging, and/or elliptical machine work
- Include 10 minutes of interval training
- 3-5 minutes of cooling down, heart rate less than 60% max

### Strength Training
- Rest day from strength training

### Stretching
- 4-6 body parts, 5-10 minutes of stretching time

## RELAXATION ROUTINE
- Choose a calming activity for at least 20 minutes

## SUPPLEMENT ROUTINE
- Take your customized multivitamin pack
- Skin moisturizer with SPF 15
- Apply a facial retinol and a beta hydroxy acid skin product daily

## DETOX ROUTINE
- Enjoy a cup of cruciferous vegetables daily
- Check/replace air filters
- Verify a mold- and mildew-free home
- Calculate your fiber intake to ensure more than 30 grams daily

# Day 2 (Tuesday)

FOOD PLAN: Vitality Foods

## Breakfast
Omelet with Veggies
Soy sausage, 1 piece, or 1 slice whole-wheat toast
Tea or coffee

## Optional Morning Snack
Nonfat cottage cheese, $1/4$ cup, with $3/4$ cup celery sticks

## Lunch
Quesadillas with Roasted Peppers and Refried Beans
Apple
Iced tea

## Afternoon Snack
Carrot and/or celery sticks, 1 cup
Hummus, 4 tbsp
Water

## Dinner
Pad Thai
Seltzer, wine, or beer

## Dessert
Nonfat, sugar-free ice cream with $1/4$ cup berries and 2–3 tbsp pecans
Hot Cocoa

## Optional Rescue Snack
Baby carrots, 1–2 cups
Nuts, 1 oz

## AGE-BUSTING FITNESS PLAN

### Aerobic Training
- 3-5 minutes of warming up
- Reach 70-85% of your max heart rate for 35-45 minutes total activity with brisk walking, jogging, or elliptical machines
- 3-5 minutes of cooling down, heart rate less than 60% max

### Strength Training
- Retest your push-up and sit-up ability
- 12 body parts, 2 sets, 10-16 reps
- Use a mixture of ball and free weight activities

### Stretching
- 4-6 body parts, 5-10 minutes of stretching time

## RELAXATION ROUTINE
- Choose a calming activity for at least 20 minutes

## SUPPLEMENT ROUTINE
- Take your customized multivitamin pack
- Skin moisturizer with SPF 15
- Apply a facial retinol and a beta hydroxy acid skin product daily

## DETOX ROUTINE
- Enjoy a cup of cruciferous vegetables daily
- Check/replace air filters
- Verify a mold- and mildew-free home
- Calculate your fiber intake to ensure more than 30 grams daily

PHASE THREE

---

# Day 3 (Wednesday)

FOOD PLAN: Vitality Foods

## Breakfast
Whole-wheat toast, 1 slice, with 1 tbsp almond butter
Soy sausage, 1 piece
Tea or coffee

## Optional Morning Snack
Edamame, ¾ cup

## Lunch
Turkey wrap
Steamed broccoli, 1 cup
Apple
Seltzer

## Afternoon Snack
Almonds, 1 oz
Water

## Dinner
Bay Scallop Stir-Fry
Brown rice, ¾ to 1 cup
Decaf green tea

## Dessert
Fruit salad with vanilla yogurt
Hot Cocoa

## Optional Rescue Snack
Veggie chicken nuggets, 4 pieces

## AGE-BUSTING FITNESS PLAN

### Aerobic Training
- 3–5 minutes of warming up
- Reach 70–85% of your max heart rate, 40 minutes with brisk walking, jogging, and/or elliptical machine work
- Include 10 minutes of interval training
- 3–5 minutes of cooling down, heart rate less than 60% max

### Strength Training
- Rest day from strength training

### Stretching
- 4–6 body parts, 5–10 minutes of stretching time

## RELAXATION ROUTINE
- Schedule a massage

## SUPPLEMENT ROUTINE
- Take your customized multivitamin pack
- Skin moisturizer with SPF 15
- Apply a facial retinol and a beta hydroxy acid skin product daily

## DETOX ROUTINE
- Enjoy a cup of cruciferous vegetables daily
- Check/replace air filters
- Verify a mold- and mildew-free home
- Calculate your fiber intake to ensure more than 30 grams daily

---

# Day 4 (Thursday)

FOOD PLAN: Vitality Foods

## Breakfast
Oatmeal with Apples and Blueberries plus 1 tbsp ground flaxseed
Tea or coffee

## Optional Morning Snack
Edamame, ¾ cup

## Lunch
Veggie burger with sliced tomato, lettuce, mustard, and whole-wheat pita bread
Mixed green salad, 2 cups
Vinaigrette Dressing, 2 tbsp
Iced tea

## Afternoon Snack
Pear
Walnuts, 1 oz
Water

## Dinner
Teriyaki Chicken with Pecan Crust
Barley with Celery, Parsley, and Mushrooms
Seltzer with a splash of orange juice

## Dessert
Cherry and Orange Juice Smoothie
Herbal tea

## Optional Rescue Snack
Sardines, 1½–3 oz
Rye crispbread, 2–3 pieces

## *AGE-BUSTING FITNESS PLAN*

### Aerobic Training
- 3-5 minutes of warming up
- Reach 70-85% of your max heart rate for 30-40 minutes total activity with brisk walking, jogging, elliptical machine options
- 3-5 minutes of cooling down, heart rate less than 60% max

### Strength Training
- 12 body parts, 1 set, 10-16 reps
- Use a mixture of ball and free weight activities

### Stretching
- 4-6 body parts, 5-10 minutes of stretching time

## RELAXATION ROUTINE
- Choose a calming activity for at least 20 minutes

## SUPPLEMENT ROUTINE
- Take your customized multivitamin pack
- Skin moisturizer with SPF 15
- Apply a facial retinol and a beta hydroxy acid skin product daily

## DETOX ROUTINE
- Enjoy a cup of cruciferous vegetables daily
- Check/replace air filters
- Verify a mold- and mildew-free home
- Calculate your fiber intake to ensure more than 30 grams daily

PHASE THREE

# Day 5 (Friday)

FOOD PLAN: Vitality Foods

**Breakfast**
Bran cereal, 1 cup, with ½ cup nonfat milk and ½ cup blueberries
Tea or coffee

**Optional Morning Snack**
Edamame, ½ cup

**Lunch**
Tuscan Grilled Shrimp and White Bean Salad
Orange
Iced tea

**Afternoon Snack**
Pecans, 1 oz
Water

**Dinner**
Gumbo
Sweet Sixteen Salad
Seltzer, wine

**Dessert**
Pear Soufflé with chocolate sauce or Raspberry Sauce
Hot Cocoa

**Optional Rescue Snack**
Veggie chicken nuggets, 4 pieces

## *AGE-BUSTING FITNESS PLAN*

### Aerobic Training
- 3-5 minutes of warming up
- Reach 70-85% of your max heart rate, 40 minutes with brisk walking, jogging, and/or elliptical machine work
- Include 10 minutes of interval training
- 3-5 minutes of cooling down, heart rate less than 60% max

### Strength Training
- Rest day from strength training

### Stretching
- 4-6 body parts, 5-10 minutes of stretching time

## RELAXATION ROUTINE
- Choose a calming activity for at least 20 minutes

## SUPPLEMENT ROUTINE
- Take your customized multivitamin pack
- Skin moisturizer with SPF 15
- Apply a facial retinol and a beta hydroxy acid skin product daily

## DETOX ROUTINE
- Enjoy a cup of cruciferous vegetables daily
- Check/replace air filters
- Verify a mold- and mildew-free home
- Calculate your fiber intake to ensure more than 30 grams daily

# Day 6 (Saturday)

FOOD PLAN: Vitality Foods

## Breakfast
Oatmeal and Flax Muffin with sugar-free apricot jam
Blueberry-Soy Milk Smoothie
Tea or coffee

## Optional Morning Snack
Hot Cocoa

## Lunch
Pasta Salad with Veggies, White Beans, and Pine Nuts
Orange
Iced tea

## Afternoon Snack
Spicy Baked Garbanzo Beans
Water

## Dinner
Leek and Shiitake Soufflé
Brown rice, 1 cup
Steamed broccoli, 1 cup, tossed with Vinaigrette, 1 tbsp
Seltzer, wine

## Dessert
Crêpes Suzette
Seltzer with a splash of orange juice

## Optional Rescue Snack
1 apple
1 oz nuts

## *AGE-BUSTING FITNESS PLAN*

### Aerobic Training
- 3-5 minutes of warming up
- Reach 70-85% of your max heart rate for 30-40 minutes total activity with brisk walking, jogging, elliptical machine options
- 3-5 minutes of cooling down, heart rate less than 60% max

### Strength Training
- 12 body parts, 2 sets, 10-16 reps
- Use a mixture of ball and free weight activities

### Stretching
- 4-6 body parts, 5-10 minutes of stretching time

## RELAXATION ROUTINE
- Choose a calming activity for at least 20 minutes

## SUPPLEMENT ROUTINE
- Take your customized multivitamin pack
- Skin moisturizer with SPF 15
- Apply a facial retinol and a beta hydroxy acid skin product daily

## DETOX ROUTINE
- Enjoy a cup of cruciferous vegetables daily
- Check/replace air filters
- Verify a mold- and mildew-free home
- Calculate your fiber intake to ensure more than 30 grams daily

PHASE THREE

# Day 7 (Sunday)

FOOD PLAN: Vitality Foods

**Breakfast**
Avocado and Broccoli Frittata
Soy sausage, 1 piece
Tea or coffee

**Optional Morning Snack**
None

**Lunch**
White Bean, Corn, and Bell Pepper Salad
Iced mint tea

**Afternoon Snack**
Air-popped popcorn, 2 cups, sprinkled with 1 tbsp brewer's yeast

**Dinner**
Sole with Almond Crust
Citrus, Fennel, and Spinach Salad
Seltzer, wine

**Dessert**
Strawberries, ½ pint, dipped in 1 oz melted semi-sweet dark chocolate, with ¼ cup
    vanilla nonfat yogurt
Herbal tea

**Optional Rescue Snack**
Almonds, 1 oz

## AGE-BUSTING FITNESS PLAN

### Aerobic Training
- Aerobic rest day
- Go for a 20–30 minute casual walk with family and friends

### Strength Training
- Rest day from strength training

### Stretching
- 4–6 body parts, 5–10 minutes of stretching time

## RELAXATION ROUTINE
- Choose a calming activity for at least 20 minutes

## SUPPLEMENT ROUTINE
- Take your customized multivitamin pack
- Skin moisturizer with SPF 15
- Apply a facial retinol and a beta hydroxy acid skin product daily

## DETOX ROUTINE
- Enjoy a cup of cruciferous vegetables daily
- Check/replace air filters
- Verify a mold- and mildew-free home
- Calculate your fiber intake to ensure more than 30 grams daily

---

# Day 8 (Monday)

FOOD PLAN: Vitality Foods

**Breakfast**
Soy sausage, 2 pieces, with ¾ to 1 cup grits
Tea or coffee

**Optional Morning Snack**
Nonfat yogurt, 4–6 oz

**Lunch**
Avocado and Shrimp Cocktail
Mixed green salad, 2 cups
Vinaigrette Dressing, 2 tbsp
Iced mint tea

**Afternoon Snack**
Pear
Walnuts, 1 oz

**Dinner**
Indian Lentils (Dhal)
Indian Rice
Raita
Steamed broccoli
Decaf tea

**Dessert**
Mango Frozen Yogurt
Mint tea

**Optional Rescue Snack**
Almonds, 1 oz

## *AGE-BUSTING FITNESS PLAN*

### Aerobic Training
- 3-5 minutes of warming up
- Reach 70-85% of your max heart rate for 40 minutes total activity with brisk walking, jogging, elliptical machine options
- Include 10 minutes of interval training
- 3-5 minutes of cooling down, heart rate less than 60% max

### Strength Training
- Rest day from strength training

### Stretching
- 4-6 body parts, 5-10 minutes of stretching time

## RELAXATION ROUTINE
- Choose a calming activity for at least 20 minutes

## SUPPLEMENT ROUTINE
- Take your customized multivitamin pack
- Skin moisturizer with SPF 15
- Apply a facial retinol and a beta hydroxy acid skin product daily

## DETOX ROUTINE
- Enjoy a soy product daily
- Skip alcohol at least 2 days per week, and limit alcohol to 1-2 servings per day
- Avoid all passive tobacco smoke
- Use a headset for the cell phone

# Day 9 (Tuesday)

FOOD PLAN: Vitality Foods

**Breakfast**
Bran cereal, 1 cup, with ½ cup berries and ½ cup nonfat milk
Tea or coffee

**Optional Morning Snack**
Blueberry, Soy Milk, and Flaxseed Smoothie

**Lunch**
Crab with Mixed Salad
Apple
Iced tea

**Afternoon Snack**
Hummus, ¼ cup, with baby carrots, 1 cup
Water

**Dinner**
Grilled Turkey Breast
Wild Rice with Red Onions and Shiitake Mushrooms
Sweet Sixteen Salad
Seltzer, wine

**Dessert**
Mixed fresh fruit with nonfat yogurt
Hot Cocoa

**Optional Rescue Snack**
Almonds, 1 oz

PHASE THREE

## *AGE-BUSTING FITNESS PLAN*

### Aerobic Training
- 3-5 minutes of warming up
- Reach 70-85% of your max heart rate for 30-40 minutes total activity with brisk walking, jogging, elliptical machine options
- 3-5 minutes of cooling down, heart rate less than 60% max

### Strength Training
- 12 body parts, 2 sets, 10-16 reps
- Use a mixture of ball and free weight activities

### Stretching
- 4-6 body parts, 5-10 minutes of stretching time

## RELAXATION ROUTINE
- Choose a calming activity for at least 20 minutes

## SUPPLEMENT ROUTINE
- Take your customized multivitamin pack
- Skin moisturizer with SPF 15
- Apply a facial retinol and a beta hydroxy acid skin product daily

## DETOX ROUTINE
- Enjoy a soy product daily
- Skip alcohol at least 2 days per week, and limit alcohol to 1-2 servings per day
- Avoid all passive tobacco smoke
- Use a headset for the cell phone

PHASE THREE

# Day 10 (Wednesday)

FOOD PLAN: Vitality Foods

## Breakfast
Oatmeal and Flaxseed Muffin with 2 tsp sugar-free apricot jam
Blueberry–Soy Milk Smoothie
Tea or coffee

## Optional Morning Snack
Nonfat yogurt, 4–6 oz
Pure water

## Lunch
Chicken wrap
Julienned Vegetables
Lemon Yogurt Dip
Orange
Iced tea

## Afternoon Snack
Pecans, 1 oz

## Dinner
Coq au Vin
Sweet Sixteen Salad
Seltzer, wine

## Dessert
Blueberry and Port Frozen Yogurt
Hot Cocoa

## Optional Rescue Snack
Sardines, 1½–3 oz can
Rye crispbread, 2

## AGE-BUSTING FITNESS PLAN

### Aerobic Training
- 3-5 minutes of warming up
- Reach 70-85% of your max heart rate for 30-40 minutes total activity with brisk walking, jogging, elliptical machine options
- Include 10 minutes of interval training
- 3-5 minutes of cooling down, heart rate less than 60% max

### Strength Training
- Rest day from strength training

### Stretching
- 4-6 body parts, 5-10 minutes of stretching time

## RELAXATION ROUTINE
- Choose a calming activity for at least 20 minutes

## SUPPLEMENT ROUTINE
- Take your customized multivitamin pack
- Skin moisturizer with SPF 15
- Apply a facial retinol and a beta hydroxy acid skin product daily

## DETOX ROUTINE
- Enjoy a soy product daily
- Skip alcohol at least 2 days per week, and limit alcohol to 1-2 servings per day
- Avoid all passive tobacco smoke
- Use a headset for the cell phone

---

# Day 11 (Thursday)

FOOD PLAN: Vitality Foods

## Breakfast
Avocado and Broccoli Frittata
Soy sausage, 1 piece
Tea or coffee

## Optional Morning Snack
Nonfat cottage cheese, ½ cup with celery sticks, 1 cup

## Lunch
Mixed Green Salad with Salmon, Apple, and Corn
Iced tea

## Afternoon Snack
Almonds, 1 oz

## Dinner
Pepperonata
Mixed green salad
Vinaigrette Dressing, 2 tbsp
Seltzer with a splash of orange juice

## Dessert
Mixed fresh fruit, 1 cup
Nonfat vanilla yogurt, ½ cup

## Optional Rescue Snack
Veggie chicken nuggets, 4 pieces

## *AGE-BUSTING FITNESS PLAN*

### Aerobic Training
- 3-5 minutes of warming up
- Reach 70-85% of your max heart rate for 30-40 minutes total activity with brisk walking, jogging, elliptical machine options
- 3-5 minutes of cooling down, heart rate less than 60% max

### Strength Training
- 12 body parts, 1 set, 10-16 reps
- Use a mixture of ball and free weight activities

### Stretching
- 4-6 body parts, 5-10 minutes of stretching time

## RELAXATION ROUTINE
- Choose a calming activity for at least 20 minutes

## SUPPLEMENT ROUTINE
- Take your customized multivitamin pack
- Skin moisturizer with SPF 15
- Apply a facial retinol and a beta hydroxy acid skin product daily

## DETOX ROUTINE
- Enjoy a soy product daily
- Skip alcohol at least 2 days per week, and limit alcohol to 1-2 servings per day
- Avoid all passive tobacco smoke
- Use a headset for the cell phone

PHASE THREE

# Day 12 (Friday)

FOOD PLAN: Vitality Foods

## Breakfast
Oatmeal with Apples and Berries plus 1 tbsp ground flaxseed
Tea or coffee

## Optional Morning Snack
Nonfat yogurt, 4–6 oz
Water

## Lunch
Veggie burger with sliced tomato, mustard, lettuce, and pita bread
Sweet Potato Fries with Cinnamon
Iced tea

## Afternoon Snack
Miso Soup

## Dinner
Cioppino
Steamed broccoli, 1 to 2 cups, tossed with Vinaigrette, 1 tbsp
Seltzer, wine

## Dessert
Nonfat, sugar-free ice cream, $\frac{1}{2}$–$\frac{3}{4}$ cup
Pecans, 2–3 tbsp
Hot Cocoa

## Optional Rescue Snack
Almonds, 1 oz

## AGE-BUSTING FITNESS PLAN

### Aerobic Training
- 3-5 minutes of warming up
- Reach 70-85% of your max heart rate for 40 minutes total activity with brisk walking, jogging, elliptical machine options
- Include 10 minutes of interval training
- 3-5 minutes of cooling down, heart rate less than 60% max

### Strength Training
- Rest day from strength training

### Stretching
- 4-6 body parts, 5-10 minutes of stretching time

## RELAXATION ROUTINE
- Choose a calming activity for at least 20 minutes

## SUPPLEMENT ROUTINE
- Take your customized multivitamin pack
- Skin moisturizer with SPF 15
- Apply a facial retinol and a beta hydroxy acid skin product daily

## DETOX ROUTINE
- Enjoy a soy product daily
- Skip alcohol at least 2 days per week, and limit alcohol to 1-2 servings per day
- Avoid all passive tobacco smoke
- Use a headset for the cell phone

PHASE THREE

---

# Day 13 (Saturday)

FOOD PLAN: Vitality Foods

## Breakfast
Oatmeal and Flaxseed Muffins
Blueberry–Soy Milk Smoothie
Tea or coffee

## Optional Morning Snack
Almonds, 1 oz

## Lunch
Tilapia with Pistachio Crust
Coleslaw
Iced tea

## Afternoon Snack
Julienned Vegetables, 1 cup
Lemon Yogurt Dip
Seltzer

## Dinner
Couscous with Chicken
Sweet Sixteen Salad
Seltzer, wine, or beer

## Dessert
Strawberries, 1/2 pint, dipped in 1 oz melted semi-sweet dark chocolate, with 1/4 cup
    vanilla nonfat yogurt
Herbal tea

## Optional Rescue Snack
Smoked oysters, 1 1/2–3 oz

## AGE-BUSTING FITNESS PLAN

### Aerobic Training
- 3-5 minutes of warming up
- Reach 70-85% of your max heart rate for 40 minutes total activity with brisk walking, jogging, elliptical machine options
- 3-5 minutes of cooling down, heart rate less than 60% max

### Strength Training
- 12 body parts, 2 sets, 10-16 reps
- Use a mixture of ball and free weight activities

### Stretching
- 4-6 body parts, 5-10 minutes of stretching time

## RELAXATION ROUTINE
- Choose a calming activity for at least 20 minutes

## SUPPLEMENT ROUTINE
- Take your customized multivitamin pack
- Skin moisturizer with SPF 15
- Apply a facial retinol and a beta hydroxy acid skin product daily

## DETOX ROUTINE
- Enjoy a soy product daily
- Skip alcohol at least 2 days per week, and limit alcohol to 1-2 servings per day
- Avoid all passive tobacco smoke
- Use a headset for the cell phone

PHASE THREE

---

# Day 14 (Sunday)

FOOD PLAN: Vitality Foods

## Breakfast
Blueberry and Tofu Pancakes
Apricot, Ginger, and Pear Sauce
Tea or coffee

## Optional Morning Snack
None

## Lunch
Black Bean Chili with Peppers and Lime
Mixed green salad, 2 cups
Vinaigrette Dressing, 2 tbsp

## Afternoon Snack
Edamame, 1 cup

## Dinner
Lobster Tails with Ginger, Garlic, and Lime
Mashed Potatoes and Cauliflower
Mixed green salad
Vinaigrette Dressing, 2 tbsp
Seltzer, wine, or beer

## Dessert
Chocolate Mousse with Grand Marnier
Champagne (to celebrate being Ten Years Younger)

## Optional Rescue Snack
Almonds, 1 oz

## AGE-BUSTING FITNESS PLAN

### Aerobic Training
- Aerobic rest day
- Take a walk with a loved one

### Strength Training
- Rest day from strength training

### Stretching
- 4–6 body parts, 5–10 minutes of stretching time

## RELAXATION ROUTINE
- Choose a calming activity for at least 20 minutes

## SUPPLEMENT ROUTINE
- Take your customized multivitamin pack
- Skin moisturizer with SPF 15
- Apply a facial retinol and a beta hydroxy acid skin product daily

## DETOX ROUTINE
- Enjoy a soy product daily
- Skip alcohol at least 2 days per week, and limit alcohol to 1–2 servings per day
- Avoid all passive tobacco smoke
- Use a headset for the cell phone

PHASE THREE

## Breakfast Recipes

# AVOCADO AND BROCCOLI FRITTATA

*A flavorful and nutrient-rich meal to start your day, or have as a light dinner.*

Serves: 4

1 teaspoon extra-virgin olive oil
2 cups broccoli florets, sliced finely
¼ teaspoon sea salt
¼ teaspoon black pepper, ground
1 teaspoon Italian herbs, dried
8 large eggs (omega-3, free-range, organic)

1 cup nonfat milk
1 small avocado, cut into ½-inch cubes
Tabasco sauce
4 tablespoons nonfat sour cream (optional)

Preheat oven to 400° F.

Heat an ovenproof sauté pan or omelet pan to medium-high heat. Add oil. Sauté broccoli, salt, pepper, and herbs for 2 minutes, stirring occasionally.

Meanwhile, whisk eggs with milk in a large bowl, then add the avocado and cooked broccoli into the egg mixture, stir, and pour back into the sauté pan. Slip onto the middle oven rack and bake until eggs are set and browned, 15 to 20 minutes.

*Serving suggestion:* Serve with soy sausage or whole-grain toast. Garnish with Tabasco sauce to taste and sour cream. For dinner, serve with Guacamole, Salsa, and either a whole-grain dish or Sweet Potato Fries.

*Per Serving*
Calories: 199 · Fiber: 2.6g · Saturated fat: 2.4g · Sodium: 317mg ·
Protein: 15.5g · Total fat: 10.3g · Carbs: 11.5g · Calories from fat: 46%

# BLUEBERRY AND TOFU PANCAKES

*Surprise! Tofu adds a wonderful, fluffy texture to pancakes. This is an easy recipe that both children and adults enjoy. You can substitute any fruit in the pancake batter; try strawberries, apricots, or pears. Serve with Apricot, Ginger, and Pear Sauce (page 292), Raspberry Sauce (page 346), or nut butter.*

Serves 6 (makes 16–20 medium pancakes)

2 cups whole-wheat pastry flour
1 cup cornmeal
2 teaspoons baking powder

¼ teaspoon sea salt
2 tablespoons maple syrup (or sugar-free maple-flavored syrup)

1 tablespoon canola oil (organic, expeller-
pressed)
1 teaspoon vanilla
3 cups calcium-fortified soy milk (or nonfat milk)

½ 14-ounce package soft tofu
1 cup blueberries
Canola oil spray

Mix flour, cornmeal, baking powder, and salt in a large bowl. In a separate bowl, combine syrup, oil, vanilla, and soy milk. Gently fold wet ingredients into dry until just mixed; batter will be a little lumpy.

Rinse tofu and pat dry. Mash tofu with a potato masher or crumble through your fingers, then gently fold into batter. Fold in blueberries.

Heat a nonstick pan or griddle over medium heat. Spray pan with oil. Pour batter into pan and cook until underside is golden; flip and cook other side.

*Per Serving*
Calories: 353 · Fiber: 9g · Saturated fat: 1g · Sodium: 345mg ·
Protein: 13g · Total fat: 11.5g · Carbs: 56g · Calories from fat: 27%

# OATMEAL AND FLAXSEED MUFFINS

*Packed with fiber, nutrients, and flavor, these are equally good for breakfast or a snack. I like these enough that I'll enjoy them for dessert, too.*

Serves: 12 (1 muffin per serving)

2 ¼ cups oats
½ cup ground flaxseed
2 teaspoons baking powder
1 teaspoon cinnamon
½ teaspoon sea salt
½ cup dried figs, chopped (or dates)
⅓ cup molasses (or ⅓ cup apple juice
with 3 tablespoons Splenda)

¾ cup calcium-fortified soy milk
3 large eggs (omega-3, free-range,
organic), beaten
¼ cup canola oil (organic, expeller-
pressed)
¾ cup unsweetened applesauce
Canola oil spray

Preheat oven to 350° F.

Mix oats, flaxseed, baking powder, cinnamon, salt, and figs in a large bowl. In another bowl, combine molasses, soy milk, eggs, oil, and applesauce. Gently fold dry ingredients into wet ingredients. Spray muffin pan with oil and pour batter into pan. Bake for 35 to 45 minutes, until a toothpick inserted into a muffin comes out clean.

*Per Serving*
Calories: 194 · Fiber: 5g · Saturated fat: 1.7g · Sodium: 198mg ·
Protein: 5g · Total fat: 4g · Carbs: 27g · Calories from fat: 37%

## Lunch Recipes

### AVOCADO AND SHRIMP COCKTAIL

*This is an easy appetizer or even a light lunch served with soup or salad.*

Serves: 4

½ pound cooked shrimp, peeled and
deveined
1 medium tomato, chopped
1 garlic clove, minced
¼ teaspoon sea salt

¼ teaspoon black pepper
1 tablespoon chopped parsley
1 medium avocado, cut into ½-inch cubes
Juice of 1 lime
Tabasco sauce

Mix shrimp with tomato, garlic, salt, pepper, and parsley. Gently mix in avocado. Divide among 4 small dishes. Sprinkle lime juice on top and add Tabasco to taste.

*Per Serving*
Calories: 132 · Fiber: 2.5g · Saturated fat: 1.1g · Sodium: 349mg ·
Protein: 13g · Total fat: 7.6g · Carbs: 5g · Calories from fat: 49%

### BLACK BEAN CHILI WITH PEPPERS AND LIME

*Lime juice and beans go well together, especially with peppers and chili.*

Serves: 4

2 tablespoons extra-virgin olive oil
1 small onion, diced
¼ teaspoon sea salt
¼ teaspoon black pepper
1 teaspoon cumin
1 teaspoon dried oregano
2 medium carrots, diced
¼ teaspoon red pepper flakes or to taste

One 8-ounce can green chiles, rinsed and
diced (or roasted bell peppers)
Two 15-ounce cans black beans, rinsed
and drained
¼ cup tomato paste
Juice of 1 or 2 limes
½ cup chopped cilantro
¼ cup plain nonfat yogurt

Heat a large saucepan over medium-high heat. Add oil, then sauté onion with salt and pepper for 2 to 3 minutes, until softened. Add cumin, oregano, carrots, and pepper flakes and cook 3 minutes, stirring occasionally. Add chiles, beans, tomato paste, and 1 cup water and stir. Reduce heat to low and simmer 10 to 12 minutes, until carrots are tender. Remove from heat and add lime juice and cilantro.

Serve in bowls, garnished with yogurt.

*Per Serving*
Calories: 203 · Fiber: 10g · Saturated fat: 1g · Sodium: 411mg ·
Protein: 10g · Total fat: 3.7g · Carbs: 33g · Calories from fat: 16%

# QUESADILLAS WITH ROASTED PEPPERS AND REFRIED BEANS

*These tortilla sandwiches are another quick and easy fiber-packed meal.*

Serves: 2

4 corn tortillas (or whole-wheat flour tortillas)
4 tablespoons nonfat refried beans
4 tablespoons shredded nonfat cheese (or soy cheese)

2 medium roasted peppers (page 235)
4 tablespoons Salsa (page 236)

Warm tortillas. Spread 2 tablespoons beans and 2 tablespoons cheese on one tortilla and top with a roasted pepper. Cover with a second tortilla. Prepare second quesadilla the same way. Heat each quesadilla in the microwave for 30 seconds, or heat in a pan over medium heat for 1 to 2 minutes on each side. Cut into quarters to serve.

*Per Serving*
Calories: 213 · Fiber: 6.5g · Saturated fat: 0.2g · Sodium: 538mg · Protein: 11g · Total fat: 1.6g · Carbs: 41g · Calories from fat: 7%

# REFRIED BEAN BURRITOS

*When looking for a quick meal, burritos come to my rescue.*
*You can easily add chicken or shrimp for a heartier lunch or dinner.*

Serves: 4 (makes 8 burritos)

8 whole-wheat flour tortillas
One 15-ounce can nonfat refried beans
1 cup Salsa (page 236)
2 cups shredded lettuce

4 tablespoons nonfat sour cream
3 medium scallions, diced
½ large avocado, mashed

Warm tortillas and refried beans. Lay one tortilla flat. Place one-eighth each of the beans, salsa, lettuce, sour cream, scallions, and avocado at bottom of tortilla. Roll up, tucking sides in. Repeat with other tortillas.

*Serving suggestion:* Serve with roasted peppers and/or Mexican Rice (page 291).

*Per Serving*
Calories: 212 · Fiber: 16g · Saturated fat: 0.7g · Sodium: 346mg · Protein: 11g · Total fat: 4.7g · Carbs: 35g · Calories from fat: 19%

**PHASE THREE**

# TUSCAN GRILLED SHRIMP AND WHITE BEAN SALAD

*This is one of Susan Golant's recipes adapted for this section.*
*The combo of salad greens, white beans, and grilled shrimp is excellent.*

Serves: 2

½ pound large shrimp, peeled and deveined

Juice of 1 lemon

3 garlic cloves, minced

⅛ teaspoon red pepper flakes or to taste

¼ teaspoon sea salt

¼ teaspoon black pepper

2 tablespoons extra-virgin olive oil

½ medium red onion, thinly sliced

2 celery stalks with leaves, diced

1 teaspoon dried thyme (or 4 sprigs fresh thyme, minced leaves only)

One 16-ounce can cannellini (or any white beans), rinsed and drained

½ cup chopped flat-leaf parsley

3 medium plum tomatoes, chopped

6 cups arugula, mixed lettuce, or baby spinach leaves

2 lemon wedges

Preheat the grill, barbecue, or broiler.

In a small bowl, marinate shrimp for at least 10 minutes with lemon juice, garlic, pepper flakes, salt, and pepper. Thread shrimp onto metal skewers or place shrimp in a grilling tray. (If using bamboo skewers, soak them in water for 15 minutes before using.) Reserve marinade.

Heat a sauté pan over medium heat, add oil, and sauté onion, celery, and thyme in the remaining shrimp marinade for 2 minutes, stirring often. Add cannellini, parsley, and tomatoes and cook 1 to 2 minutes. Set aside.

Grill or broil shrimp for approximately 3 minutes on each side or until shrimp are pink.

To serve, place a bed of arugula, spinach leaves, or mixed lettuce on each plate. Spoon the hot bean salad mixture on top, stirring sauce into leaves. Add grilled shrimp and serve with a lemon wedge.

*Per Serving*
Calories: 481 · Fiber: 12g · Saturated fat: 2.5g · Sodium: 521mg ·
Protein: 35g · Total fat: 15g · Carbs: 46g · Calories from fat: 32%

# WHITE BEAN, CORN, AND BELL PEPPER SALAD

*Served with hearty whole-grain bread, olive oil for dipping, and a glass of
crisp white wine, this salad reminds me of eating lunch outside on a terrace in Italy.
The salad keeps well in the refrigerator for a few days.*

Serves: 4

One 15-ounce can white beans, rinsed and
    drained
½ medium red onion, diced
2 scallions, diced
1 large red bell pepper, diced
1 large yellow bell pepper, diced
One 15-ounce can corn, rinsed and
    drained

¼ teaspoon sea salt
⅛ teaspoon black pepper
2 tablespoons extra-virgin olive oil
2 tablespoons red wine vinegar
½ teaspoon Dijon mustard
1 garlic clove, minced
4 tablespoons chopped basil
4 large romaine lettuce leaves, torn

Combine beans, onion, scallions, bell peppers, corn, salt, and black pepper.
Whisk oil, vinegar, mustard, garlic, and basil and toss with salad. Serve on a bed
of romaine.

*Per Serving*
Calories: 410 · Fiber: 6g · Saturated fat: 1.2g · Sodium: 185mg ·
Protein: 13g · Total fat: 10.4g · Carbs: 69g · Calories from fat: 22%

## Dinner Recipes

## BAY SCALLOP STIR-FRY

*A scallop dish with wonderful colors. You can substitute
shrimp or diced chicken for the scallops.*

Serves: 4

1 teaspoon canola oil
2 cups sliced shiitake mushrooms
4 cups sliced broccoli florets
2 medium red bell peppers, sliced
2 cups snow peas, trimmed
1 pound bay scallops

Canola oil spray (organic, expeller-
    pressed)
1 tablespoon rice vinegar
2 tablespoons low-sodium soy sauce
⅛ teaspoon cayenne or to taste
2 teaspoons sesame oil
¼ cup chopped cilantro (or basil)

PHASE THREE

*(continued)*

Heat a sauté pan over medium-high heat. Add oil, then sauté mushrooms until soft, 2 to 3 minutes, stirring occasionally. Add broccoli, bell peppers, and snow peas and sauté another 2 to 3 minutes, until nearly cooked. Remove from pan and set aside.

Rinse scallops and pat dry. Spray sauté pan with oil for 2 to 3 seconds. Heat pan for 20 seconds over medium-high heat, then sear scallops for 90 seconds on each side, until lightly golden. Add vegetables to pan. Stir in rice vinegar, soy sauce, cayenne, and sesame oil. Cover and simmer for 30 seconds. Garnish with chopped cilantro.

*Serving suggestion:* Serve with brown rice, soba noodles, or any whole-grain side dish.

*Per Serving*
Calories: 243 · Fiber: 7g · Saturated fat: 0.6g · Sodium: 487mg ·
Protein: 25g · Total fat: 5g · Carbs: 27g · Calories from fat: 17%

# COQ AU VIN

*Coq au Vin is a traditional French meal that is flavorful, hearty, and fragrant.*
Serves: 4

| | |
|---|---|
| 1 tablespoon extra-virgin olive oil | 4 skinless, boneless chicken breasts |
| 1 medium onion, chopped | (about 5 ounces each) |
| 1 teaspoon sea salt | 2 tablespoons whole-wheat flour |
| 2 cups sliced mushrooms | 1 cup dry white wine |
| ½ teaspoon dried thyme | 1 cup low-sodium vegetable broth |
| ½ teaspoon dried oregano | ½ pound red potatoes, cut into ½-inch |
| 4 medium carrots, chopped | cubes |
| 2 cups chopped celery | 2 bay leaves |
| 4 garlic cloves, minced | ½ cup chopped parsley |
| | 2 cups chopped cabbage |

Heat a large stockpot over medium-high heat, add oil, and sauté onion with salt, mushrooms, thyme, and oregano for 2 minutes. Add carrots, celery, and garlic and cook 1 minute, stirring occasionally. Push veggies to the edges of the pot and sauté chicken breasts until lightly golden. Stir flour into vegetables, then add wine, broth, potatoes, bay leaves, parsley (reserving 1 tablespoon for garnish), and cabbage. Stir and simmer, covered, 45 minutes.

Remove bay leaves and ladle into large bowls. Garnish with parsley.

*Serving suggestion:* Accompany with a mixed salad.

*Per Serving*
Calories: 383 · Fiber: 7.2g · Saturated fat: 1.3g · Sodium: 849mg ·
Protein: 38g · Total fat: 7.5g · Carbs: 25g · Calories from fat: 17%

# GRILLED TURKEY BREAST

*This is a simple, tasty dinner. Turkey breast meat is very low in saturated fat and high in quality protein. Rosemary is packed with anti-aging compounds and imparts a wonderful flavor.*

Serves: 2

1 tablespoon extra-virgin olive oil
3 garlic cloves, minced
1 teaspoon dried rosemary
¼ teaspoon sea salt

Juice of ½ lemon
Two 6-ounce skinless, boneless turkey
breast portions

Combine oil, garlic, rosemary, salt, and lemon juice and marinate turkey for 30 minutes. Grill about 8 to 10 minutes on one side, then turn, drizzle with a few spoonfuls of marinade, and grill for another 8 to 10 minutes until done.

*Per Serving*
Calories: 219 · Fiber: 0.5g · Saturated fat: 1.5g · Sodium: 69mg ·
Protein: 34g · Total fat: 7g · Carbs: 3g · Calories from fat: 30%

# GUMBO

*Gumbo is easy to make and keeps well in the refrigerator for a few days. You can make gumbo with shrimp, chicken, turkey, or scallops.*

Serves: 4

1 tablespoon extra-virgin olive oil
1 medium onion, chopped
¼ teaspoon sea salt
¼ teaspoon black pepper
2 cups low-sodium vegetable broth
(or chicken stock)
4 cups okra, trimmed and cut into 1-inch
pieces
4 medium plum tomatoes, chopped

4 garlic cloves, minced
One 15-ounce can black-eyed peas,
drained and rinsed
One 15-ounce can corn kernels (or 1 cup
cooked brown rice)
1 pound shrimp, shelled and deveined
1 teaspoon filé powder
Tabasco sauce

Heat a large stockpot over medium-high heat, add oil, and sauté onion with salt and pepper until soft. Add broth, 3 cups water, okra, tomatoes, and garlic and bring to a boil. Then reduce heat to medium and simmer for 10 minutes. Add black-eyed peas, corn, and shrimp and simmer until shrimp are pink and cooked through, 4 to 5 minutes. Remove from heat and stir in filé powder

*(continued)*

(do not boil after adding filé or gumbo will become stringy). Serve in bowls and add Tabasco to taste.

*Per Serving*
Calories: 526 · Fiber: 7.5g · Saturated fat: 1.2g · Sodium: 603mg · Protein: 38g · Total fat: 10g · Carbs: 77g · Calories from fat: 16%

# INDIAN LENTILS (DHAL)

*Lentils with curry spices create a fragrant side dish.*
*Combined with rice and a vegetable, they make a wonderful meal.*

Serves: 4

| | |
|---|---|
| 1 cup lentils | 3 teaspoons curry powder |
| One 4-ounce can stewed, chopped, or puréed tomatoes | ⅛ teaspoon sea salt |

Bring lentils and 2 cups water to a boil, add tomatoes, and then simmer until lentils are tender but not soft, about 25 to 35 minutes. Add curry powder and salt and serve.

*Variation:* Make your own curry seasoning and omit curry powder. While lentils and tomatoes are cooking, heat 2 teaspoons canola oil in a pan and add ½ teaspoon whole cumin seeds, ⅛ teaspoon cardamom, 1 bay leaf, 1 whole clove, 1 cinnamon stick, ¼ teaspoon red pepper flakes (or to taste), ¼ teaspoon turmeric, and ⅛ teaspoon ground cumin. Cook 2 to 3 minutes until fragrant, stirring occasionally. Add spice mixture and salt to lentils while they simmer. Remove bay leaf to serve.

*Per Serving*
Calories: 199 · Fiber: 6.2g · Saturated fat: 0.4g · Sodium: 78mg · Protein: 12.5g · Total fat: 3.5g · Carbs: 31g · Calories from fat: 16%

# LEEK AND SHIITAKE SOUFFLÉ

*Soufflés are spectacular dinner entrées and much easier to make than most people realize. Much of the preparation can be done in advance. The trick is folding the sautéed vegetables gently into the egg whites to enable the soufflé to rise properly.*

Serves: 4

| | |
|---|---|
| 2 tablespoons extra-virgin olive oil | ¼ teaspoon black pepper |
| 2 medium leeks, white part only, cleaned and finely diced (or 1 onion, finely diced) | 1 teaspoon Italian seasoning |
| | 2 cups shiitake mushrooms, stemmed and finely diced |
| ¼ teaspoon sea salt | 2 tablespoons whole-wheat pastry flour |

4 garlic cloves, minced
½ cup dry white wine
½ cup calcium-fortified soy milk (or non-
    fat milk)
¼ cup chopped basil
½ cup grated nonfat mozzarella or Swiss
    cheese (or soy cheese)

5 egg yolks (omega-3, free-range, organic)
8 egg whites
2 slices whole-wheat bread, toasted and
    processed into crumbs (1 cup)
2 tablespoons slivered almonds
4 basil sprigs

Preheat oven to 400° F. Heat a sauté pan over medium-high heat, add oil, and sauté leeks with salt, pepper, and herbs for 2 to 3 minutes, until soft. Add mushrooms and cook, stirring occasionally, until mushrooms are soft, about 3 minutes. Stir in flour and garlic and cook 2 minutes, stirring occasionally. Pour in wine, stir to mix, and cook until thickened. Add soy milk and cook, stirring, until sauce is the consistency of heavy cream. Remove from heat and mix in basil, cheese, and egg yolks.

Whip egg whites until stiff. Fold bread crumbs into egg whites. Stir about ¼ cup of the egg-white mixture into the vegetables, then gently fold the vegetable mixture into the remaining egg-white mixture, a quarter at a time. Be careful not to overmix the egg-white mixture or the soufflé will not rise.

Spray a soufflé dish with oil and pour in egg-white and vegetable mixture. Sprinkle almonds on top and bake on the middle rack of the oven for 30 minutes, until top is golden and a toothpick inserted into the center comes out clean. Remove from the oven, garnish with basil sprigs, and serve immediately.

*Per Serving*
Calories: 326 · Fiber: 4.2g · Saturated fat: 2g · Sodium: 547mg ·
Protein: 24g · Total fat: 10g · Carbs: 31g · Calories from fat: 28%

# LOBSTER TAILS WITH GINGER, GARLIC, AND LIME

*This is a recipe we enjoy for a treat. Spiny lobsters have less fat and are lower in mercury than northeastern lobsters, so choose warm-water species when available. Lobster is a healthy and delicious dinner option, especially if you serve it with this sauce rather than melted butter.*

Serves: 4

4 medium lobster tails (4 to 8 ounces
    each)
3 tablespoons extra-virgin olive oil
1 tablespoon grated ginger
6 garlic cloves, minced

¼ teaspoon sea salt
⅛ teaspoon black pepper
1 teaspoon Italian seasoning
Juice of 1 lime

*(continued)*

Preheat grill or broiler.

With scissors, remove the soft undershell of the lobster tails. Gently separate the sides of the shell from the lobster meat, leaving lobster in the shell. Insert a metal skewer through the center length of the lobster tail to keep it straight and prevent curling while cooking. (If using bamboo skewers, shorten to the length of the lobster tail or soak in water for 15 minutes to prevent burning.)

Mix oil, ginger, garlic, salt, pepper, Italian seasoning, and lime juice in a bowl. Spoon about 2 tablespoons of sauce over each lobster tail, gently pushing sauce down the sides of the tail. Marinate at least 5 and up to 30 minutes.

Grill about 12 minutes with belly facing up, or broil in pan 5 to 6 inches from heat. Drizzle with remaining sauce.

*Per Serving (6-ounce tail)*
Calories: 354 · Fiber: 0.2g · Saturated fat: 1.7g · Sodium: 780mg ·
Protein: 47g · Total fat: 14g · Carbs: 9g · Calories from fat: 36%

# PAD THAI

*The mélange of tamarind, sugar, peanuts, bean sprouts, shrimp, and lime is a signature of Thai cuisine. The classic version of this dish is served with fried rice noodles. Far healthier is to serve this meal with soba noodles or brown rice. You can find tamarind, Thai basil, and soba noodles in most Asian food stores.*

Serves: 4

1 pound small shrimp, peeled and deveined (or one 14-ounce package firm tofu, cut into small cubes)
4 garlic cloves, minced
1/4 cup low-sodium vegetable broth
2 tablespoons tamarind liquid or sauce, or 1 tablespoon tamarind paste (mixed with 1 tablespoon water)
1 teaspoon low-sodium soy sauce
1/4 teaspoon red pepper flakes or to taste
10 ounces soba noodles, cooked (or 3 cups cooked brown rice)
3 teaspoons canola oil (organic, expeller-pressed)

2 large eggs (omega-3, free-range, organic), beaten
1 tablespoon grated ginger
2 medium carrots, grated or shredded
1 medium red bell pepper, cut into thin strips
3 cups bean sprouts, rinsed, drained, and patted dry
1 recipe Spicy Peanut Sauce (page 237)
10 Thai or regular basil leaves, chopped
1/4 cup roasted peanuts, chopped
2 scallions, chopped
Juice of 1 or 2 limes

In a deep bowl, combine shrimp, garlic, broth, tamarind, soy sauce, and red pepper flakes and marinate 15 to 20 minutes. Cook soba noodles in boiling water until nearly done, drain, rinse with cold water to stop the cooking process, and set aside.

Heat a large wok or skillet over medium-high heat and add 1 teaspoon oil and eggs. Scramble eggs; when cooked, remove from pan and set aside. Add remaining 2 teaspoons oil to the wok and sauté ginger and carrots for 2 minutes, stirring often. Add shrimp and marinade and continue to cook, stirring, until shrimp are nearly done, 3 to 4 minutes. Add bell pepper and 1 cup of bean sprouts and cook 1 minute. Remove from heat.

To serve, heat peanut sauce, mix sauce with noodles, and spoon onto a platter. Spoon stir-fry over noodles. Garnish with scrambled egg, basil, peanuts, scallions, and remaining bean sprouts. Drizzle lime juice on each portion.

*Per Serving*
Calories: 626 · Fiber: 10.5g · Saturated fat: 2.8g · Sodium: 485mg ·
Protein: 41g · Total fat: 21g · Carbs: 72g · Calories from fat: 29%

# TERIYAKI CHICKEN WITH PECAN CRUST

*This teriyaki marinade and pecan crust works well
with chicken, shrimp, or fish.*

Serves: 2

1 tablespoon low-sodium soy sauce
1 tablespoon sherry
1 tablespoon rice vinegar
1 tablespoon sugar-free maple-flavored
   syrup (or regular maple syrup)
2 teaspoons grated ginger

2 skinless, boneless chicken breasts
   (about 5 ounces each)
½ cup pecans, toasted and finely ground
½ teaspoon sea salt
⅛ teaspoon black pepper
Olive oil spray

Preheat oven to 400° F.

Mix soy sauce, sherry, vinegar, syrup, and 1 teaspoon of ginger in a bowl, add chicken, and marinate for at least 15 minutes, turning a couple of times.

Mix ground pecans with salt, pepper, and remaining ginger in a shallow dish. Coat chicken in pecan mixture. Spray ovenproof pan with olive oil spray; place chicken on pan and spray top of chicken. Bake 20 minutes, until golden.

*Serving suggestions:* Serve with Roasted Beets, Carrots, and Parsnips (page 291), Barley with Celery, Parsley, and Mushrooms (page 230), or your favorite whole grain.

*Per Serving*
Calories: 412 · Fiber: 3g · Saturated fat: 1.7g · Sodium: 378mg ·
Protein: 43g · Total fat: 22g · Carbs: 8g · Calories from fat: 48%

# TOMATOES AND ARTICHOKE HEARTS WITH SALMON AND SOBA NOODLES

*I've prepared this dish dozens of times for cooking demos.*
*It is easy to make, delicious, and popular.*

Serves: 4

1 tablespoon canola oil (organic, expeller-
   pressed
1 medium onion, diced
¼ teaspoon sea salt
¼ teaspoon black pepper
1 teaspoon Italian seasoning
¼ cup dry red wine (or vegetable broth or
   water)
2 cups artichoke hearts, quartered (or
   one 15-ounce can, drained and rinsed)
3 cups cherry tomatoes, halved
4 garlic cloves, minced

½ cup chopped basil
½ cup chopped parsley
Canola oil spray
1 pound coho salmon (or any wild-caught
   Alaskan salmon)
¼ teaspoon sea salt
2 tablespoons dried dill
12 ounces soba noodles (or whole-wheat
   or fiber-enriched pasta)
Juice of 1 lemon
2 tablespoons slivered almonds

Bring a pot of water to boil for soba noodles. Then heat a sauté pan, add oil, and sauté onion with salt and pepper until translucent. Add Italian seasoning and reduce heat to medium. Add wine and stir, then add artichoke hearts and cook 2 minutes. Add tomatoes and garlic, ¼ cup basil, and ¼ cup parsley. Set aside.

Spray another pan with oil and heat over medium-high heat. Add the salmon and sprinkle with 1 tablespoon dill and half the salt. Cook 4 to 5 minutes, turn salmon, sprinkle with remaining dill and salt, and cook 4 to 5 minutes more, until done.

While vegetables and salmon are cooking, cook soba noodles in boiling water until al dente. Drain noodles and place on a platter. Mix half the sautéed vegetables with the noodles, then top with the remaining vegetables. Place salmon on top and drizzle with lemon juice. Garnish with almonds and remaining basil and parsley.

*Per Serving*
Calories: 527 · Fiber: 11g · Saturated fat: 2.3g · Sodium: 578mg ·
Protein: 46g · Total fat: 13g · Carbs: 58g · Calories from fat: 21%

## Salad Recipes

# CITRUS, FENNEL, AND SPINACH SALAD

*This salad brings lovely flavors together. It makes a great side dish, or you can add white beans and serve as a light lunch.*

Serves: 4

Salt
1 small fennel bulb
1 tablespoon lemon juice
1 large pink or red grapefruit
1 large orange, peeled, segments
   separated

¼ cup chopped mint
1 teaspoon sugar (or 1 packet Splenda)
4 cups spinach leaves, rinsed and dried
1 medium red onion, thinly sliced
One 15-ounce can white beans, drained
   and rinsed (optional)

Bring a pot of water to boil with a dash of salt. Cut fennel into thin slices, mix with lemon juice (to prevent browning), and drop fennel into boiling water. Boil for 2 to 3 minutes until tender but firm; don't overcook. Drain and plunge into ice water until chilled. Place in a bowl.

Cut grapefruit in half. Cut out citrus segments between the membranes and place in a bowl with the fennel. Cut orange segments in half and add to the bowl. Squeeze remaining juice from grapefruit into bowl. Add mint and sugar and stir.

Place spinach, onion, and beans (if using) in a salad bowl. Add fennel-citrus mixture and toss.

*Per Serving*
Calories: 210 · Fiber: 10g · Saturated fat: 0.1g · Sodium: 63mg ·
Protein: 13g · Total fat: 0.7g · Carbs: 42g · Calories from fat: 3%

# JULIENNED VEGETABLES

*Flash-cook vegetables to create great snacks and hors d'oeuvres.*
*Toss with mustard vinaigrette and serve as a side dish,*
*or skip the dressing and serve with dip.*

Serves: 4

2 cups broccoli florets, julienned
2 cups julienned carrots
1 cup cauliflower florets, julienned

1 cup asparagus, cut into 3-inch lengths
1 medium red bell pepper, julienned

Bring several quarts of water to a boil. Add broccoli, carrots, and cauliflower. After 30 seconds add asparagus and pepper. Cook another 30 seconds until tender but firm. Drain veggies and immediately immerse in ice water to stop the cooking process.

*Per Serving*
Calories: 64 · Fiber: 5.2g · Saturated fat: 0g · Sodium: 43mg ·
Protein: 4g · Total fat: 0.5g · Carbs: 14g · Calories from fat: 7%

# LEMON YOGURT DIP

*This dip goes well with vegetables and steamed artichokes.*

Serves: 6

1 cup plain nonfat yogurt
½ cup lemon juice
¼ teaspoon dried dill (or 1 teaspoon chopped fresh dill)

½ teaspoon honey (or ½ packet Splenda)
⅛ teaspoon sea salt
2 tablespoons nonfat sour cream

Drain any liquid from the top of the yogurt. Mix yogurt, lemon juice, dill, honey, salt, and sour cream in a bowl. Chill and serve.

*Variation:* Drain the yogurt for a few hours in a cheesecloth-lined strainer. This makes it thicker, and you won't need to add the sour cream.

*Per Serving*
Calories: 44 · Fiber: 0.1g · Saturated fat: 0g · Sodium: 123mg ·
Protein: 3g · Total fat: 0.1g · Carbs: 8g · Calories from fat: 2%

PHASE THREE

# RASPBERRY VINAIGRETTE SALAD DRESSING

*This is a delicate dressing. Make a double batch; it lasts for a week in the refrigerator.*
*With the seeds it has more fiber and nutrients, but it is crunchy!*

Makes: 1 ½ cups (twelve 2-tablespoon servings)

1 cup raspberries (thawed if frozen)
½ cup red wine or balsamic vinegar
½ cup extra-virgin olive oil
¼ teaspoon sea salt

½ cup mint
1 tablespoon maple syrup (or 1 tablespoon
    Splenda)

Combine in a blender and pulse until smooth.

*Per Serving*
Calories: 96 · Fiber: 1g · Saturated fat: 1g · Sodium: 47mg (2 tablespoons) ·
Protein: 0.1g · Total fat: 9g · Carbs: 4g · Calories from fat: 84%

# SWEET SIXTEEN SALAD

*This salad combines multiple nutrients and flavors from my list of*
*Sweet Sixteen Vitality Foods. It's also a bigger serving, as I suggest at least*
*3 cups of salad per person to increase your anti-aging food intake*
*and quell your hunger before digging into the entrée.*

Serves: 2

4 cups mixed greens
2 cups red cabbage, shredded or chopped
4 tablespoons Vinaigrette Dressing
    (page 233)
½ cup cherry tomatoes, halved

2 scallions, chopped
¼ cup shelled edamame, cooked (or any
    cooked bean)
2 tablespoons chopped pecans, walnuts,
    or sliced almonds

Toss greens and cabbage with dressing. Mix in tomatoes, scallions, and beans.
Garnish with chopped nuts and serve.

*Per Serving*
Calories: 266 · Fiber: 5.5g · Saturated fat: 2.6g · Sodium: 115mg ·
Protein: 5.5g · Total fat: 21g · Carbs: 18g · Calories from fat: 66%

PHASE THREE

## Side Dish Recipes

# COLESLAW

*This is a fresh break from regular creamy coleslaw. Here you'll enjoy the crisp flavors of apple, mint, and lemon mixed with the crunchy texture of grated cabbage and carrots.*

Serves: 4

2 cups grated red cabbage
3 medium carrots, grated
1 medium apple, grated
Juice of 1 lemon

2 teaspoons walnut oil (or extra-virgin olive oil)
2 tablespoons chopped mint

Combine cabbage, carrots, and apple. Add lemon juice and oil and toss. Stir in mint and serve.

*Per Serving*
Calories: 80 · Fiber: 4g · Saturated fat: 0.4g · Sodium: 24mg ·
Protein: 1.4g · Total fat: 2.7g · Carbs: 14g · Calories from fat: 28%

# MASHED POTATOES AND CAULIFLOWER

*Cauliflower makes a terrific addition to regular mashed potatoes. Most of the potato nutrients are in the skin, so please don't peel them.*

Serves: 4

1 pound russet potatoes, unpeeled, cut into 1-inch cubes
1 pound cauliflower, cut into 1-inch cubes
¼ teaspoon sea salt

⅛ teaspoon black pepper
¼ cup nonfat milk, heated

Bring a pot of water to a boil. Boil potatoes 15 minutes, then add cauliflower and boil another 8 minutes. Drain.

Process potatoes and cauliflower in a food processor until smooth. Add salt and pepper to taste. Add milk and process briefly.

*Per Serving*
Calories: 112 · Fiber: 5.1g · Saturated fat: 0.1g · Sodium: 175mg ·
Protein: 5.3g · Total fat: 0.6g · Carbs: 23g · Calories from fat: 18%

PHASE THREE

## Condiment Recipes

### BEAN DIP WITH SALSA

*Bean dip is great with vegetables. You can also serve it with
whole-grain tortillas or whole-wheat pita bread cut into triangles.*

Serves: 4

¼ cup minced onion
1 teaspoon extra-virgin olive oil
¼ teaspoon sea salt
2 medium tomatoes, chopped
One 15-ounce can nonfat refried beans

¼ teaspoon cumin
⅛ teaspoon cayenne or to taste
¼ cup chopped cilantro (or parsley)
¼ cup nonfat sour cream
Cilantro sprigs

To serve cold, mix all ingredients except cilantro sprigs in a bowl, garnish with
cilantro sprigs, and serve. To serve warm, heat a sauté pan over medium heat,
add oil, and cook onion for 2 minutes. Add tomatoes, beans, cumin, and
cayenne and heat another 2 minutes, until bubbling. Stir in chopped cilantro.
Garnish with cilantro sprigs and serve.

*Per Serving*
Calories: 132 · Fiber: 6g · Saturated fat: 0.2g · Sodium: 574mg ·
Protein: 6g · Total fat: 1.4g · Carbs: 22g · Calories from fat: 10%

## Dessert Recipes

### BERRY, SOY MILK, AND FLAXSEED SMOOTHIE

*Great with breakfast, for a snack, or as dessert.*

Serves: 2 (2-cup servings)

2 cups calcium-fortified soy milk
1 cup frozen berries (blueberries,
    raspberries, cherries, etc.)

2 tablespoons flaxseed, ground
1 to 2 packets Splenda (optional)
2 tablespoons port (optional)

Combine ingredients in a blender and process until smooth.

*Per Serving*
Calories: 210 · Fiber: 7.5g · Saturated fat: 0.9g · Sodium: 145mg ·
Protein: 9g · Total fat: 7.5g · Carbs: 24g · Calories from fat: 31%

PHASE THREE

## CHERRY-FLAXSEED SMOOTHIE

*Great with breakfast, for a snack, or as dessert.*

Serves: 2 (2-cup servings)

1 ½ cups calcium-fortified vanilla soy milk  
2 cups frozen cherries

1 cup nonfat yogurt  
2 tablespoons flaxseed, ground

Combine ingredients in a blender and process until smooth.

*Per Serving*  
Calories: 294 · Fiber: 6g · Saturated fat: 1g · Sodium: 188mg ·  
Protein: 14.5g · Total fat: 7.5g · Carbs: 45g · Calories from fat: 22%

## CRÊPES SUZETTE

*This is a delicious dessert with a spectacular presentation.*  
*The crêpes and sauce can be made in advance and assembled when needed.*  
*Serve at a party or special event.*

Serves: 4 (2 crêpes per serving)

1 cup whole-wheat pastry flour  
1 cup calcium-fortified soy milk (or nonfat milk)  
Zest and juice from 3 oranges (about ½ cup grated zest and 1 ¼ cups juice)  
⅛ teaspoon sea salt  
3 large eggs (omega-3, free-range, organic)

Canola oil spray (organic, expeller-pressed)  
1 teaspoon kuzu powder (or cornstarch)  
¼ cup maple syrup (or ¼ cup apple juice with 2 tablespoons Splenda)  
1 tablespoon canola oil (organic, expeller-pressed)  
6 ½ tablespoons Grand Marnier

To make crêpes, mix flour, milk, 1 teaspoon zest, salt, and eggs. Spray a crêpe pan or small nonstick skillet with oil and heat over medium-high heat. Pour ⅛ cup batter into pan and tip pan to coat bottom. Cook crêpe until underside is golden, about 30 seconds, then flip and continue cooking on the other side for about 20 seconds.

To make sauce, dissolve kuzu in orange juice in a saucepan. Add remaining zest, syrup, oil, and 2 tablespoons Grand Marnier and cook over medium heat until just bubbling. Reduce heat and simmer until sauce thickens to the consistency of thin syrup. Set aside.

To serve, warm a serving platter in a 200° oven. Reheat orange sauce in a pan until bubbling. Dip crêpes into sauce one at a time using tongs, then fold crêpes in half twice to form triangles. Place crêpes on warmed platter. Pour remaining sauce over crêpes. Heat remaining 4½ tablespoons Grand Marnier in another saucepan until it just barely starts to bubble; don't overcook or all the alcohol will evaporate. Carefully ignite the heated Grand Marnier in the saucepan with a match or lighter and pour immediately over the crêpes.

*Variation:* You can substitute 1 teaspoon orange extract for the Grand Marnier in the sauce and skip the flambéing.

*Per Serving*
Calories: 323 · Fiber: 4.5g · Saturated fat: 1g · Sodium: 154mg ·
Protein: 10g · Total fat: 6.7g · Carbs: 45g · Calories from fat: 18%

# PEAR SOUFFLÉ

*Pears are wonderful when baked. This is a light, flavorful dessert,
with a terrific presentation for company or for a special occasion.*

Serves: 6

2 teaspoons almond oil (or canola or any other nut oil)
2 medium Bosc pears, cored and cut into ¼-inch cubes
⅛ teaspoon sea salt
⅓ cup almonds, finely ground
2 tablespoons brown sugar (or 6 packets of Splenda)

2 tablespoons rum (or brandy or cognac) (optional)
3 egg yolks (omega-3, free-range, organic)
6 egg whites
¼ cup sugar
2 tablespoons water
Canola oil spray (organic, expeller-pressed)

Preheat oven to 400° F.

Heat a saucepan over medium-high heat, add oil, then add pears and salt and sauté for 2 minutes, until pears just start to soften. Stir in almond flour, brown sugar, and optional rum, and cook, stirring occasionally, for 2 minutes. Remove from heat, let cool until lukewarm, then stir in egg yolks.

Beat egg whites until they form soft peaks. Meanwhile, combine sugar and water in another saucepan. Cook over medium-high heat for 2 to 3 minutes, until bubbling; remove from heat before it caramelizes. Carefully pour heated sugar syrup into egg whites while beating at high speed for 1 minute. (Use caution, as the syrup can splatter and burn.)

Gently fold the pear mixture into the sweetened egg whites. Don't overmix or the soufflé won't rise.

PHASE THREE

*(continued)*

Spray a soufflé dish with oil. Pour soufflé mixture into dish. Bake for 30 minutes, until the top is golden and a toothpick inserted in the center comes out clean. Serve immediately.

*Serving suggestion:* Garnish with a drizzle of melted semi-sweet chocolate or raspberry sauce.

*Per Serving*
Calories: 211 · Fiber: 2.5g · Saturated fat: 1g · Sodium: 71mg · Protein: 6.5g · Total fat: 7.5g · Carbs: 26g · Calories from fat: 32%

---

# PUMPKIN PUDDING

*Very easy to make, tasty, and popular with guests.*

Serves: 4

1 cup calcium-fortified soy milk
One 15-ounce can pumpkin purée
8 ounces soft tofu
½ cup maple syrup (or ½ cup apple juice with 4 tablespoons Splenda)

½ teaspoon sea salt
1 teaspoon cinnamon
¼ teaspoon ground cloves

Preheat oven to 375° F. Combine ingredients in a blender or food processor and process until smooth. Pour into individual oven-safe bowls or a pie plate. For pie plate, bake for 40 to 45 minutes, until a toothpick inserted in the center comes out clean. For individual bowls, bake for 35 to 40 minutes. Cool and refrigerate at least 30 minutes before serving.

*Per Serving*
Calories: 151 · Fiber: 4.5g · Saturated fat: 0.6g · Sodium: 20mg · Protein: 7g · Total fat: 3.7g · Carbs: 26g · Calories from fat: 20%

---

# RASPBERRY SAUCE

*I love this sauce with chocolate desserts, drizzled over fruit, pancakes, or sorbet, and poured over crêpes—delicious!*

Serves: 4 (¼ cup per serving)

2 ½ cups fresh or frozen raspberries
⅓ cup sugar (or ¼ cup Splenda)
⅛ teaspoon sea salt

2 teaspoons port
Juice of 1 lemon

Heat raspberries, sugar, and salt in a saucepan over medium-high heat until bubbling. Mash raspberries, reduce heat to medium, and simmer 5 minutes.

Remove from heat and pour through a sieve or strainer over a bowl. Stir and push raspberry mixture through the mesh to remove seeds. Pour raspberry sauce back into the saucepan and add wine and lemon juice with seedless raspberry sauce. Cook over medium heat, stirring, until thickened, 5 to 10 minutes. Serve hot or chilled.

*Per Serving*
Calories: 121 · Fiber: 1g · Saturated fat: 0g · Sodium: 78mg ·
Protein: 1g · Total fat: 0.4g · Carbs: 29g · Calories from fat: 3%

# Sticking with It

The Ten Years Younger Program is more than something you follow for just ten weeks. It's a lifestyle for the long haul that yields tremendous benefits, including longevity and vitality. Once in a blue moon, someone wins the longevity lottery—inheriting an incredible set of genes that guarantees long life and vitality regardless of lifestyle choices. Much more likely, we have to earn these rewards.

## Succeeding on the Program

Optimal aging doesn't come on a silver platter, nor is it a gimmick too good to be true. The science surrounding it has grown tremendously in the last few years, but you have to be willing to adopt an approach that matches your built-in need to succeed.

Throughout *Ten Years Younger*, I've suggested numerous diet and lifestyle changes that will make you look and feel younger. But sometimes it's hard to motivate yourself to alter ingrained habits. Yet during the past ten years I've given more than 500 presentations to lay audiences on how to live better. And I know people can turn their lives around because I've seen it thousands of times with my patients. Here are a few simple rules for sticking with the Ten Years Younger changes I advocate, especially when it comes to eating.

## Don't Hold Back

While some people may do well taking baby steps, many others improve by making drastic changes. And they feel better faster, too. Contrary to popular medical opinion, studies have shown that motivated patients (people who are willing to make big changes for big benefits) find dramatic diet changes as acceptable as more modest ones. Even more striking is the fact that they appear to stick with these dramatic changes better than they do with less drastic adjustments. So I encourage you to dive right into the Ten Years Younger Program—momentum can propel you through the challenging early phases and help you stick with the changes over the long haul.

## Learn to Read Food Labels

Many people are already interested in nutrition and read the labels on packaged foods. But do they understand what they're reading? Unfortunately not—and it may not be their fault. Food labels deceive more than half the people who read them. Foods labeled "Lower Fat" are usually still very high in fat. "Organic" doesn't mean sugar free. "No Cholesterol" can mean the contents are still packed with those nasty trans fats. After reading this book, you should have the tools and knowledge to decipher labels, look out for Aging Accelerators, and avoid them.

## Ask for Help

In counseling my patients, I've found that you'll be vastly more successful if you sit down with your partner (preferably *not* over a meal) and talk about your personal health goals. After ensuring that he or she understands what you're after, ask for help in achieving those goals. You might say, "Will you help me get fit? I want to look and feel better. I need to go to the gym every day, and I have to get the ice cream, potato chips, and pizza out of the house. Can you help me with this?" A request like this will probably be met with support and success. On the other hand, you're unlikely to be successful if you tell your partner what he or she can or can't do. "That was your last burger and fries" will get you nowhere fast!

Getting others involved is a critical step. Family participation can make or break your compliance with a new health regimen, especially if your partner does the shopping or cooking. Cooking is easier when the family chef has only one meal to prepare. Plus it lessens the stigma of changing diets when your whole family shifts its eating habits together. Besides, what's healthy for you will be good for them too!

### Have a Plan

Clinical studies of motivated people who want to change their eating habits have found that having specific meal plans in hand (customized to your food preferences and social habits) is effective in improving diets for more than a year. That means motivated people need direction and healthy recipes to succeed in the long term. The demand for recipes led me to write my first book, *The 28-Day Antioxidant Diet Program,* and to go through a chef internship at the Four Seasons restaurant in Seattle. Part III of *Ten Years Younger* provides you with everything you need to begin the program and tackle it on a day-by-day basis. You've most likely already perused the weekly meal and exercise plans as well as the recipes. Now it's time to put them into action!

## Can We Really Slow Aging?

Of course we can! You inherited twenty-three pairs of chromosomes; this is your genetic makeup. But the messages encoded in your genes are not set in stone—they're not destiny! *You get to choose how you express them.* Your current life is one expression of your genetic potential. But you are free to experiment and try other lifestyles—ones that can enhance your health, fitness, and emotional well-being.

The good news is that *you actually get to choose* how you age. In *Ten Years Younger* I've done my best to show you how to make better choices. The rest is up to you. I wish you well on your journey toward vitality and optimal health!

# SATURATED FAT CONTENT

| Item (serving size) | Cal. | Sat. Fat | Item (serving size) | Cal. | Sat. Fat |
|---|---|---|---|---|---|
| **Seafood** | | | **Meat** | | |
| Catfish (6 oz) | 115 | 1.5 | Bacon (4 strips) | 140 | 4.0 |
| Clams (6 oz) | 300 | 0.4 | Bologna (2 slices, 1½ oz) | 180 | 5.0 |
| Cod (6 oz) | 218 | 0.3 | Bratwurst (1) | 300 | 9.0 |
| Crab, canned (3 oz) | 220 | 0.3 | Cheeseburger, large | 580 | 12.0 |
| Crab cakes (2) | 318 | 4.4 | Hamburger (6 oz) | 490 | 14.0 |
| Grouper (6 oz) | 201 | 0.5 | Hamburger, lean (6 oz) | 467 | 12.5 |
| Lobster, spiny (6 oz) | 285 | 0.6 | Hot dog | 140 | 6.0 |
| Mahi mahi (6 oz) | 218 | 0.5 | Pork chop (6 oz) | 280 | 6.0 |
| Mussels (3 oz meat) | 170 | 0.8 | Salami, beef (3 oz) | 450 | 13.0 |
| Oysters (3 oz meat) | 72 | 0.6 | Sausage (6 oz) | 550 | 15.0 |
| Salmon, Atlantic, | | | Steak, sirloin (6 oz) | 316 | 4.0 |
| farmed (6 oz) | 400 | 5.0 | Steak, prime rib (6 oz) | 692 | 24.0 |
| Salmon, Atlantic, | | | | | |
| wild (6 oz) | 360 | 2.4 | **Other Fast Food** | | |
| Salmon, coho, wild (6 oz) | 278 | 2.0 | Chicken nuggets | 430 | 5.0 |
| Salmon, pink, wild, | | | French fries (large) | 577 | 8.0* |
| canned (3 oz) | 110 | 1.0 | Pizza, Sicilian (2 slices) | 590 | 13.2 |
| Sardines, canned (3 oz) | 215* | 1.5 | Pizza supreme (2 slices) | 820 | 12.5 |
| Scallops (6 oz) | 300 | 0.4 | Sandwich, ham and | | |
| Shrimp (6 oz) | 200 | 0.5 | cheese | 790 | 13.0 |
| Sole (6 oz) | 155 | 0.5 | Sandwich, chicken (reg) | 500 | 8.5 |
| Trout (6 oz) | 300 | 2.1 | Sandwich, roast beef | 473 | 9.0 |
| Tuna, albacore (3 oz) | 128 | 0.8 | Taco, beef (2) | 520 | 12.0 |
| Tuna, bluefin (6 oz) | 360 | 3.2 | Taco, chicken (2) | 410 | 8.0 |
| Tunafish sandwich (1) | 533 | 4.0 | | | |
| | | | **Appetizers** | | |
| **Poultry (6 oz)** | | | Chicken wings (6 oz) | 607 | 10.0 |
| Chicken, breast, fried | 319 | 3.0 | Nachos (7) | 570 | 13.0 |
| Chicken, breast, baked | 230 | 2.0 | Onion rings (med) | 450 | 8.0 |
| Chicken, leg, fried | 208 | 3.5 | | | |
| Turkey, breast, baked | 200 | 2.0 | **Dairy** | | |
| Turkey, leg, baked | 270 | 2.2 | Cheddar (1 oz) | 112 | 6.0 |

NOTE: Most of the data in Appendixes A, B, C and D is derived from the USDA National Nutrient Database. Portions listed are typical serving sizes. For more information, visit their Web site: www.nal.usda.gov/fnic/foodcomp/search/index.html.

| Item (serving size) | Cal. | Sat. Fat |
|---|---|---|
| Cottage cheese, whole-milk (½ cup) | 120 | 3.0 |
| Cottage cheese, low-fat (½ cup) | 90 | 1.0 |
| Cottage cheese, nonfat (½ cup) | 80 | 0.2 |
| Egg, regular | 75 | 1.6 |
| Egg, omega-3 enriched | 75 | 1.0 |
| Egg, white only | 17 | 0.0 |
| Egg, scrambled | 101 | 2.2 |
| Brie cheese | 100 | 6.0 |
| Gouda (1 oz) | 105 | 5.0 |
| Mozzarella, part skim (1 oz) | 80 | 2.7 |
| Whole milk (1 cup) | 149 | 5.0 |
| 2% milk (1 cup) | 137 | 3.0 |
| 1% milk (1 cup) | 118 | 1.8 |
| Nonfat milk (1 cup) | 86 | 0.3 |
| Cream (2 tbsp) | 100 | 6.0 |
| Half and half (2 tbsp) | 40 | 2.0 |
| Soy creamer (2 tbsp) | 40 | 0.1 |
| Yogurt, whole-milk (1 cup) | 160 | 4.5 |
| Yogurt, low-fat (1 cup) | 145 | 3.0 |
| Yogurt, nonfat (1 cup) | 120 | 0.1 |

**Spreads**

| | | |
|---|---|---|
| Almond butter (1 tbsp) | 95 | 1.0 |
| Butter (1 tbsp) | 100 | 7.0 |
| Guacamole (1 tbsp) | 21 | 0.5 |
| I Can't Believe It's Not Butter (1 tbsp) | 90 | 4.0* |
| Margarine (1 tbsp) | 100 | 3.5* |
| Mayonnaise (1 tbsp) | 100 | 2.0 |
| Parkay (1 tbsp) | 60 | 1.5 |
| Peanut butter (1 tbsp) | 100 | 1.5 |
| Smart Balance (1 tbsp) | 45 | 1.5 |

**Oils**

| | | |
|---|---|---|
| Almond oil (1 tbsp) | 120 | 1.0 |
| Canola oil (1 tbsp) | 116 | 1.0 |
| Corn oil (1 tbsp) | 120 | 2.0 |
| Olive oil (1 tbsp) | 120 | 2.0 |

**Nuts**

| | | |
|---|---|---|
| Almonds (1 oz) | 170 | 1.1 |
| Cashews (1 oz) | 163 | 2.6 |
| Peanuts (1 oz) | 166 | 2.0 |
| Pecans (1 oz) | 201* | 1.7 |
| Walnuts (1 oz) | 185 | 1.7 |

**Snacks**

| | | |
|---|---|---|
| Corn chips (1½ oz) | 240 | 2.5 |
| Potato chips (1½ oz) | 230 | 4.0 |
| Popcorn, air-popped (3 cups) | 108 | 0.2 |
| Popcorn, oil-popped (3 cups) | 142 | 7.9 |
| Tortilla chips (1½ oz) | 260 | 2.0 |
| Tortilla chips, baked (1½ oz) | 180 | 1.5 |

**Breakfast**

| | | |
|---|---|---|
| Cinnabon (1) | 670 | 14.0 |
| Croissant (1) | 350 | 11.0 |
| Danish, apple (1) | 197 | 6.0 |
| Muffin (1 sm) | 200 | 3.0 |
| Scone, cinnamon | 530 | 13.0 |

**Dressings (2 Tbsp)**

| | | |
|---|---|---|
| Vinaigrette | 125 | 2.0 |
| Ranch | 120 | 2.5 |
| Blue cheese | 120 | 3.0 |
| Thousand Island | 116 | 2.0 |
| Caesar | 156 | 2.6 |

**Desserts**

| | | |
|---|---|---|
| Carrot cake (1 slice) | 270 | 1.5 |
| Cheese cake (1 slice) | 271 | 7.0 |
| Chocolate cake (1 slice) | 270 | 5.0 |
| Chocolate chip cookie (1) | 250 | 8.0 |
| Cream puff (1) | 335 | 5.0 |
| Donut, glazed (1) | 491 | 7.0 |
| Fudge brownies (1) | 260 | 2.0 |
| Ice cream (1 cup) | 520 | 18.0 |
| Ice cream, nonfat (1 cup) | 200 | 0.5 |
| M&M's (2 oz) | 270 | 8.0 |
| Reese's Peanut Butter Cup (2 oz) | 260 | 6.0 |
| Snickers (2 oz bar) | 280 | 14.0 |
| White cake (1 slice) | 270 | 4.0 |

*May include trans fats

# FIBER CONTENT

| Item (serving size) | Fiber (grams) | Item (serving size) | Fiber (grams) |
|---|---|---|---|
| **Fruits** | | Brussels sprouts (1 cup) | 3.3 |
| Apple (1 med) | 3.3 | Cabbage (1 cup shredded) | 2.0 |
| Apple juice (8 oz) | 0.0 | Carrots (1 cup) | 3.6 |
| Applesauce (⅔ cup) | 2.9 | Cauliflower (1 cup) | 2.5 |
| Apricot (3 med) | 2.4 | Celery (1 cup, chopped) | 1.6 |
| Banana (1 med) | 3.0 | Eggplant, raw (1 cup) | 2.8 |
| Blackberries (½ cup) | 3.8 | Green beans (1 cup) | 3.7 |
| Blueberries, fresh (½ cup) | 1.8 | Lettuce (1 cup chopped) | 1.0 |
| Blueberries, frozen (½ cup) | 2.1 | Mixed vegetables, frozen (1 cup) | 4.0 |
| Cherries, fresh (10) | 1.5 | Okra, cooked (1 cup) | 4.0 |
| Dates (½ cup) | 7.1 | Onions (½ cup, chopped) | 1.5 |
| Grapes (1 cup) | 1.0 | Peas (1 cup) | 7.4 |
| Grapefruit (½) | 1.8 | Peppers (½ cup, chopped) | 1.3 |
| Mango (1 med) | 3.0 | Potato, baked, with skin (1 med) | 3.8 |
| Melon (1 cup cubed) | 1.4 | Potato, baked, no skin (1 med) | 2.3 |
| Orange (1 med) | 3.1 | Potato, french fries (1 med serv) | 4.0 |
| Peach (1 med) | 1.5 | Potato, mashed (1 cup) | 3.0 |
| Pear (1 med) | 5.1 | Potato salad (1 cup) | 2.5 |
| Pineapple (1 cup diced) | 2.2 | Pumpkin (½ cup) | 3.8 |
| Plum (2 med) | 2.0 | Spinach, raw (1 cup) | 0.7 |
| Prunes (2) | 2.0 | Spinach, cooked (1 cup) | 4.3 |
| Raisins (⅓ cup) | 3.5 | Squash, cooked (1 cup) | 2.5 |
| Raspberries, fresh (½ cup) | 4.0 | Sweet potato, no skin (1 med) | 6.0 |
| Raspberries, frozen (½ cup) | 5.5 | Sweet potato, with skin (1 med) | 4.0 |
| Strawberries, fresh (½ cup) | 1.7 | Tomato, fresh (1 med) | 1.5 |
| Watermelon (1 cup) | 0.6 | Tomato, cooked (1 cup) | 1.7 |
| | | | |
| **Vegetables** | | **Beans (legumes) cooked** | |
| Artichoke (1 med whole) | 6.5 | Baked beans (1 cup) | 10.4 |
| Artichoke hearts (½ cup) | 4.5 | Broad beans (1 cup) | 37.0 |
| Asparagus (½ cup, 6 spears) | 1.7 | Black beans (1 cup) | 15.0 |
| Avocado (½ med) | 6.5 | Kidney beans (1 cup) | 16.5 |
| Beets (1 cup) | 3.5 | Lentils (1 cup) | 15.6 |
| Broccoli (1 cup, chopped) | 2.3 | Lima beans (1 cup) | 13.2 |

| Item (serving size) | Fiber (grams) |
|---|---|
| Navy beans (1 cup) | 19.1 |
| Pinto beans (1 cup) | 15.4 |
| Soy beans, green, boiled (1 cup) | 07.6 |
| Soybeans, dry roasted (1 cup) | 13.9 |
| Tofu (½ block) | 0.4 |
| | |
| **Grain Products cooked** | |
| Barley, hulled (1 cup) | 8 |
| Barley, pearl (1 cup) | 6 |
| Corn, yellow (1 cup) | 4.6 |
| Popcorn (1 cup) | 1.2 |
| Rice, white (1 cup) | 0.6 |
| Rice, brown (1 cup) | 3.5 |
| Rice, wild (1 cup) | 3.0 |
| Rice pilaf (1 cup) | 1.2 |
| Soba (1 cup) | 7.6 |
| Soba white noodles (1 cup) | 2.0 |
| Spaghetti, (1 cup) | 2.4 |
| Spaghetti, whole-wheat (1 cup) | 7.0 |
| Spaghetti, multigrain (1 cup) | 4.0 |
| Tortillas, corn (2 med) | 3.0 |
| Tortillas, white flour (2 med) | 2.8 |
| | |
| **Breads** | |
| Bagel (1) | 0.6 |
| Bread, white (1 slice) | 0.6 |
| Bread, whole-wheat (1 slice) | 2.0 |
| Bread, 7-grain (1 slice) | 1.8 |
| Bread, pumpernickel (1 slice) | 3.0 |
| Biscuits, white flour (1) | 0.5 |
| Corn bread, from mix (1 piece) | 1.4 |
| Pita bread, regular (1 pocket) | 1.3 |
| Pita bread, oat bran (1 pocket) | 3.6 |
| Pita bread, whole-wheat (1 pocket) | 4.7 |
| | |
| **Crackers and Chips** | |
| Corn chips (2 oz) | 1.9 |
| Potato chips (2 oz) | 2.0 |
| Rye crispbread (3 oz) | 4.8 |
| Soda crackers (4) | 0.4 |
| Tortilla chips (2 oz) | 2.5 |
| Wheat Thins (1 oz) | 0.9 |

| Item (serving size) | Fiber (grams) |
|---|---|
| **Cereal** | |
| Kellogg's Raisin Bran | 7.3 |
| Kellogg's bran flakes | 6.7 |
| Cheerios | 3.6 |
| Honey Nut Cheerios | 1.8 |
| Cocoa Puffs | 0.7 |
| Corn flakes | 0.5 |
| Grits | 0.5 |
| Oatmeal | 4.0 |
| Rice Krispies | 0.1 |
| Shredded wheat | 5.6 |
| Special K | 0.7 |
| Total | 3.5 |
| Wheaties | 3.0 |
| Frosted Wheaties | 0.8 |
| | |
| **Nuts and seeds** | |
| Almonds (1 oz) | 3.3 |
| Almond butter (1 tbsp) | 0.7 |
| Brazil nuts (1 oz) | 2.1 |
| Cashews (1 oz) | 0.9 |
| Corn nuts (1 oz) | 2.0 |
| Filberts (1 oz) | 2.7 |
| Flaxseed (1 tbsp) | 3.4 |
| Hazelnuts (1 oz) | 2.7 |
| Macadamia (1 oz) | 2.3 |
| Mixed nuts (1 oz) | 2.5 |
| Peanuts (1 oz) | 2.2 |
| Peanut butter (1 tbsp) | 2.6 |
| Pecans (1 oz) | 2.7 |
| Sunflower seeds (1 oz) | 2.6 |
| Walnuts (1 oz) | 1.9 |
| | |
| **Snacks and Bars** | |
| Harvest Bar | 2.0 |
| Nature Valley Bar | 2.0 |
| Kellogg's Bran Bar | 5.0 |
| Luna Bar | 4.0 |
| | |
| **Meat, Poultry, Seafood** | |
| Any | 0.0 |

# APPENDIX C

# SOURCES OF CALCIUM

| Item (serving size) | Calcium content (mg) | Item (serving size) | Calcium content (mg) |
|---|---|---|---|
| Yogurt (8 oz) | 415 | Oatmeal, instant, calcium-fortified (1 pkt) | 163 |
| Cow's milk (8 oz) | 300 | Oatmeal, regular (1 cup) | 20 |
| Soy or rice milk, calcium-fortified (8 oz) | 300 | Tofu (½ cup) | 130 |
| Orange juice, calcium fortified (8 oz) | 300 | Navy beans, cooked (1 cup) | 128 |
| Edamame (1 cup) | 261 | Garbanzo beans (1 cup) | 80 |
| Sardines in tomato sauce (3.5 oz) | 240 | Almonds (1 oz) | 75 |
| Cheddar cheese (1 oz) | 204 | Carrots (1 cup) | 35 |
| Broccoli, cooked (1 cup) | 175 | Brown rice (1 cup) | 20 |
| Kale and other cooked greens (1 cup) | 100–150 | Whole-wheat bread (1 slice) | 20 |
| Seaweed, hijiki or wakame, dry (1 sheet) | 100–160 | Cottage cheese (½ cup) | 69 |

# SOURCES OF OMEGA-3 FATS

## BEST CHOICES

The following are high in omega-3s, fairly low in saturated fat, and low in mercury. Enjoy up to 3 to 5 servings per week. All are based on a 3-oz serving, unless noted.

|  | Omega-3s (grams) | Saturated Fat (grams) |
|---|---|---|
| Herring, Atlantic | 2.1 | 2.6 |
| Mussels | 0.7 | 0.8 |
| Oysters | 0.6 | 0.6 |
| Salmon, Atlantic, wild | 2.2 | 1.3 |
| Salmon, coho, Pacific, wild | 2.4 | 1.4 |
| Sardines, water-packed | 1.9 | 1.5 |
| Sole or flounder | 0.5 | 0.4 |
| Trout, rainbow, wild | 1.2 | 1.6 |
| Trout, rainbow, farmed | 1.2 | 2.1 |
| Whitefish | 1.8 | 1.2 |

## GOOD CHOICES

The following are low in mercury but also relatively low in omega-3 fats. They aren't as good as salmon or sole, but they're better protein sources than chicken or turkey breast. Enjoy up to 2 to 3 servings per week.

|  | Omega-3s (grams) | Saturated Fat (grams) |
|---|---|---|
| Calamari (squid) | 0.3 | 0.4 |
| Catfish, channel, farmed | 0.2 | 1.8 |
| Clams | 0.3 | 0.2 |
| Cod, Atlantic | 0.3 | 0.3 |
| Crabs, Dungeness (fresh) | 0.4 | 0.2 |
| Halibut | 0.5 | 0.4 |
| Lobster, spiny | 0.5 | 0.3 |
| Shrimp | 0.5 | 0.3 |
| Mahi mahi | 0.1 | 0.2 |
| Pollock | 0.5 | 0.2 |
| Scallops | 0.15 | 0.05 |
| Tilapia | 0.1 | 0.5 |

## LIMIT YOUR INTAKE

The following are moderately high in mercury (more than 0.2 parts per million), so limit consumption of these to not more than 2 or 3 servings monthly. In general, largemouth fish are higher in mercury levels.

|  | Omega-3s (grams) | Saturated Fat (grams) |
|---|---|---|
| Bass (including Chilean sea bass) | 0.9 | 0.7 |
| Bluefish | 0.9 | 1.2 |
| Grouper | 0.3 | 0.3 |
| Lobster, Maine | 0.1 | 0.1 |
| Salmon, Atlantic, farmed | 2.3 | 2.5 |
| Tuna, albacore (has the lowest mercury content among types of tuna) | 0.9 | 0.9 |
| Tuna, bluefin | 1.5 | 1.6 |
| Tuna, yellowfin | 0.3 | 0.3 |

## AVOID

The following are high in mercury (greater than 0.5 parts per million). Avoid these fish as much as possible.

- King mackerel
- Marlin
- Shark
- Swordfish
- Tilefish

# THE MULTIVITAMIN SNAPSHOT SUMMARY

What to look for when choosing a multivitamin

| Ingredient | Dosing Range | Comments |
| --- | --- | --- |
| Iron | 0 mg or 8–20 mg | 0 for men and women without menses; 8–20 mg for menstruating women |
| Vitamin A (as retinol or retinyl) | 3,000–5,000 IU | |
| Vitamin A (as mixed carotenoids) | 3,000–15,000 IU | Mixed beta-carotene, lycopene, lutein, zeaxanthin, alpha-carotene, cryptoxanthin |
| Thiamin ($B_1$) | 15–50 mg | |
| Riboflavin ($B_2$) | 10–30 mg | |
| Niacin ($B_3$) | 30–100 mg | Mixture of niacin and niacinamide |
| Pantothenic acid ($B_5$) | 50–100 mg | |
| Pyridoxine ($B_6$) | 10–50 mg | Homocysteine elevations may require higher doses. |
| Cobalamin ($B_{12}$) | 100–1,000 mcg | Homocysteine elevations may require higher doses. Stomach-acid-blocking meds decrease absorption. |
| Biotin | 300–1,200 mcg | Higher dosages needed with blood sugar regulation problems |
| Folic acid | 600–4,000 mcg | Homocysteine elevations may require higher doses. |
| Vitamin C (calcium ascorbate) | 250–1,000 mg | |
| Vitamin D | 400–1,200 IU | Higher dosages needed with advancing age and with bone density loss, and without sun exposure |
| Vitamin E (with mixed d-alpha, gamma, and delta tocopherols) | 50–150 IU | Dosages >150 IU are warranted for various indications, but may lower HDL levels. |
| Vitamin K | 75–100 mcg | |

| Ingredient | Dosing Range | Comments |
|---|---|---|
| Calcium (as a chelate) | 0–100 mg | Can be dosed separately from a multivitamin (total needs vary from 800 to 1,500 mg daily) |
| Magnesium (as a chelate) | 0–100 mg | Can be dosed separately from a multivitamin (total needs vary from 400 to 800 mg daily) |
| Iodine (from kelp) | 75–200 mcg | |
| Chromium (nicotinate) | 100–400 mcg | 400–800 mcg daily for blood sugar control |
| Manganese | 3–10 mg | |
| Molybdenum | 100–150 mcg | |
| Selenium | 100–200 mcg | Caution: Dosages > 500 mcg daily may be toxic |
| Zinc (glycinate or amino acid chelate) | 15–25 mg | Taking more than 40–50 mg daily long-term can cause gastrointestinal irritation |
| Copper | 2 mg | Zinc and copper should be in a 10:1 to 15:1 ratio |
| Boron | 1–2 mg | |

# WEEKLY SHOPPING LISTS

To help you shop, we've listed recipe ingredients for Phases One, Two, and Three. Only you know how many people you'll be cooking for in your household and whether you have dinner guests. You get to determine how much to buy. Items are organized week by week according to where you will find them in the grocery store.

## Phase One, Week 1, Shopping List

Salmon, wild-caught, fresh or frozen
Sole, fresh or frozen
Shrimp, peeled and deveined
Mussels, in the shell
Scallops, sea or bay
Chicken breasts, boneless (5 oz each)
Tofu, firm
Tofu, extra firm
Tofu, silken or soft
Bell pepper, green
Bell pepper, red
Bell pepper, orange or yellow
Broccoli
Cabbage, green
Carrots
Cauliflower
Celery
Cherry tomatoes
Cucumber
Japanese eggplant
Leeks
Mixed salad greens
Mushrooms
Onion, red
Onion
Potatoes
Scallions (green onions)
Shiitake mushrooms, fresh
Spinach, fresh
Sweet potatoes
Apples
Banana, frozen
Orange
Cantaloupe
Lime
Lemon
Strawberries, fresh
Berries, frozen
Ice cream, nonfat, sugar-free

Frozen yogurt, vanilla, nonfat
Cilantro, fresh
Dill weed, fresh
Garlic cloves
Ginger root
Mint leaves, fresh
Parsley, flat-leaf, fresh
Thai basil (or regular)
Eggs (omega-3, free-range, organic)
Soy milk (or nonfat milk)
Soy creamer
Tomato paste
Pasta sauce, jarred (or see page 237)
Vegetable broth, low-sodium
Balsamic vinegar
Canola oil, organic expeller-pressed
Canola oil spray
Chili paste with garlic
Dijon mustard
Kuzu root powder (or corn starch)
Olive oil spray
Olive oil, extra virgin
Oyster sauce
Rice vinegar
Sesame oil
Soy Sauce, low-sodium
Sweetened chili sauce for Thai Cabbage Rolls
Brown sugar (or Splenda)
Sugar (or Splenda)
Maple syrup (or apple juice)
Chocolate chips, dark, semi-sweet
Cocoa powder, unsweetened
Peanut butter, old-fashioned
Black pepper, ground
Cayenne
Cinnamon, ground
Italian seasoning
Oregano, dried
Paprika

Rosemary, dried
Sea salt
Thyme, dried
Brown rice
Soba noodles (buckwheat)
Wild rice
Almonds
Cashews
Pecans

Sliced almonds
Grand Marnier
Red wine, dry
White wine, dry
Sherry
Seltzer, unsweetened
Tea, herbal
Tea, green or black decaf
Coffee, espresso (or for filter)

## Phase One, Week 2

Snapper fillets
Tilapia fillets, fresh or frozen
Shrimp, peeled and deveined
Mussels, in the shell
Chicken breasts, skinless, boneless
  (5 oz ea)
Tofu, extra-firm
Miso paste
Avocado
Bell pepper, red
Broccoli
Cabbage, green or red
Carrots
Celery
Mixed salad greens
Mushrooms
Onion
Onion, red
Onion, sweet
Scallions (green onions)
Shiitake mushrooms, fresh
Spinach, fresh
Tomatoes
Apple
Banana, frozen
Berries, frozen
Blueberries, frozen (or other berries)
Mango, fresh or frozen
Mixed fresh fruit (for fruit salad)
Orange, organic
Strawberries, fresh
Peas, frozen
Mixed vegetables, frozen or fresh
Ice cream, nonfat, sugar-free
Basil
Cilantro, fresh
Gingerroot
Garlic cloves
Lime
Lemon
Parsley, flat-leaf, fresh
Eggs, omega-3, free range, organic
Milk, nonfat (or soy milk)

Mozzarella cheese, reduced fat
Parmesan cheese
Sour cream, nonfat
Yogurt, vanilla, nonfat
Yogurt, nonfat, plain
Pasta sauce, jarred
Roasted bell peppers, fresh or canned
Tomato paste, canned
Canola oil, organic expeller-pressed
Canola oil spray
Dijon mustard
Olive oil, extra-virgin
Olive oil spray
Chili paste with garlic
Kuzu root powder (or corn starch)
Rice vinegar
Red wine vinegar
Soy sauce, low-sodium
Whole-wheat pastry flour (or whole-
  wheat flour)
Chocolate chips, dark, semi-sweet
Cocoa powder, unsweetened
Milk, evaporated nonfat
Sugar (or Splenda)
Vanilla extract
Black pepper
Cayenne pepper
Italian seasoning
Oregano, dried
Paprika
Sea salt
Rosemary, dried
Saffron
Thyme, dried
Brown rice
Barley, hulled or pearled
Popcorn (air-popped or without
  butter/trans fat)
Soba noodles (buckwheat)
Whole-wheat bread
Whole-wheat spaghetti noodles
Whole-wheat tortillas
Wild rice

Cashews
Hazelnuts
Pecans
Pistachio nuts
Slivered almonds
Grand Marnier

Port
Red wine, dry
Sake (rice wine) or white wine, dry
White wine, dry
Seltzer, unsweetened

## Phase Two, Week 3

Mahi-mahi, fresh or frozen
Crab meat, fresh or canned
Shrimp, large, peeled and deveined
Sea scallops, fresh or frozen
Chicken breasts, skinless, boneless
    (5oz ea)
Tofu, silken or soft
Bell pepper, green
Bok choy
Beets
Parsnips
Cabbage
Carrots
Celery
Broccoli
Green beans
Snow peas
Button mushrooms, whole
Shiitake mushrooms, fresh
Mixed salad greens
Cherry tomatoes
Tomatoes
Bell pepper, green
Bell pepper, red
Bell pepper, orange or yellow
Onion, red
Onion
Scallions (green onions)
Tomatoes
Zucchini
Apples
Green apples
Orange, organic
Mango, fresh
Peaches, fresh or frozen
Pineapple, fresh or canned
Strawberries, fresh
Raspberries, fresh or frozen
Cherries, frozen
Berries, fresh
Mixed fruit, fresh
Ice cream, nonfat, sugar-free
Lime
Lemon
Ginger root
Garlic cloves

Cilantro, fresh
Parsley, flat-leaf, fresh
Eggs, omega-3, free-range, organic
Sour cream, nonfat
Soy milk (or nonfat milk)
Yogurt, nonfat, vanilla
Yogurt, nonfat, plain
Orange juice, with pulp
Black beans, canned (or cooked)
Cannellini beans, canned
Vegetable broth, low-sodium
Applesauce, unsweetened
Canola oil, organic expeller-pressed
Olive oil, extra virgin
Olive oil spray
Balsamic vinegar
Dijon mustard
Tabasco
Sesame oil
Rice vinegar
Soy sauce, low-sodium
Kuzu root powder (or corn starch)
Brown sugar (or Splenda)
Maple syrup
Tapioca, quick-cooking
Chocolate chips, dark, semi-sweet
Cocoa powder, unsweetened
Cayenne
Paprika
Sea salt
Black pepper, ground
Italian seasoning
Oregano, dried
Rosemary, dried
Thyme
Brown rice
Wild rice
Barley, hulled or pearled
Corn tortillas, fresh or frozen, soft
Whole-wheat pasta or fiber-enriched
    pasta
Whole-wheat bread
Granola, low-fat
Pecans
Pine nuts
Hazelnuts

Slivered almonds
Sherry
White wine, dry
Red wine, dry
Grand Marnier

Port
Seltzer, unsweetened
Tea, herbal
Tea, green or black decaf
Coffee, espresso or filter

## Phase Two, Week 4

Salmon, wild-caught, fresh or frozen
Sole, fresh or frozen
Shrimp, peeled and deveined
Chicken breasts, skinless, boneless
  (5 oz ea)
Bok choy
Broccoli
Cabbage, green
Carrots
Celery
Cauliflower
Snow peas
Bibb lettuce
Cucumber
Fennel bulb
Tomatoes
Avocado
Bell pepper, red
Onion, red
Onion
Scallions (green onions)
Salad greens, mixed
Poblano peppers or other chiles
Potatoes
Mango, fresh or frozen
Strawberries, fresh
Blueberries, frozen
Mixed fruit, fresh
Peas, frozen
Corn kernels, frozen or fresh
Ice cream, nonfat, sugar-free
Lime
Lemon
Gingerroot
Garlic cloves
Cilantro, fresh
Mint, fresh
Eggs, omega-3, free range, organic
Sour cream, nonfat
Soy milk (or nonfat milk)
Yogurt, nonfat, plain
Yogurt, vanilla, nonfat
Tomato paste, canned
Black beans, canned (or cooked)
Garbanzo beans, canned (or cooked)

Vegetable broth, low-sodium
Roasted bell peppers, fresh or canned
Canola oil, organic expeller-pressed
Canola oil spray
Olive oil, extra-virgin
Olive oil spray
Balsamic vinegar
Tabasco
Sesame oil
Rice vinegar
Soy sauce, low-sodium
Oyster sauce
Sugar (or Splenda)
Maple syrup (or Splenda)
Chocolate chips, dark, semi-sweet
Cocoa powder, unsweetened
Vanilla extract
Dried fruit (figs, dates, raisins)
Baking powder
Brewer's yeast
Cayenne
Cinnamon powder
Cumin seed
Cumin powder
Paprika
Saffron
Sea salt
Black pepper, ground
Oregano, dried
Brown rice
Brown basmati rice
Cornmeal, coarse
Whole-wheat pita bread
Whole-wheat tortillas
Whole-wheat bread
Whole-wheat couscous
Pecans
Slivered almonds
Red wine, dry
Sherry
Grand Marnier
Port
Seltzer, unsweetened
Tea, mint
Tea, green or black decaf

## Phase Three, Week 5

Salmon, wild-caught, fresh or frozen
Sole, fresh or frozen
Shrimp, peeled and deveined
Bay scallops, fresh or frozen
Chicken breasts, skinless, boneless
    (5 oz ea)
Bean sprouts
Bell pepper, red
Broccoli
Fennel bulb
Cabbage, red
Carrots
Celery
Cherry tomatoes
Snow peas
Mixed salad greens
Mushrooms
Shiitake mushrooms, fresh
Spinach, fresh
Cherry tomatoes
Leeks
Okra, fresh or frozen
Onion, red
Onion
Scallions (green onions)
Tomatoes
Orange
Grapefruit, pink
Bosc pear
Mixed fruit, fresh
Strawberries, fresh
Cherries, frozen
Corn, frozen or canned
Berries, fresh
Berries, mixed, frozen
Raspberries, frozen
Ice cream, nonfat, sugar-free
Lime
Lemon
Gingerroot
Garlic cloves
Basil leaves
Cilantro, fresh
Mint, fresh
Parsley, flat-leaf, fresh
Thai basil (or regular)
Eggs, omega-3, free range, organic
Soy milk (or nonfat milk)
Yogurt, nonfat, plain
Yogurt, nonfat, vanilla
Mozzarella cheese, nonfat

Orange juice, with pulp
Artichoke hearts, in water
Black-eyed peas, canned (or cooked)
White beans, canned (or cooked)
Vegetable broth, low-sodium
Canola oil, organic expeller-pressed
Canola oil spray
Olive oil, extra virgin
Olive oil spray
Almond oil
Balsamic vinegar
Tabasco
Sesame oil
Rice vinegar
Soy sauce, low-sodium
Kuzu powder (or corn starch)
Chili paste
Tamarind paste or liquid
Whole-wheat pastry flour (or whole-
    wheat flour)
Brown sugar (or Splenda)
Sugar (or Splenda)
Maple syrup (or apple juice)
Chocolate chips, dark, semi-sweet
Cocoa powder, unsweetened
Peanut butter, natural
Cayenne
Crushed pepper flakes (optional)
Dill weed, dried
Gumbo filé
Sea salt
Black pepper, ground
Italian seasoning
Oregano, dried
Brown rice
Barley, hulled or pearled
Soba noodles (buckwheat)
Whole-wheat bread
Almonds
Ground flaxseed
Peanuts, roasted
Pecans
Slivered almonds
Sherry
Grand Marnier
Port
Rum
White wine, dry
Seltzer, unsweetened
Tea, herbal
Tea, green or black, decaf

## Phase Three, Week 6

Lobster tails, fresh or frozen (8 oz ea)
Salmon, wild-caught, fresh or frozen
Shrimp, peeled and deveined
Mussels, in the shell
Sea or bay scallops, fresh or frozen
Chicken breasts, skinless, boneless
    (5 oz ea)
Turkey breasts, skinless, boneless
    (6 oz ea)
Tofu, silken or soft
Broccoli
Cabbage, green
Cabbage, red
Carrots
Celery
Cherry tomatoes
Cauliflower
Fennel bulb
Shiitake mushrooms, fresh
Mushrooms
Mixed salad greens
Cucumber
Tomatoes
Bell pepper, green
Bell pepper, red
Bell pepper, orange or yellow
Onion, red
Onion
Scallions (green onions)
Potatoes, red
Potatoes
Zucchini
Orange
Mango, fresh or frozen
Mixed fruit, fresh
Strawberries, fresh
Blueberries, frozen
Edamame (fresh or frozen/shelled or
    unshelled)
Ice cream, nonfat, sugar-free
Peas, frozen
Lime
Lemon
Gingerroot
Garlic cloves
Cilantro, fresh
Parsley, flat-leaf, fresh
Soy milk (or nonfat milk)
Yogurt, nonfat, plain
Yogurt, nonfat, vanilla

Pasta sauce, canned (or homemade)
Tomatoes, chopped, canned
White beans, canned (or cooked)
Lentils, dried
Vegetable broth, low-sodium
Canola oil, organic expeller-pressed
Olive oil, extra-virgin
Balsamic vinegar
Dijon mustard
Soy sauce, low-sodium
Tabasco
Whole-wheat pastry flour or
    whole-wheat flour
Sugar (or Splenda)
Maple syrup (or apple juice)
Chocolate chips, dark, semi-sweet
Cocoa powder, unsweetened
Vanilla extract
Dried fruit (figs, raisins, etc)
Cinnamon powder
Cumin seeds
Cumin powder
Curry powder
Italian herbs
Paprika
Saffron
Sea salt
Black pepper, ground
Italian seasoning
Oregano, dried
Rosemary, dried
Thyme
Bay leaves
Brown basmati rice
Wild rice
Whole-wheat pasta (or fiber enriched)
Couscous, whole grain
Pecans
Pine nuts
Slivered almonds
Champagne
Red wine, dry
White wine, dry
Grand Marnier
Port
Seltzer, unsweetened
Tea, herbal
Tea, mint
Espresso (or strong coffee)

# ACKNOWLEDGMENTS

It gives me pleasure to extend my deepest and most heartfelt appreciation to all the people who have helped me to create this book.

Many thanks are owed to my agent, Matthew Guma with Inkwell Management, who has been a great source of guidance throughout the production of this book. Likewise, I feel very blessed to have worked with Susan Golant, a very talented writer, who has artfully edited this book and helped to transform technical aspects into lively discussion. She also interviewed subjects from my Ten Years Younger Study and painted their stories into this book beautifully. I owe a special thanks to Ann Campbell, senior editor at Broadway Books with Random House, who appreciated what this book offered and has endeavored to make it clear, practical, and powerful.

I am grateful to the staff at two hospital libraries that have been extremely helpful in aiding my review of several thousand medical journal articles. At Morton Plant Hospital in Clearwater, Florida, I would like to thank Karen Roth and the many hospital volunteers. At Providence St. Peter Hospital in Olympia, Washington, I would like to thank Edean Berglund, Kathy Wagner, and Lewis Daniell.

I feel fortunate to have worked in the kitchens of two wonderful restaurants in Seattle, Washington. I want to thank the staff at Café Flora, a vegetarian gourmet restaurant, and especially the executive chef, Catherine Geier, for welcoming me into their restaurant. I'm also grateful to the staff at the Four Seasons hotel and restaurants in Seattle, Washington, and their executive chef at the time, Kerry Sear, for inviting me to do an internship in their kitchen and pastry stations.

My clinical colleagues have been very supportive of my desire to pursue work apart from seeing patients in our clinics over the years. Thanks

ML1

to my former workmates at Group Health Cooperative's Olympia Medical Center in Olympia, Washington, and at the Turley Family Health Center with Morton Plant Mease Health Care in Clearwater, Florida. I also need to extend special thanks to current co-workers who have helped to create the Carillon Executive Health Program as well as the recent Ten Years Younger Study Program, including Howard Drenth, Glenda Fahey, Gil Peri, Angie Presby, Karen Reich, Kerri Vowels, and Wendy Weaver.

I am very grateful to the founders of Functional Medicine, and in particular Dr. Jeffrey Bland, who showed me how to see beyond the simple model of diagnosing and treating diseases and directed me toward assessing and promoting optimal wellness for every patient. Identifying optimal function has become a cornerstone of my medical evaluation process thanks to this organization.

Group Health Cooperative, the Morton Plant Hospital Foundation, St. Anthony's Health Care, and the American Heart Association have generously sponsored my research projects over many years. The experience with my co-investigators has been invaluable, and I am grateful in particular to Colleen Hawes, Sharon Phillips, Douglas Schocken, M.D., Julia Sokoloff, M.D., Carol Weideman, and Gordon Wheat, M.D.

Several medical colleagues critiqued earlier versions of this book and helped to make it both practical and based upon evidence. In particular, I'd like to thank Fleur Sack, M.D., and Joseph Pellicer, M.D., for their feedback.

My wife, Nicole, has been extremely supportive of the work involved in researching, creating recipes for, and writing this book. My sons, Lucas and Marcos, have freely given me the time to study and write, and have been willing recipe testers over the years. I have also had numerous friends and family members who have generously edited recipes and my written materials for years.

Lastly, I want to thank my many patients in Tucson, Arizona; in Olympia, Washington; in the Tampa Bay, Florida, region; and at the Pritikin Longevity Center for their encouragement in creating this book. They have helped me to convert this technical information into everyday words that empower people along a path toward health and vitality.

# A NOTE ABOUT REFERENCES

For a detailed bibliography and list of references supporting the research and concepts presented in this book, please visit my Web site, www. tenyearsyounger.net, and select the Reference option.

# INDEX OF RECIPE TITLES

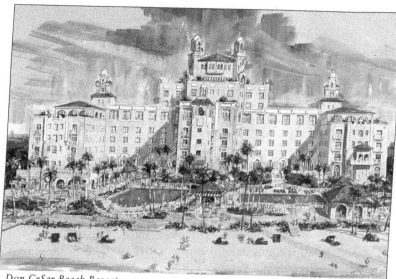

*Don CeSar Beach Resort*

## Win a Romantic and Healthy Getaway!!

Turn a romantic getaway into an experience that will help you jumpstart a healthy life together. Win a two night stay at the renowned luxury resort, Don CeSar Beach Resort, A Loews Hotel, in St. Pete Beach, Florida, complete with a comprehensive "couples" health and lifestyle evaluation with Dr. Steven Masley, Medical Director of Carillon Executive Health and author of *Ten Years Younger*.

Visit **www.tenyearsyounger.net** for official rules and entry details.

No purchase is necessary. Open to legal U.S. Residents 21 and older. Winners selected by random drawing. Sweepstakes commences on January 1, 2007. All electronic entries must be received no later than 5:00 p.m. on June 30, 2007. Void outside of the U.S. or wherever prohibited or restricted by law.

*For additional information on health,*
*wellness, skin care, supplements,*
*or to contact Dr. Steven Masley, visit*
*www.tenyearsyounger.net or www.drmasley.com*

# ABOUT THE AUTHOR

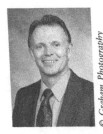

**Steven Masley, M.D.,** is a physician, a nutritionist, and the former medical director of the Pritikin Longevity Center® in Aventura, Florida. Currently medical director of the acclaimed Carillon Executive Health Program for St. Anthony's Hospital in St. Petersburg, Florida, he is also a clinical assistant professor at the University of South Florida.

www.drmasley.com